Endoscopic Ultrasound-Guided Diagnosis and Treatment of Gastrointestinal Diseases

Endoscopic Ultrasound-Guided Diagnosis and Treatment of Gastrointestinal Diseases

Editor

Manol Jovani

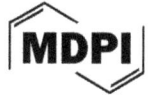

Basel • Beijing • Wuhan • Barcelona • Belgrade • Novi Sad • Cluj • Manchester

Editor
Manol Jovani
SUNY Downstate University
Brooklyn, NY
USA

Editorial Office
MDPI
St. Alban-Anlage 66
4052 Basel, Switzerland

This is a reprint of articles from the Special Issue published online in the open access journal *Journal of Clinical Medicine* (ISSN 2077-0383) (available at: https://www.mdpi.com/journal/jcm/special_issues/Ultrasound_Guided).

For citation purposes, cite each article independently as indicated on the article page online and as indicated below:

Lastname, A.A.; Lastname, B.B. Article Title. *Journal Name* **Year**, *Volume Number*, Page Range.

ISBN 978-3-7258-0195-4 (Hbk)
ISBN 978-3-7258-0196-1 (PDF)
doi.org/10.3390/books978-3-7258-0196-1

© 2024 by the authors. Articles in this book are Open Access and distributed under the Creative Commons Attribution (CC BY) license. The book as a whole is distributed by MDPI under the terms and conditions of the Creative Commons Attribution-NonCommercial-NoDerivs (CC BY-NC-ND) license.

Contents

About the Editor vii

Tong Ye, Ye Zong, Guiping Zhao, Anni Zhou, Bing Yue, Haiying Zhao and Peng Li
Role of Endoscopy in Esophageal Tuberculosis: A Narrative Review
Reprinted from: *J. Clin. Med.* **2022**, *11*, 7009, doi:10.3390/jcm11237009 1

Dushyant Singh Dahiya, Mohammad Al-Haddad, Saurabh Chandan, Manesh Kumar Gangwani, Muhammad Aziz, Babu P. Mohan, et al.
Artificial Intelligence in Endoscopic Ultrasound for Pancreatic Cancer: Where Are We Now and What Does the Future Entail?
Reprinted from: *J. Clin. Med.* **2022**, *11*, 7476, doi:10.3390/jcm11247476 12

Jun Liang Teh and Anthony Yuen Bun Teoh
Techniques and Outcomes of Endoscopic Ultrasound Guided—Pancreatic Duct Drainage (EUS-PDD)
Reprinted from: *J. Clin. Med.* **2023**, *12*, 1626, doi:10.3390/jcm12041626 27

Michelle Baliss, Devan Patel, Mahmoud Y. Madi and Ahmad Najdat Bazarbashi
EUS-Guided Vascular Interventions
Reprinted from: *J. Clin. Med.* **2023**, *12*, 2165, doi:10.3390/jcm12062165 41

John B. Doyle and Amrita Sethi
Endoscopic Ultrasound-Guided Biliary Drainage
Reprinted from: *J. Clin. Med.* **2023**, *12*, 2736, doi:10.3390/jcm12072736 55

Alexander M. Prete and Tamas A. Gonda
Endoscopic Ultrasound-Guided Local Ablative Therapies for the Treatment of Pancreatic Neuroendocrine Tumors and Cystic Lesions: A Review of the Current Literature
Reprinted from: *J. Clin. Med.* **2023**, *12*, 3325, doi:10.3390/jcm12093325 63

Jagoda Oliwia Rogowska, Łukasz Durko and Ewa Malecka-Wojciesko
The Latest Advancements in Diagnostic Role of Endosonography of Pancreatic Lesions
Reprinted from: *J. Clin. Med.* **2023**, *12*, 4630, doi:10.3390/jcm12144630 84

Da Yeon Ryoo, Bryn Koehler, Jennifer Rath, Zarine K. Shah, Wei Chen, Ashwini K. Esnakula, et al.
A Comparison of Single Dimension and Volume Measurements in the Risk Stratification of Pancreatic Cystic Lesions
Reprinted from: *J. Clin. Med.* **2023**, *12*, 5871, doi:10.3390/jcm12185871 107

Navkiran Randhawa, Ahamed Khalyfa, Rida Aslam, M. Christopher Roebuck, Mahnoor Inam and Kamran Ayub
Endoscopic Ultrasound-Guided Botox Injection for Refractory Anal Fissure
Reprinted from: *J. Clin. Med.* **2022**, *11*, 6207, doi:10.3390/jcm11206207 119

Sebastian Stefanovic, Helena Degroote and Pieter Hindryckx
Reduction of Lams-Related Adverse Events with Accumulating Experience in a Large-Volume Tertiary Referral Center
Reprinted from: *J. Clin. Med.* **2023**, *12*, 1037, doi:10.3390/jcm12031037 125

Ken Ishii, Yuji Fujita, Eisuke Suzuki, Yuji Koyama, Seitaro Tsujino, Atsuki Nagao, et al.
The Efficacy and Safety of EUS-Guided Gallbladder Drainage as a Bridge to Surgery for Patients with Acute Cholecystitis
Reprinted from: *J. Clin. Med.* **2023**, *12*, 2778, doi:10.3390/jcm12082778 135

Marco Spadaccini, Maria Cristina Conti Bellocchi, Benedetto Mangiavillano, Alberto Fantin, Daoud Rahal, Erminia Manfrin, et al.
Secondary Tumors of the Pancreas: A Multicenter Analysis of Clinicopathological and Endosonographic Features
Reprinted from: *J. Clin. Med.* **2023**, *12*, 2829, doi:10.3390/jcm12082829 . . . . **144**

About the Editor

Manol Jovani

Dr. Jovani has international experience with the treatment of gastrointestinal diseases, since he trained and conducted research in Italy (University of Bologna and University of Milan) and in the United States (Harvard University and Johns Hopkins University). Dr. Jovani is a therapeutic endoscopist with formal training in epidemiology and biostatistics. He has authored/coauthored over 70 peer-reviewed articles and book chapters. Among these are two international clinical practice guidelines from the European Society of Gastrointestinal Endoscopy (ESGE). He has served on committees of the American Society of Gastrointestinal Endoscopy (ASGE), the American Gastroenterological Society (AGA), and the European Society of Gastrointestinal Endoscopy (ESGE), in addition to serving as an award-winning reviewer for popular peer-reviewed journals in the field of endoscopy (*Gastrointestinal Endoscopy and VideoGIE*). He is member of the American Society of Gastrointestinal Endoscopy (ASGE), the American Gastroenterological Association (AGA), American College of Gastroenterology (ACG), the European Society of Gastrointestinal Endoscopy (ESGE), the New York Society for Gastrointestinal Endoscopy (NYSGE), and the World Endoscopy Organization (WEO). His interests include therapeutic endoscopic ultrasound, third space endoscopy, and bariatric endoscopy.

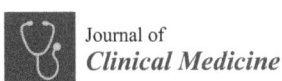

Review

Role of Endoscopy in Esophageal Tuberculosis: A Narrative Review

Tong Ye, Ye Zong, Guiping Zhao, Anni Zhou, Bing Yue, Haiying Zhao * and Peng Li *

Department of Gastroenterology, Beijing Friendship Hospital, Capital Medical University, Beijing 100050, China
* Correspondence: zhybfhxhk@163.com (H.Z.); lipeng@ccmu.edu.cn (P.L.)

Abstract: Esophageal tuberculosis (ET) is a rare infectious disease of the gastrointestinal tract. Awareness of ET is deficient due to its low incidence. Unexplained dysphagia and upper gastrointestinal bleeding are the most common symptoms of ET. The prognosis is generally good if patients are diagnosed properly and receive anti-tubercular treatment promptly. However, ET is difficult to differentiate from other diseases. Endoscopic techniques such as esophagogastroduodenoscopy (EGD), endoscopic ultrasonography (EUS), contrast-enhanced harmonic endoscopic ultrasonography (CH-EUS), elastography, and endoscopic ultrasound–guided fine-needle aspiration (EUS-FNA) improve the diagnosis of ET. Thus, the characteristics of ET and other difficult-to-detect diseases according to EGD and EUS were summarized. Intriguingly, there is no literature relevant to the application of CH-EUS and elastography in ET. The authors' research center was first in introducing CH-EUS and elastography into the field of ET. The specific manifestation of ET based on CH-EUS was discovered for the first time. Correlative experience and representative cases were shared. The role of endoscopy in acquiring esophageal specimens and treatment for ET was also established. In this review, we aim to introduce a promising technology for the diagnosis and treatment of ET.

Keywords: endoscopy ultrasonography; contrast-enhanced harmonic endoscopic ultrasonography; elastography; endoscopic ultrasound-guided fine-needle aspiration; esophageal tuberculosis

1. Introduction

Esophageal tuberculosis (ET) is a rare disease, accounting for around 0.15% in the necrotic tissue of subjects with tuberculosis and about 0.07–3.00% for subjects with gastrointestinal tuberculosis [1,2]. To date, with the resurgence of tuberculosis, the incidence of ET has gradually increased [3]. However, the diagnosis of ET remains challenging because its clinical features are often nonspecific and variable. It may be mistaken for esophageal carcinoma and could lead to unnecessary surgery [2]. Following a definite diagnosis and treatment with anti-tuberculosis therapy, the patient will become asymptomatic after 6 months and obtain endoscopy healing at 1-year follow-up [2–6], which is widely divergent from malignancy. Despite the optimistic prognosis of ET, it could become life-threatening in some cases, for example, massive bleeding resulting from aortoesophageal fistula [5]. Therefore, prompt and explicit diagnosis has always been the essential and challenging aspect of ET.

Esophagogastroduodenoscopy (EGD) could observe the morphology of the lesion directly. Endoscopic ultrasonography (EUS) can detect the echogenic characteristics of the lesion, different layers of the esophageal wall, and para-esophageal organs and tissues. Additionally, EUS is able to guide fine-needle aspiration to obtain extra-esophageal tissue such as an infected lymph node [7]. Contrast-enhanced harmonic endoscopic ultrasonography (CH-EUS) delineates the vascular distribution and blood perfusion of the target organs via an agent injected into the superficial median cubital vein. The hemodynamic state of blood vessels is described by CH-EUS with high resolution, which is helpful in distinguishing benign from malignant [8,9]. Elastography has been developed as a qualitative and

Citation: Ye, T.; Zong, Y.; Zhao, G.; Zhou, A.; Yue, B.; Zhao, H.; Li, P. Role of Endoscopy in Esophageal Tuberculosis: A Narrative Review. *J. Clin. Med.* **2022**, *11*, 7009. https://doi.org/10.3390/jcm11237009

Academic Editors: Ewa Małecka-Wojciesko and Manol Jovani

Received: 22 September 2022
Accepted: 17 November 2022
Published: 27 November 2022

Publisher's Note: MDPI stays neutral with regard to jurisdictional claims in published maps and institutional affiliations.

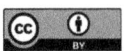

Copyright: © 2022 by the authors. Licensee MDPI, Basel, Switzerland. This article is an open access article distributed under the terms and conditions of the Creative Commons Attribution (CC BY) license (https://creativecommons.org/licenses/by/4.0/).

quantitative technique for the assessment of elasticity of different tissues. Previous studies revealed the advantage of elastography in the differential diagnosis of lymph nodes [10–12].

Thus, in this article, we summarize recent literature on the application of endoscopy techniques in ET, share several representative cases, and highlight the experience of diagnosis of ET in our research center.

2. Classification and Clinical Manifestation

According to absence or presence of extraesophageal tubercular lesions, tubercle bacilli's involvement in the esophagus can be classified as primary or secondary [13]. The differences between primary and secondary esophageal tuberculosis are listed in Table 1. The majority of ET is secondary in adjacent tuberculosis lesions, such as extension of mediastinal lymph nodes, pulmonary, laryngeal, or Pott's spine or, less commonly, through hematogenous spread [3,14–17]. Primary ET occurs when patients swallow sputum or food contaminated with tubercle bacilli. However, primary ET very rarely occurs due to multiple efficacious esophageal protective mechanisms such as stratified squamous epithelium, saliva, and mucus [18].

Table 1. Differences between primary and secondary esophageal tuberculosis.

Classification	Primary Esophageal Tuberculosis	Secondary Esophageal Tuberculosis	Reference
Frequency	Rare	Common	[18]
Extraesophageal tubercular lesions	Absence	Present	[13]
Etiology	Swallow sputum or food contaminated with tubercle bacilli	Invasion of adjacent extraesophageal tubercular lesions	[3,14–18]

The symptoms of ET are variable and depend on the endoscopic morphology. Dysphagia is the main symptom and can be caused by several factors, such as obstruction of intrinsic pseudotumor on account of fibrosis formation or extrinsic compression of infected mediastinal lymph nodes. Upper gastrointestinal tract hematemesis is often caused by damage of blood vessels at the base of an ulcer or artery–esophageal fistula. Respiratory symptoms such as cough and wheezing are the result of a tracheoesophageal fistula. Anorexia, fatigue, night sweats, low-grade fever, and weight loss are common tuberculemia symptoms [19–27].

3. Manifestations of ET According to Upper GI Endoscopy

ET has multiple morphological types according to EGD which can be summarized as follows: ulcerations, eminence lesions, fistula, stricture, and traction diverticula (Table 2). The most common morphology is mid-esophageal linear ulcerations with irregular infiltrated margins and grayish membranous necrotic base [17,22,28]. ET ulcerations usually occur in the mid-esophagus. Tuberculosis-infected lymph nodes are primarily located in the subcarinal region and always intrude into the esophagus on the same level and therefore result in the formation of mid-esophageal ulcerations [21,28]. Deep and large ulcerations have a bleeding tendency and usually present with recent petechiae. Sometimes, ulcerations invade the aorta and start a lethal hemorrhage [5,17]. When encountering unexplained upper gastrointestinal bleeding, the possibility of ET should also be taken into consideration. Nevertheless, the specificity of morphology was inferior; when ulcerations are observed in the upper or middle esophagus, in addition to ET, Crohn's disease and Behçet's disease should also be considered. To differentiate these diseases, other symptoms should be taken into account. For instance, Crohn's disease has representative ileocecal longitudinal, discontinuous, and cobblestone ulcerations [29] and extra-intestinal damage in joints, skin, and eyes, or oral mucosa [30]. Behçet's disease causes ulcers in the mouth, eyes, and genitals [31,32].

Table 2. Role of different types of endoscopies in the diagnosis of esophageal tuberculosis.

	Types of Endoscopy		Features of Esophageal Tuberculosis	Reference
	EGD		Ulcerations, eminence lesions, fistula, stricture, traction diverticula	[5,6,17,18,21,22,28,33,34]
EUS	Esophageal wall		Thickening esophageal wall with vague boundary	[17,18]
	Tuberculosis Lymph node	Phase I	Homogeneous and hypoechoic mass	[1,6,17,18]
		Phase II	Heterogeneous which presents as hyperechoic foci or strands on hypoechoic background	
		Phase III	Heterogeneous hyperechoic mixed hypoechoic mass with indistinct adventitia, occasionally partially matting	
	CH-EUS		Hypo-enhancement compared with the surrounding tissues	
	Elastography		Green	

EGD: esophagogastroduodenoscopy; EUS: endoscopy ultrasonography; CH-EUS: contrast-enhanced harmonic endoscopic ultrasonography.

Eminence lesions comprise intrinsic protruding lesions and extrinsic bulge compression (Figures 1a and 2a). The surface of eminence lesions can be smooth, with ulcerations, fistula, or diverticula [6,18]. Using EGD, the granular form appears as scattered verrucous grayish nodules accompanied by ulcers or erosions. The hypertrophic form refers to when the esophageal wall is fibrotic and forms a pseudotumor [33]. Carina lymph nodes are deposited under trachea bifurcation, close to the mid-esophagus. In addition to causing ulcers, carina lymph nodes also compress the esophagus, and present as extrinsic eminence [21]. Moreover, mediastinal fibrosis can compress the esophagus and lead to extrinsic bulges or traction diverticula [34]. Once protruding lesions block and cause the stricture of the lumen, patients will experience varying degrees of dysphagia, especially with confusing symptoms such as weight loss, making differential diagnosis from malignancy more difficult.

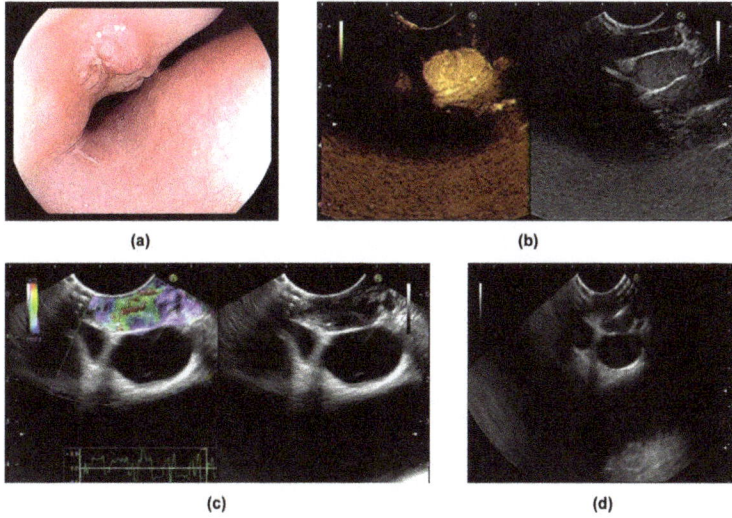

Figure 1. Manifestations of Case 1: (a) manifestations of the lesion according to EGD; (b) the lesion was hypo-enhanced according to CH-EUS; (c) the lesion was soft according to elastography; (d) EUS-FNA for the lesion.

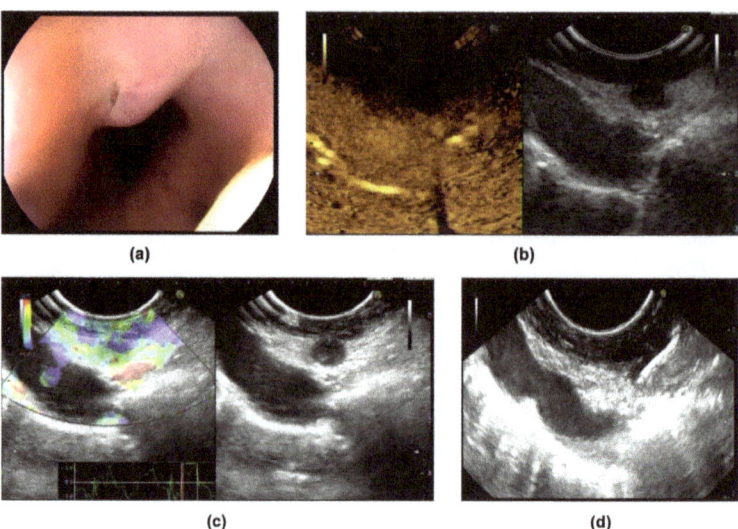

Figure 2. Manifestations of Case 2: (**a**) manifestations of the lesion according to EGD; (**b**) the lesion was hypo-enhanced according to CH-EUS; (**c**) the lesion was soft according to elastography; (**d**) EUS-FNA for the lesion.

Tuberculous lesions encroach on and result in the formation of an abnormal communication between the esophagus and trachea. A double-barreled appearance can be seen when using endoscopy (Figure 3a,b). Meanwhile, the fistulous opening can be observed near the carina using bronchoscopy. A tracheoesophageal fistula can increase the risk of aspiration pneumonia, as reported previously [5]. This double-barreled appearance may resemble fistula tracts caused by aggressive fungal infection or esophageal carcinoma. Histopathology and pathogeny can be relied on to confirm the diagnosis [35,36].

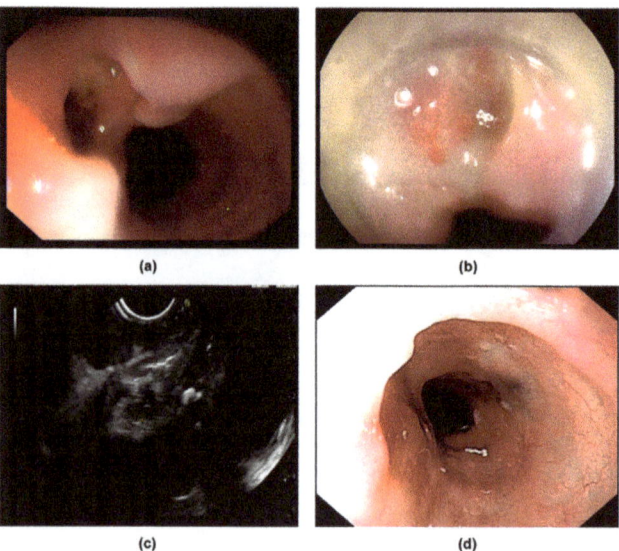

Figure 3. Manifestations of Case 4: (**a**,**b**) manifestations of the lesion according to EGD; (**c**) the lesion as shown by EUS; (**d**) changes shown by using endoscopy after drug treatment.

4. Manifestations of ET According to EUS

EUS has unique advantages in the diagnosis of ET [17,18] (Table 2). It can depict the echogenic characteristics of a tuberculosis lesion, different layers of the esophageal wall, and periesophageal tissue, and the relationship between them. Moreover, endoscopic ultrasound-guided fine-needle aspiration (EUS-FNA) can acquire deep biopsy tissues for further examination [37].

In most cases, ET is caused by the rupture of infected mediastinal lymph nodes to the esophagus. The esophageal wall thickens, and the boundary between the surrounding lesions becomes vague [17,18].

The features of a tuberculosis lymph node when using EUS depend on its stage of development [17]. Lymphoid hyperplasia is the first phase when lymph nodes try to clear the invading mycobacterium tuberculosis via lymphoid tissue hyperplasia. In this phase, hyperplastic lymphocytes and a small amount of caseation concurrence are shown as homogeneous and hypoechoic by EUS. Then, caseous necrosis is further aggravated and leaves hyperechoic foci or strands on heterogeneous hypoechoic background which represent calcification or fibrosis, respectively. Moreover, the adventitia of the lymph nodes is destroyed, and lymph nodes fuse with each other, which appears as indistinct adventitia with partial matting. Overall, based on EUS, the characteristics of lymph nodes can be summarized as heterogeneous, predominantly hypoechoic mass with local hyperechoic foci or strands, indistinct adventitia, and occasionally partial matting (Figures 1b, 2b and 3c) [1,6,18].

Both ET and carcinoma manifest as hypoechoic masses encroaching into various layers of the esophageal wall. Nevertheless, esophageal carcinoma is a hypoechoic mass derived from the epithelial layer, infiltrating from the inside to the outside [38,39]. Most ET is secondary to mediastinal lymph nodes, which are invaded externally. Benign esophageal submucosal tumors (SMTs) are easily identified from ET. Benign esophageal SMTs, such as esophageal leiomyoma, originate from the esophageal lamina propria or mucosal muscle layer with homogeneous hypoechoic lesion, regular boundaries, and normal mediastinal lymph nodes. Furthermore, the echo of malignant esophageal SMTs, such as leiomyosarcoma, is heterogeneous hypoechoic with irregular margins and malignant lymph nodes [40–42]. Malignant lymph nodes present as spherical, hypoechoic, and sharply demarcated [42].

Sarcoidosis is a non-caseous necrotic granulomatous lesion involving multiple organs and systems, particularly affecting both lungs, and hilar and mediastinal lymph nodes. Some experts have proposed that sarcoidosis could be easily differentiated from ET by using EUS because sarcoidosis-associated mediastinal lymph nodes are isoechoic, well margined, and clustered [43,44]. Other experts have suggested that EUS findings for sarcoidosis-associated lymph nodes were nonspecific [45].

The incidence of esophageal Crohn's disease is 0.3–10% [46]. It is difficult to distinguish Crohn's disease from ET using EUS [46]. Only one case regarding Crohn's disease reported that the esophageal wall thickened to 15.4 mm and presented as heterogeneous echo with strand-like hyperechoic areas using EUS. Five layers of the esophageal wall were destroyed. The extra-esophageal lymph nodes were hypoecho and enlarged to 3–4 mm [47]. Differential diagnosis should also refer to whether patients have typical ulcers in the ileocecum or whether there are extra-intestinal manifestations. Unfortunately, there is nothing in the literature on the application of EUS in Behçet's disease.

5. Manifestations of ET According to CH-EUS and Elastography

CH-EUS was performed in two cases in our research center. Both lesions featured hypo-enhancement compared with the surrounding tissues (Figures 1b and 2b) (Table 2). Mechanically, hypo-enhancement reflects a deficiency of blood supply, which corresponds to Stage II or above when the lymph nodes undergo caseous necrosis. Caseous granuloma is always detected in infected lymph nodes which are in Stage II or a more severe stage. In fact, granuloma was found in Cases 1–4 which we will introduce later. Using elastography, images of two lesions were mainly green, showing that both lesions were soft

(Figures 1c and 2c) (Table 2). The characteristics of ET when using CH-EUS and elastography are worth further evaluation.

6. Role of Endoscopy in Acquiring Esophageal Specimens

A definite diagnosis of ET ultimately relies on pathologic and pathogenic investigations of the esophageal specimens. Common methods to obtain biopsy specimens include using biopsy forceps to remove regional esophageal mucosa and using EUS-FNA to obtain a strip of tissue from deep tissues (Figures 1 and 2d) (Table 3). The specimens acquired by biopsy forceps or EUS-FNA are conserved in formalin. The first choice is acquiring esophageal mucosal tissues with biopsy forceps. The positivity rate may be elevated by multi-point deep biopsy. Obtaining samples at the edge of the ulceration is secure and sufficient. Indications of EUS-FNA are listed as follows: 1. The lesion originates from the submucosa or outside the digestive tract; 2. Routine biopsy by forceps was negative, but ET is still highly suspected.

The histopathological specialty of typical tuberculosis granuloma shows central caseous necrosis, surrounded by a radial arrangement of epithelioid cells, with scattered Langhans giant cells. Lots of lymphocytes and fibrous connective tissue can be viewed around the nodule, whereas classical tuberculosis granuloma is uncommon in clinical practice, the emergence of epithelioid cells, multinucleated giant cells along with caseous necrosis is sufficient for diagnosis [25,48]. One study proposed that even if there was no caseous necrosis, ET could be diagnosed [28]. In addition, other than tuberculosis granuloma, Crohn's disease, sarcoidosis, syphilis, and fungal infections also manifest as granuloma. Consequently, it is still difficult to differentiate ET from other granulomatous diseases [26,49,50]. Endoscopy techniques could provide more information for definite diagnosis of ET.

Table 3. Role of endoscopy in acquiring esophageal specimens and different testing methods.

Classification	Function	Testing Methods		Reference
Biopsy forceps	Removing regional esophageal mucosa	Histopathology: tuberculosis granuloma		[25,28,48]
		Etiology	Ziehl-Neelsen staining	[51–55]
EUS-FNA	Obtaining strip of tissue from deep tissues		Cultures	[51–53]
			Polymerase chain reaction	[3,5,48,56]

EUS-FNA: endoscopic ultrasound-guided fine-needle aspiration.

Taking secretions from the center of the ulcer may be beneficial to the detection of pathogens. Ziehl–Neelsen staining is recommended to discover acid-fast bacilli (AFB). To our knowledge, Ziehl–Neelsen staining has a limited sensitivity between 40–60% [51–53], and only shows positive in <25% patients [54,55]; furthermore, 75% cases with extrapulmonary disease could not recognize acid-fast bacilli [53]. Cultures for AFB enjoyed an impressive sensitivity and specificity, recorded as 80% and 98%, respectively. However, it takes a great deal of time, about 6 to 8 weeks, to cultivate mycobacterium tuberculosis [51–53]. The molecular biology technique such as polymerase chain reaction (PCR) is reliable and worthwhile in the diagnosis of ET [3,5,48]. PCR is faster than culture, and the sensitivity of PCR is similar to culture [48,56]. Forceps biopsy and EUS-FNA provide sufficient histological specimens for PCR.

7. Medication and Endoscopic Treatment

A standard nine-month course of treatment consists of four drugs (isoniazid, rifampicin, ethambutol, and pyrazinamide) for two months and two drugs (isoniazid and rifampicin) for seven months. Multidrug resistance of mycobacterium tuberculosis has gradually been acquired increasing attention from the scientific community. Biopsy forceps and EUS-FNA are expected to acquire biopsy specimens for multidrug-resistance detection. For example, rolling circle amplification (RCA) is a fast, highly sensitive, and highly specific molecular biology technique (96.6% and 89.5%, respectively) for detecting multidrug-resistant mycobacterium tuberculosis. The identification of multidrug-resistant bacteria will improve therapeutic efficacy and optimize treatment outcomes [57–59].

If traditional drug treatment is not effective, endoscopic intervention such as the closure of fistula can be performed. Recently, an associated case illustrated successful closure of the fistula with a 12 mm over-the-scope clip (OTSC) [60]. A cap was attached to the tip of the endoscope; then an OTSC was deposited on the tissue in the cap, and a vacuum was generated through endoscopic suction to pull the tissue around the fistula into the cap. The success rate of OTSC was 33–77%. [61–63]. The epithelialization of the fistula is speculated to make it difficult to heal. Argon plasma coagulation (APC) can be utilized to burn the epithelialized mucosa before clipping, which may be more conducive to the healing of the fistula [64] (Table 4).

Table 4. Endoscopic treatment of esophageal tuberculosis.

Endoscopic Treatment	Function	Reference
Biopsy forcep/EUS-FNA	Acquire biopsy specimens for multidrug-resistance detection	[57–59]
Over-the-scope clip	Closure of fistula	[60–63]
Argon plasma coagulation	De-epithelialization prior to closure	[64]

EUS-FNA: endoscopic ultrasound-guided fine-needle aspiration.

8. Case Reports

We retrospectively analyzed medical records from 2013 to 2022 from Beijing Friendship Hospital and screened a total of four patients who were diagnosed with ET (Table 5). The chief complaint in all patients was dysphagia. None of them had AIDS, syphilis, hepatitis, post-transplantation status, or other diseases that led to being immunocompromised. CH-EUS and elastography was performed in two cases. Enlarged mediastinal lymph node and thickening of the middle esophageal wall were detected in all of the cases, which were considered as secondary ET. There were two cases that presented as eminence lesions. (1) A 1.5 × 1.5 cm protruding lesion was found in Case 1, which was 28 cm from the incisor. The surface mucosa of the lesion was uneven with central depression (Figure 1a). EUS showed that the mediastinum mass was mainly hypo-echoic mixed with hyper-echo, and the boundary between the mass and the esophageal wall was vague. Using CH-EUS, it was found that the mass was hypo-enhanced (Figure 1b). The lesion was soft according to elastography (Figure 1c). Then, EUS-FNA was performed (Figure 1d). (2) An elevated submucosal lesion with fissure-like changes in the surface was found in Case 2 (Figure 2a). The lesion was 0.8 × 0.8 cm and 25 cm from the incisor. EUS indicated that the hypoechoic lesions violated the esophageal wall (lymph nodes were considered). CH-EUS also showed hypo-enhancement (Figure 2b), and elastography revealed that the lesion was soft (Figure 2c). EUS-FNA was performed to puncture the extra-esophageal hypoechoic lesions from the mid-esophagus (Figure 2d). (3) Multiple ulcers with esophageal stricture were shown in Case 3. Scattered ulcers were detected in the esophageal mucosa within 18 cm of the incisor with white moss on the bottom. Then, we carefully passed through the stricture using an extra slim scope and circumferential mucosal ulcers with nodular changes extending to the cardia emerged. (4) A 1.0 × 2.5 cm longitudinal fistula with pus overflowing in the anterior esophageal wall at 27–29 cm from the incisor was demonstrated in Case 4. A granule-like tissue was seen at the base of the fistula, and no lichen was attached at the base. The surface of the fistula and the surrounding mucosa were red (Figure 3a,b). EUS revealed a heterogeneous hypoechoic background with hyperechoic strands which were detected under the carina and were fused with each other (Figure 3c).

Table 5. Case summary.

No.	Age	Sex	EGD	EUS	CH-EUS	Elastography	Histopathology	PCR/Ziehl-Neelsen Staining
1	28	Female	Eminence	Hypoechoic with hyperechoic	Hypo-enhancement	Soft	Granuloma	Negative/Negative
2	67	Male	Eminence	Hypoechoic	Hypo-enhancement	Soft	Granuloma	Negative/Negative
3	63	Female	Ulcerated stricture	-	-	-	Granuloma	-/-
4	68	Male	Fistula	Hypoechoic with hyperechoic	-	-	Granuloma	-/-

EGD: esophagogastroduodenoscopy; EUS: endoscopic ultrasonography; CH-EUS: contrast-enhanced harmonic endoscopic ultrasonography; PCR: polymerase chain reaction.

The pathological results discovered granuloma in all patients. PCR and Ziehl-Neelsen staining were performed on two patients, but the results were all negative. Finally, diagnostic anti-tuberculosis therapy was conducted. After 9 months of drug treatment, four patients were asymptomatic. After 1-year follow-up, all of the lesions had disappeared and left scars on the esophageal mucosa according to endoscopy (Figure 3d).

9. Discussion

ET can occur in immunocompromised or immunocompetent hosts. If the patient has a history of TB exposure and symptoms of dysphagia or upper gastrointestinal bleeding, ET should be considered, especially when: (1) mid-esophageal ulcerations, protuberant lesions, or fistulas are detected with EGD; (2) EUS shows a thickened esophageal wall with destruction. Mediastinal lymph nodes were primarily low echo mixed with high echo, adventitia blurred, mutually fused, or had a close relationship with the esophagus; (3) hypo-enhancement is revealed by CH-EUS; and (4) elastography reveals that the lesions are soft.

Although the morphological specificity of ET is poor according to EGD, other techniques could make up for this defect. EUS is expected to improve the differential diagnostic accuracy of ET from carcinoma and SMTs. In addition, CH-EUS and elastography are able to provide supplementary information. Certainly, diagnosis of ET ultimately depends on pathological and pathogenic evidence. Esophageal mucosal tissue can be acquired by biopsy forceps. Deep biopsy tissue such as infected lymph nodes can be obtained with the aid of EUS-FNA. Endoscopic techniques can also be used to detect multidrug-resistant mycobacterium tuberculosis and close the fistula with OTSC and APC.

Due to the low incidence of ET and the fact that CH-EUS has not been widely used in clinical practice, the deficiency of this article lies in its sample size being inadequate. As the sample size expands, there is a posssibility that ET lesions could manifest as iso- or hyper-enhanced according to CH-EUS. Mechanically, the blood supply of Stage I lymph nodes was normal or even abundant compared with the surrounding tissues. Nonetheless, we speculate that hypo-enhancement accounts for the majority because most patients have progressed to Stage II or a more severe stage when they first seek medical treatment. We need to expand the sample size and study the role of CH-EUS in differential diagnosis of ET from other diseases in the near future.

Endoscopists could protect themselves from the following aspects when encountering suspected ET patients. First, the endoscopy center should be divided into clean area or contaminated area. It is necessary to reduce the movement of people and instruments between different areas. Second, endoscopists should wear caps, protective clothes, masks, double gloves and shoe covers. Finally, disposable accessories should be used whenever possible. Items that must be reused should be strictly sterilized. The environment should also be sterilized after the endoscopic procedure.

Future investigations of ET could focus on the following topics. First, future studies should focus on describing more in detail EUS and CH-EUS features of ET and their potential differentiation from carcinoma, SMTs, sarcoidosis, Crohn's disease, and Behçet's disease. Second, the pathological and pathogenic detection method of higher sensitivity and specificity needs to be developed. Third, the therapeutic effects of endoscopy in ET, such as the closure of a fistula, deserve further exploration. In conclusion, endoscopic techniques play crucial roles in the diagnosis of ET. The development of endoscopic techniques such as CH-EUS is expected to improve the diagnostic accuracy of ET.

Author Contributions: Conceptualization, H.Z. and P.L.; resources, B.Y.; writing—original draft preparation, T.Y.; writing—review and editing, Y.Z., G.Z., and A.Z.; supervision, H.Z. and P.L.; funding acquisition, P.L. All authors have read and agreed to the published version of the manuscript.

Funding: This research was funded by Capital's Funds for Health Improvement and Research, grant number 2020-2-2026.

Institutional Review Board Statement: Not applicable.

Informed Consent Statement: Not applicable.

Data Availability Statement: Not applicable.

Conflicts of Interest: The authors declare no conflict of interest.

References

1. Nie, D.; Li, J.; Liu, W.; Wu, Y.; Ji, M.; Wang, Y.; Li, P.; Zhang, S. Esophagomediastinal fistula due to secondary esophageal tuberculosis: Report of two cases. *J. Int. Med. Res.* **2021**, *49*, 3000605211023696. [CrossRef] [PubMed]
2. de Cossío, S.; Labrador, B.; Yarza, R.; Corbella, L.; Fernández-Ruiz, M. Oesophageal ulcer: An uncommon presentation of tuberculous lymphadenitis mimicking an oesophageal carcinoma. *Gastroenterol. Hepatol.* **2020**, *43*, 133–134. [CrossRef] [PubMed]
3. Peixoto, P.C.; Ministro, P.S.; Sadio, A.D.; Cancela, E.M.; Araújo, R.N.; Machado, J.L.; Castanheira, A.H.; Silva, A.T.; Nunes, R.D.; Carvalho, M.T.; et al. Esophageal tuberculosis: An unusual cause of dysphagia. *Gastrointest. Endosc.* **2009**, *69*, 1173–1176. [CrossRef] [PubMed]
4. Elosua Gonzalez, A.; Macias Mendizabal, E.; Saldana Duenas, C.; Fernández-Urién Sainz, I.; Vila Costas, J.J. Esophageal tuberculosis: A cause of dysphagia we should be aware of. *Gastrointest. Endosc.* **2018**, *88*, 964–965. [CrossRef]
5. Abid, S.; Jafri, W.; Hamid, S.; Khan, H.; Hussainy, A. Endoscopic features of esophageal tuberculosis. *Gastrointest. Endosc.* **2003**, *57*, 759–762. [CrossRef] [PubMed]
6. Xiong, J.; Guo, W.; Guo, Y.; Gong, L.; Liu, S. Clinical and endoscopic features of esophageal tuberculosis: A 20-year retrospective study. *Scand. J. Gastroenterol.* **2020**, *55*, 1200–1204. [CrossRef] [PubMed]
7. Rana, S.; Bhasin, D.; Rao, C.; Srinivasan, R.; Singh, K. Tuberculosis presenting as Dysphagia: Clinical, endoscopic, radiological and endosonographic features. *Endosc. Ultrasound.* **2013**, *2*, 92–95. [CrossRef] [PubMed]
8. Kitano, M.; Sakamoto, H.; Komaki, T.; Kudo, M. New techniques and future perspective of EUS for the differential diagnosis of pancreatic malignancies: Contrast harmonic imaging. *Dig. Endosc.* **2011**, *23* (Suppl. 1), 46–50. [CrossRef]
9. Kitano, M.; Yoshida, T.; Itonaga, M.; Tamura, T.; Hatamaru, K.; Yamashita, Y. Impact of endoscopic ultrasonography on diagnosis of pancreatic cancer. *J. Gastroenterol.* **2019**, *54*, 19–32. [CrossRef]
10. Cui, X.-W.; Chang, J.-M.; Kan, Q.-C.; Chiorean, L.; Ignee, A.; Dietrich, C.F. Endoscopic ultrasound elastography: Current status and future perspectives. *World J. Gastroenterol.* **2015**, *21*, 13212–13224. [CrossRef]
11. Janssen, J.; Dietrich, C.; Will, U.; Greiner, L. Endosonographic elastography in the diagnosis of mediastinal lymph nodes. *Endoscopy* **2007**, *39*, 952–957. [CrossRef] [PubMed]
12. Xu, W.; Shi, J.; Zeng, X.; Li, X.; Xie, W.-F.; Guo, J.; Lin, Y. EUS elastography for the differentiation of benign and malignant lymph nodes: A meta-analysis. *Gastrointest. Endosc.* **2011**, *74*, 1001–1009, quiz 115 e1–e4. [CrossRef] [PubMed]
13. Singh, A.; Mittal, D.; Jain, V.; Kabra, S.K.; Agarwala, S. Primary Esophageal Tuberculosis. *Indian J. Pediatr.* **2021**, *88*, 947. [CrossRef] [PubMed]
14. Danna, B.J.; Harvey, A.W.; Woc-Colburn, L.E. Esophageal Tuberculosis—A Mass of Confusion. *Am. J. Med.* **2020**, *133*, e589–e590. [CrossRef]
15. Fahmy, A.R.; Guindi, R.; Farid, A. Tuberculosis of the oesophagus. *Thorax* **1969**, *24*, 254–256. [CrossRef]
16. Eng, J.; Sabanathan, S. Tuberculosis of the esophagus. *Dig. Dis. Sci.* **1991**, *36*, 536–540. [CrossRef]
17. Puri, R.; Khaliq, A.; Kumar, M.; Sud, R.; Vasdev, N. Esophageal tuberculosis: Role of endoscopic ultrasound in diagnosis. *Dis. Esophagus* **2012**, *25*, 102–106. [CrossRef]
18. Zhu, R.; Bai, Y.; Zhou, Y.; Fang, X.; Zhao, K.; Tuo, B.; Wu, H. EUS in the diagnosis of pathologically undiagnosed esophageal tuberculosis. *BMC Gastroenterol.* **2020**, *20*, 291. [CrossRef]
19. Ramakantan, R.S.P. Dysphagia due to mediastinal fibrosis in advanced pulmonary tuberculosis. *AJR Am. J. Roentgenol.* **1990**, *154*, 61–63. [CrossRef]
20. Porter, J.C.F.J.; Freedman, A.R. Tuberculosis bronchoesophageal fistulae in patients infected with the HIV virus Three case reports and review. *Clin. Infect. Dis.* **1994**, *9*, 954–957. [CrossRef]

21. Rana, S.S.; Sharma, V.; Bhasin, D.K. An unusual cause of dysphagia. *Clin. Gastroenterol. Hepatol.* **2015**, *13*, e43–e44. [CrossRef] [PubMed]
22. Fagundes, R.B.; Dalcin, R.P.; Rocha, M.P.; Moraes, C.C.; Carlotto, V.S.; Wink, M.O. Esophageal tuberculosis. *Endoscopy* **2007**, *39* (Suppl. 1), E149. [CrossRef] [PubMed]
23. Nagi, B.; Lal, A.; Kochhar, R.; Bhasin, D.K.; Gulati, M.; Suri, S.; Singh, K. Imaging of esophageal tuberculosis: A review of 23 cases. *Acta Radiol.* **2003**, *44*, 329–333. [PubMed]
24. Devarbhavi, H.C.; Alvares, J.F.; Radhikadevi, M. Esophageal tuberculosis associated with esophagotracheal or esophagomediastinal fistula: Report of 10 cases. *Gastrointest. Endosc.* **2003**, *57*, 588–592. [CrossRef]
25. Fujiwara, Y.; Osugi, H.; Takada, N.; Takemura, M.; Lee, S.; Ueno, M.; Fukuhara, K.; Tanaka, Y.; Nishizawa, S.; Kinoshita, H. Esophageal tuberculosis presenting with an appearance similar to that of carcinoma of the esophagus. *J. Gastroenterol.* **2003**, *38*, 477–481. [CrossRef]
26. Jain, S.K.; Kumar, N.; Das, D.K. Esophageal tuberculosis. Endoscopic cytology as a diagnostic tool. *Acta Cytol.* **1999**, *43*, 1085–1090. [CrossRef]
27. Fang, H.-Y.; Lin, T.-S.; Cheng, C.-Y.; Talbot, A.R. Esophageal tuberculosis: A rare presentation with massive hematemesis. *Ann. Thorac. Surg.* **1999**, *68*, 2344–2346. [CrossRef]
28. Jain, S.K.; Jain, S.; Jain, M.; Yaduvanshi, A. Esophageal tuberculosis: Is it so rare? Report of 12 cases and review of the literature. *Am. J. Gastroenterol.* **2002**, *97*, 287–291. [CrossRef]
29. Limsrivilai, J.; Shreiner, A.B.; Pongpaibul, A.; Laohapand, C.; Boonanuwat, R.; Pausawasdi, N.; Pongprasobchai, S.; Manatsathit, S.; Higgins, P.D. Meta-Analytic Bayesian Model For Differentiating Intestinal Tuberculosis from Crohn's Disease. *Am. J. Gastroenterol.* **2017**, *112*, 415–427. [CrossRef]
30. Laass, M.W.; Roggenbuck, D.; Conrad, K. Diagnosis and classification of Crohn's disease. *Autoimmun Rev.* **2014**, *13*, 467–471. [CrossRef]
31. Yazici, Y.; Hatemi, G.; Bodaghi, B.; Cheon, J.H.; Suzuki, N.; Ambrose, N.; Yazici, H. Behcet syndrome. *Nat. Rev. Dis. Primers* **2021**, *7*, 67. [CrossRef] [PubMed]
32. Sakakibara, Y.; Nakazuru, S.; Akasaka, T.; Ishida, H.; Mita, E. A case of Behcet's disease with esophageal ulcers. *Gastrointest. Endosc.* **2019**, *89*, 430–431. [CrossRef] [PubMed]
33. Wang, S.-H.; Lin, C.-K.; Chang, Y.-C.; Lee, T.-H.; Chung, C.-S. An atypical infection of the esophagus mimicking malignancy. *Gastrointest Endosc.* **2018**, *88*, 765–766. [CrossRef] [PubMed]
34. Park, S.H.; Chung, J.P.; Kim, I.J.; Park, H.J.; Lee, K.S.; Chon, C.Y.; Park, I.S.; Kim, K.W.; Lee, D.Y. Dysphagia due to mediastinal tuberculous lymphadenitis presenting as an esophageal submucosal tumor: A case report. *Yonsei Med. J.* **1995**, *36*, 386–391. [CrossRef]
35. Kim, B.-W.; Cho, S.-H.; Rha, S.-E.; Choi, H.; Choi, K.-Y.; Cha, S.-B.; Choi, M.-G.; Chung, I.-S.; Sun, H.-S.; Park, D.-H. Esophagomediastinal fistula and esophageal stricture as a complication of esophageal candidiasis: A case report. *Gastrointest. Endosc.* **2000**, *52*, 772–775. [CrossRef]
36. Guccion, J.G.; Ortega, L.G. Trichomoniasis complicating esophageal intramural pseudodiverticulosis: Diagnosis by transmission electron microscopy. *Ultrastruct. Pathol.* **1996**, *20*, 101–107. [CrossRef] [PubMed]
37. von Bartheld, M.B.; van Kralingen, K.W.; Veenendaal, R.A.; Willems, L.N.; Rabe, K.F.; Annema, J.T. Mediastinal-esophageal fistulae after EUS-FNA of tuberculosis of the mediastinum. *Gastrointest. Endosc.* **2010**, *71*, 210–212. [CrossRef] [PubMed]
38. Klamt, A.L.; Neyeloff, J.L.; Santos, L.M.; Mazzini, G.D.S.; Campos, V.J.; Gurski, R.R. Echoendoscopy in Preoperative Evaluation of Esophageal Adenocarcinoma and Gastroesophageal Junction: Systematic Review and Meta-analysis. *Ultrasound Med. Biol.* **2021**, *47*, 1657–1669. [CrossRef]
39. Pfau, P.R.; Perlman, S.B.; Stanko, P.; Frick, T.J.; Gopal, D.V.; Said, A.; Zhang, Z.; Weigel, T. The role and clinical value of EUS in a multimodality esophageal carcinoma staging program with CT and positron emission tomography. *Gastrointest. Endosc.* **2007**, *65*, 377–384. [CrossRef]
40. Codipilly, D.C.; Fang, H.; Alexander, J.A.; Katzka, D.A.; Ravi, K. Subepithelial esophageal tumors: A single-center review of resected and surveilled lesions. *Gastrointest. Endosc.* **2018**, *87*, 370–377. [CrossRef]
41. Pesenti, C.; Bories, E.; Caillol, F.; Ratone, J.; Godat, S.; Monges, G.; Poizat, F.; Raoul, J.; Ries, P.; Giovannini, M. Characterization of subepithelial lesions of the stomach and esophagus by contrast-enhanced EUS: A retrospective study. *Endosc. Ultrasound* **2019**, *8*, 43–49. [CrossRef]
42. Palazzo, L.; Landi, B.; Cellier, C.; Cuillerier, E.; Roseau, G.; Barbier, J.-P. Endosonographic features predictive of benign and malignant gastrointestinal stromal cell tumours. *Gut* **2000**, *46*, 88–92. [CrossRef] [PubMed]
43. Crombag, L.M.M.; Mooij-Kalverda, K.; Szlubowski, A.; Gnass, M.; Tournoy, K.G.; Sun, J.; Oki, M.; Ninaber, M.K.; Steinfort, D.P.; Jennings, B.R.; et al. EBUS versus EUS-B for diagnosing sarcoidosis: The International Sarcoidosis Assessment (ISA) randomized clinical trial. *Respirology* **2022**, *27*, 152–160. [CrossRef] [PubMed]
44. Oki, M.; Saka, H.; Ando, M.; Tsuboi, R.; Nakahata, M.; Oka, S.; Kogure, Y.; Kitagawa, C. Transbronchial vs transesophageal needle aspiration using an ultrasound bronchoscope for the diagnosis of mediastinal lesions: A randomized study. *Chest* **2015**, *147*, 1259–1266. [CrossRef] [PubMed]
45. Michael, H.; Ho, S.; Pollack, B.; Gupta, M.; Gress, F. Diagnosis of intra-abdominal and mediastinal sarcoidosis with EUS-guided FNA. *Gastrointest. Endosc.* **2008**, *67*, 28–34. [CrossRef]

46. Laube, R.; Liu, K.; Schifter, M.; Yang, J.L.; Suen, M.K.; Leong, R.W. Oral and upper gastrointestinal Crohn's disease. *J. Gastroenterol. Hepatol.* **2018**, *33*, 355–364. [CrossRef]
47. Lou, G.C.; Yang, J.M.; Huang, W.; Zhang, J.; Zhou, B. Esophageal Crohn's disease. *Endoscopy* **2009**, *41* (Suppl. 2), E257. [CrossRef]
48. Fujiwara, T.; Yoshida, Y.; Yamada, S.; Kawamata, H.; Fujimori, T.; Imawari, M. A case of primary esophageal tuberculosis diagnosed by identification of Mycobacteria in paraffin-embedded esophageal biopsy specimens by polymerase chain reaction. *J. Gastroenterol.* **2003**, *38*, 74–78. [CrossRef]
49. Aydin, A.; Tekin, F.; Ozutemiz, O.; Musoğlu, A. Value of endoscopic ultrasonography for diagnosis of esophageal tuberculosis: Report of two cases. *Dig. Dis. Sci.* **2006**, *51*, 1673–1676. [CrossRef]
50. Ni, B.; Lu, X.; Gong, Q.; Zhang, W.; Li, X.; Xu, H.; Zhang, S.; Shao, Y. Surgical outcome of esophageal tuberculosis secondary to mediastinal lymphadenitis in adults: Experience from single center in China. *J. Thorac. Dis.* **2013**, *5*, 498–505.
51. Kotanidou, A.; Andrianakis, I.; Mavrommatis, A.; Politis, P.; Roussos, C.; Bellenis, I. Mediastinal mass with Dysphagia in an elderly patient. *Infection* **2003**, *31*, 178–180. [CrossRef] [PubMed]
52. Garg, S.K.; Tiwari, R.P.; Tiwari, D.; Singh, R.; Malhotra, D.; Ramnani, V.K.; Prasad, G.; Chandra, R.; Fraziano, M.; Colizzi, V.; et al. Diagnosis of tuberculosis: Available technologies, limitations, and possibilities. *J. Clin. Lab. Anal.* **2003**, *17*, 155–163. [CrossRef] [PubMed]
53. Mitchison, D.A. The diagnosis and therapy of tuberculosis during the past 100 years. *Am. J. Respir. Crit. Care Med.* **2005**, *171*, 699–706. [CrossRef] [PubMed]
54. Damtew, B.; Frengley, D.; Wolinsky, E.; Spagnuolo, P.J. Esophageal tuberculosis: Mimicry of gastrointestinal malignancy. *Rev. Infect. Dis.* **1987**, *9*, 140–146. [CrossRef] [PubMed]
55. Mert, A.; Tabak, F.; Ozaras, R.; Tahan, V.; Öztürk, R.; Aktuglu, Y. Tuberculous lymphadenopathy in adults: A review of 35 cases. *Acta Chir. Belg.* **2002**, *102*, 118–121. [CrossRef]
56. Rubinstein, B.M.; Pastrana, T.; Jacobson, H.G. Tuberculosis of the esophagus. *Radiology* **1958**, *70*, 401–403. [CrossRef]
57. Chen, X.; Wang, B.; Yang, W.; Kong, F.; Li, C.; Sun, Z.; Jelfs, P.; Gilbert, G.L. Rolling circle amplification for direct detection of rpoB gene mutations in Mycobacterium tuberculosis isolates from clinical specimens. *J. Clin. Microbiol.* **2014**, *52*, 1540–1548. [CrossRef]
58. Murray, C.J.; Ikuta, K.S.; Sharara, F.; Swetschinski, L.; Aguilar, G.R.; Gray, A.; Han, C.; Bisignano, C.; Rao, P.; Wool, E.; et al. Global burden of bacterial antimicrobial resistance in 2019: A systematic analysis. *Lancet* **2022**, *399*, 629–655. [CrossRef]
59. Chakaya, J.; Khan, M.; Ntoumi, F.; Aklillu, E.; Fatima, R.; Mwaba, P.; Kapata, N.; Mfinanga, S.; Hasnain, S.E.; Katoto, P.D.; et al. Global Tuberculosis Report 2020—Reflections on the Global TB burden, treatment and prevention efforts. *Int. J. Infect. Dis.* **2021**, *113* (Suppl. 1), S7–S12. [CrossRef]
60. Bassi, M.; Ferrari, M.; Ghersi, S.; Livi, V.; Dabizzi, E.; Trisolini, R.; Cennamo, V. Dual aspect endoscopic evidence of tuberculous bronchoesophageal fistula: Successful closure from the esophagus. *Endoscopy* **2020**, *52*, E378–E380. [CrossRef]
61. Surace, M.; Mercky, P.; Demarquay, J.-F.; Gonzalez, J.-M.; Dumas, R.; Ah-Soune, P.; Vitton, V.; Grimaud, J.; Barthet, M. Endoscopic management of GI fistulae with the over-the-scope clip system (with video). *Gastrointest. Endosc.* **2011**, *74*, 1416–1419. [CrossRef] [PubMed]
62. Law, R.; Song, L.M.W.K.; Irani, S.; Baron, T.H. Immediate technical and delayed clinical outcome of fistula closure using an over-the-scope clip device. *Surg. Endosc.* **2015**, *29*, 1781–1786. [CrossRef] [PubMed]
63. Sulz, M.C.; Bertolini, R.; Frei, R.; Semadeni, G.-M.; Borovicka, J.; Meyenberger, C. Multipurpose use of the over-the-scope-clip system ("Bear claw") in the gastrointestinal tract: Swiss experience in a tertiary center. *World J. Gastroenterol.* **2014**, *20*, 16287–16292. [CrossRef] [PubMed]
64. Sonomura, J.; Shimizu, T.; Taniguchi, K.; Lee, S.W.; Tanaka, R.; Imai, Y.; Honda, K.; Kawai, M.; Tashiro, K.; Uchiyama, K. Esophago-bronchial fistula treated by the Over-The-Scope-Clipping (OTSC) system with argon beam electrocoagulation: A case report. *Medicine* **2021**, *100*, e24494. [CrossRef]

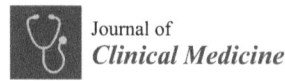

Review

Artificial Intelligence in Endoscopic Ultrasound for Pancreatic Cancer: Where Are We Now and What Does the Future Entail?

Dushyant Singh Dahiya [1,*], Mohammad Al-Haddad [2], Saurabh Chandan [3], Manesh Kumar Gangwani [4], Muhammad Aziz [5], Babu P. Mohan [6], Daryl Ramai [6], Andrew Canakis [7], Jay Bapaye [8] and Neil Sharma [2,9,10]

1. Department of Internal Medicine, Central Michigan University College of Medicine, Saginaw, MI 48601, USA
2. Division of Gastroenterology and Hepatology, Indiana University School of Medicine, Indianapolis, IN 46202, USA
3. Division of Gastroenterology and Hepatology, CHI Creighton University Medical Center, Omaha, NE 68131, USA
4. Department of Internal Medicine, The University of Toledo Medical Center, Toledo, OH 43614, USA
5. Department of Gastroenterology, The University of Toledo Medical Center, Toledo, OH 43614, USA
6. Division of Gastroenterology and Hepatology, University of Utah School of Medicine, Salt Lake City, UT 84132, USA
7. Division of Gastroenterology and Hepatology, University of Maryland School of Medicine, Baltimore, MD 21201, USA
8. Department of Internal Medicine, Rochester General Hospital, Rochester, NY 14621, USA
9. Parkview Cancer Institute, Fort Wayne, IN 46845, USA
10. Interventional Oncology & Surgical Endoscopy Programs (IOSE), Parkview Health, Fort Wayne, IN 46845, USA
* Correspondence: dush.dahiya@gmail.com; Tel.: +1-(678)-602-1176

Abstract: Pancreatic cancer is a highly lethal disease associated with significant morbidity and mortality. In the United States (US), the overall 5-year relative survival rate for pancreatic cancer during the 2012–2018 period was 11.5%. However, the cancer stage at diagnosis strongly influences relative survival in these patients. Per the National Cancer Institute (NCI) statistics for 2012–2018, the 5-year relative survival rate for patients with localized disease was 43.9%, while it was 3.1% for patients with distant metastasis. The poor survival rates are primarily due to the late development of clinical signs and symptoms. Hence, early diagnosis is critical in improving treatment outcomes. In recent years, artificial intelligence (AI) has gained immense popularity in gastroenterology. AI-assisted endoscopic ultrasound (EUS) models have been touted as a breakthrough in the early detection of pancreatic cancer. These models may also accurately differentiate pancreatic cancer from chronic pancreatitis and autoimmune pancreatitis, which mimics pancreatic cancer on radiological imaging. In this review, we detail the application of AI-assisted EUS models for pancreatic cancer detection. We also highlight the utility of AI-assisted EUS models in differentiating pancreatic cancer from radiological mimickers. Furthermore, we discuss the current limitations and future applications of AI technology in EUS for pancreatic cancers.

Keywords: artificial intelligence; endoscopic ultrasound; pancreatic cancer; chronic pancreatitis; autoimmune pancreatitis

1. Introduction

Pancreatic cancer has been identified as the seventh leading cause of cancer-related death worldwide [1]. Pancreatic ductal adenocarcinoma (PDAC), an invasive mucin-producing neoplasm with an intense stromal desmoplastic reaction, is the most common (90%) subtype of pancreatic cancer [2,3]. The median age at diagnosis for pancreatic cancer is about 70 years. PDAC is slightly more common in males compared to females on a global scale (age-standardized incidence rate of 5.5 per 100,000 in men vs. 4 per 100,000 in women) [4,5]. Current estimates by the National Cancer Institute (NCI) predict

62,210 new cases of pancreatic cancer in the US in 2022, representing 3.2% of all new cancer diagnoses [6].

Most patients with pancreatic cancer lack obvious clinical signs and symptoms until they have advanced-stage disease. Furthermore, traditional imaging techniques such as computer tomography (CT) and magnetic resonance imaging (MRI) may not be able to detect small or premalignant pancreatic lesions. Therefore, an early diagnosis is often difficult to establish. Hence, due to a late initial presentation, patients often have advanced-stage disease with widespread metastasis, leading to poor clinical outcomes and high mortality rates [3,7]. In the US, the age-adjusted death rate for pancreatic cancer was noted to be 11.1 per 100,000 men and women per year between 2015–2019 [6]. However, it is worth noting that the 5-year relative survival rate for pancreatic cancer in the US has continued to rise from 3.2% in the 1970s to 11.5% for the 2012–2018 period, reflecting possible improvements in diagnostic and management strategies [6].

Endoscopic ultrasound (EUS) has the greatest specificity and sensitivity for the diagnosis of pancreatic lesions and, in particular, pancreatic cancer. Recently, biopsies via EUS have shifted from fine-needle aspiration (FNA) to fine-needle biopsy (FNB). EUS combined with FNB has a specificity and sensitivity greater than 90% for the detection of pancreatic cancer [8,9]. However, EUS does not have widespread availability and utilization due to the need for additional training, a steep learning curve, operator dependence, the cost of equipment, and the need for sedation.

Over the years, gastroenterologists have typically relied on individualized manual analysis and the interpretation of EUS and cross-sectional radiographic images to diagnose, classify, and plan interventions for patients with gastrointestinal (GI) neoplasms [10]. This has inevitably led to significant variability in diagnosis based on clinical proficiency, expertise, and individual bias. However, recently, AI has gained immense popularity in GI, particularly for luminal and pancreaticobiliary disorders, due to its ability to analyze large sets of data with a high degree of accuracy [11]. AI algorithms not only assist with the rapid diagnosis of GI neoplasms but also reduce inter-observer variability, decrease rates of misdiagnosis, and standardize the interpretation of radiological and histopathological images, leading to accurate diagnosis and improvements in clinical outcomes [10–12].

EUS is the imaging modality of choice for pancreatic cancers and is preferred over conventional CT scans and MRIs due to its high diagnostic yield and negative predictive value [13]. In current literature, numerous AI models have been successfully integrated with EUS [14]. This has led to the early detection of pancreatic cancer, thereby expediting management, reducing the risk of mortality, and decreasing the overall healthcare burden on individuals and healthcare systems across the globe [15,16]. In this comprehensive review, we focus our discussion on AI and its application in EUS for the detection and differentiation of pancreatic neoplasms from other disease entities such as chronic pancreatitis (CP) and autoimmune pancreatitis (AIP). Furthermore, we also highlight the limitations and future applications of AI technology in EUS for pancreatic cancers.

2. Discussion

2.1. Artificial Intelligence and Its Utility in Gastroenterology

AI is a highly complex integration of computer systems and software to design computer algorithms that display the properties of critical thinking and intelligence (Figure 1) [12]. In a broader sense of the term, AI aims to replicate human intelligence with learning abilities and complex problem-solving skills. Since it was first described by John McCarthy in 1956, AI algorithms have undergone a major transformation from artificial narrow intelligence (ANI), which was primarily designed to perform simple predetermined tasks, to artificial general intelligence (AGI) and superintelligence, which can analyze large quantities of data and solve complex problems accurately [17,18]. The three major branches of AI that are slowly revolutionizing clinical practice include machine learning (ML), artificial neural networks (ANNs), and expert systems (ES).

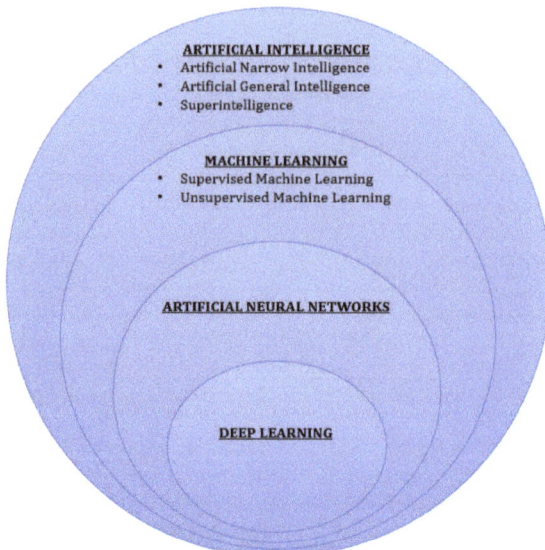

Figure 1. Types of artificial intelligence.

ML is a branch of AI that allows software applications to attain efficiency in predicting outcomes of interest without explicit programming, using already available historical data as input [19]. It can be further subdivided into supervised and unsupervised learning. Supervised ML provides data in the form of input–output pairs, wherein the input is the descriptor and the output is the outcome of interest [20]. On the other hand, unsupervised ML identifies specific groups with common features within the dataset without prior knowledge of the significance of the data [20]. In 2006, AI technology had a major breakthrough with deep learning (DL), a subset of ML [21]. DL mimics the human neuronal network as it combines multiple nonlinear processing layers wherein the original data is abstracted layer-by-layer, and different levels of the abstract features are obtained and used for target detection, classification, or segmentation [21]. The primary advantage of DL over ML is that it requires minimal human intervention to generate the output of interest [21].

ANNs are a set of interconnected computers and algorithms consisting of inputs, weights, bias/threshold, and outputs that mimic human neuroanatomy [22]. However, they differ from DL due to a lower number of hidden layers within the network. In ANNs, each computing unit essentially functions as a 'neuron' and is connected to other computing units, building a highly complex network [20]. Through this network, signals travel to reach the output layers, traversing through multiple hidden layers [20]. As the ANNs are trained with the help of training data, the weights of the interneuron connections are adjusted to optimize output data and increase efficacy [22].

ES is a computing system capable of solving complex problems with reasoning based on current knowledge, emulating the decision-making capacity of a human expert [23]. These systems are designed to mimic clinical reasoning and judgment and have the capability to express conclusions as a probability based on input data [24]. Currently, it takes many years and a large dataset to develop a single ES capable of delivering decisions on a single output of interest or diagnosis [24]. Hence, the utilization of ES in clinical medicine is very limited. However, as AI technology continues to improve, ES may soon find widespread use in clinical medicine.

AI has found widespread application in GI, particularly for endoluminal and pancreaticobiliary disorders. It helps to significantly improve diagnostic accuracy, limit errors, standardize the interpretation of radiological and histopathological images, and establish plans for interventions [11]. Major areas of utilization of AI within GI include:

1. Application in Premalignant Lesions: Esophagogastroduodenoscopy (EGD) and colonoscopy are pivotal procedures in diagnosing upper and lower premalignant GI lesions. However, there is significant variability in premalignant lesion detection due to the endoscopists' skill level. To standardize and improve the quality of EGDs and colonoscopies, AI-assisted models have been utilized. In current literature, two randomized controlled trials (RCTs) have compared the endoscopic performance for the diagnosis of premalignant lesions between AI-assisted and non-AI-assisted models. The WISENSE system, which used deep convolutional neural networks (CNNs) and deep reinforcement learning, reported lower rates of blind spots (5.86% vs. 22.46%, $p < 0.001$) during EGD for upper GI lesions compared to the non-AI-assisted control group [25]. The authors ultimately concluded that the WISENSE system significantly improved the quality of EGDs [25]. Another RCT by Wang et al. noted a significantly higher adenoma detection rate (ADR; 29.1% vs. 20.3%, $p < 0.001$) and mean number of adenomas per patient (0.53 vs. 0.31, $p < 0.001$) for diagnostic colonoscopy for an AI-mediated real-time automatic polyp detection system that provided audio-visual alerts upon polyp detection compared to diagnostic colonoscopies without the assistance of an AI system [26].

2. Application in Malignant Lesions: AI can help gastroenterologists accurately determine the prognosis of malignant GI neoplasms compared to conventional non-AI models [27–30]. A study by Gohari et al. compared the accuracy of prediction of survival rates for patients with colorectal cancer between an ANN AI-assisted model and Cox regression models [27]. The authors noted that the ANN model had more accurate predictions of survival for colon (89% vs. 78.6%) and rectal (82.7% vs. 70.7%) cancer patients compared to the Cox regression models [27]. Biglarian et al. compared the accuracy of prediction of distant metastasis for colorectal cancer between an ANN AI-assisted model and logistic regression models [28]. The authors observed that the ANN model had higher accuracy in predicting distant metastasis (area under the receiver operating characteristic curve (AUROC): 0.82 vs. 0.77) compared to the logistic regression models [28]. Another study by Nilsaz-Dezfouli et al. demonstrated the utility of a single time-point feed-forward ANN AI-assisted model to predict the probability of survival for gastric cancer patients at 1, 2, 3, 4, and 5 years after surgery [29]. The authors concluded that the prediction of survival for the ANN model was consistently accurate (88.7–90.2%), with sensitivity and specificity ranging from 70.2–92.5% and 66.7–96.2%, respectively [29]. Furthermore, DL algorithms have also found applications in the detection and treatment of GI malignancies [31–33]. A systematic review and meta-analysis of five RCTs (4354 patients) that assessed the performance of a DL computer-aided polyp detection system for the detection of colorectal neoplasia noted a significantly higher pooled adenoma detection rate (36.6% vs. 25.2%, RR 1.44; 95% confidence interval (CI) 1.27–1.62; $p < 0.01$; $I^2 = 42\%$) and adenomas detected per colonoscopy (58% vs. 36%, RR 1.70; 95% CI 1.53–1.89; $p < 0.01$; $I^2 = 33\%$) for the AI-assisted model compared to the control group [31]. From a treatment perspective, DL models can predict clinical response to chemotherapy and radiation with high accuracy ($\geq 80\%$) [32,33].

3. Application in Inflammatory Lesions: Numerous studies have investigated the use of AI-assisted models to identify a wide spectrum of inflammatory lesions. For identifying patients with inflammatory bowel disease (IBD), the support vector machine (SVM) model, a type of machine learning algorithm, had diagnostic accuracy, sensitivity, and specificity ranging from 80–100%, 80–95.2%, and 92.4–93.6%, respectively, using endoscopic or wireless capsule endoscopy (WCE) images as input data [20]. The SVM model has also been used to detect ulcerative disease (peptic ulcers, ulcers from Crohn's disease, NSAID-induced ulcers, and unexplained ulcers) with high accuracy (74–96.3%), sensitivity (75–100%), and specificity (73.3–100%) [20]. Furthermore, a study by Cui et al. used an adaptive threshold classifier AI-assisted model on 7218 small bowel WCE images to identify lymphangiectasia with a diagnostic

accuracy of 97.9% [20]. Another study by Wu et al. used the Rustboost AI-assisted model on small bowel WCE images from 10 patients to identify individuals with a hookworm infection with the accuracy, sensitivity, and specificity of 78.2%, 77.2%, and 77.9%, respectively [20]. In patients with celiac disease, the diagnostic accuracy of AI-assisted models ranges from 76.7–99.6% [20].

4. Application in Gastrointestinal Bleeding: GI bleeding is a common medical emergency associated with significant morbidity and mortality. In the current literature, twelve studies have assessed the use of AI-assisted models to detect small bowel bleeding using WCE images/videos as input data [20,34–43]. Of these, six studies using an SVM AI-assisted model to identify patients with small bowel bleeding reported diagnostic accuracy ranging from 91.8–99.6% [35–37,39–41]. Additionally, five studies that utilized various AI-assisted models, such as multilayer perceptron network (MLP), probabilistic neural network, joint diagonalization principal component analysis, and CNN reported diagnostic accuracy ranging from 87.4–98% [20,34,38,42,43]. However, a study by Jung et al. that utilized a color spectrum transformation AI-assisted model to identify small bowel GI bleeding using WCE images as input data had a diagnostic accuracy of only 30% but a sensitivity and specificity of 94.9% and 96.1%, respectively [20].

5. Application in Hepatology: The utilization of AI-assisted models to detect liver fibrosis, non-alcoholic fatty liver disease (NAFLD), and esophageal varices has increased exponentially in recent years. Seven studies that used AI-assisted models to detect liver fibrosis associated with viral hepatitis (hepatitis B and C viruses) reported diagnostic accuracy of $\geq 84.4\%$ [20]. The diagnostic accuracy of AI-assisted models from six studies that aimed to identify individuals with NAFLD ranged from 79% to 89% [20]. Two studies that used MLP and random forest AI-assisted models to detect esophageal varices noted a diagnostic accuracy of 87.8% and 0.82 (AUROC), respectively [20]. Overall, these AI models identified their target factor with $\geq 80\%$ accuracy.

2.2. Utilization of Artificial Intelligence in Endoscopic Ultrasound for the Detection of Pancreatic Cancer

In the US, the incidence and prevalence of pancreatic cancer continue to rise [6]. It is currently the third leading cause of cancer mortality and soon will be the second, behind lung cancer [10]. Despite these rising trends, there are no definitive guidelines on pancreatic cancer screening in average-risk individuals. Imaging modalities such as CT scans and MRIs are often used to aid the diagnosis of pancreatic cancer, but EUS is considered far superior due to its higher diagnostic yield and ability to obtain high-quality images [44]. However, there are some limitations to conventional EUS, such as low sensitivity in differentiating benign from malignant intraductal papillary mucinous neoplasms (IPMNs) and low specificity in differentiating chronic pancreatitis (CP) from malignant pancreatic lesions [44–46]. Furthermore, EUS is highly operator-dependent, and therefore, less experienced endoscopists may not be able to appreciate the subtle differences between CP and pancreatic cancer due to the presence of concomitant scarring and calcification secondary to the presence of chronic inflammation [44–46].

Numerous studies have been performed to assess and compare the diagnostic accuracy of non-AI and AI-augmented models of EUS for pancreatic cancer (Table 1). A retrospective study of 50 patients with IPMN, which used EUS images as input data for a DL algorithm, reported the sensitivity, specificity, and accuracy of 95.7%, 92.6%, and 94.0%, respectively, for malignant IPMNs [47]. This far exceeded the accuracy of human diagnosis [56.0%] [47]. Another retrospective study by Zhang et al. utilized SVM for EUS images from 216 patients to assess the ability of the SVM AI-assisted model to differentiate normal tissue from pancreatic cancer [48]. All 216 of these patients underwent EUS-guided fine-needle aspiration (EUS-FNA) and pathologic analysis to correlate findings with the definitive diagnosis [48]. The authors concluded that the SVM model had the accuracy, sensitivity, and specificity of 98%, 94.3%, and 99.5%, respectively [48]. Therefore, it could be used as a rapid, non-invasive test for pancreatic cancer screening [48]. Ozkan et al. conducted a retrospective study to develop a high-performance computer-aided diagnosis (CAD) system with image processing and pattern recognition abilities using ANNs [49]. The input data for the ANN was collected from EUS images of 332 patients. which were classified into three groups based on patient age (<40, 40–60, and >60 years old) [49]. The authors observed that the CAD system performed significantly better, with a sensitivity of 83.3%, specificity of 93.3%, and diagnostic accuracy of 87.5% when the images were classified according to the patient's age, reflecting the importance of age in aiding the diagnosis of pancreatic cancer [49]. Furthermore, in a systematic review of 11 studies examining the role of AI-assisted EUS models in diagnosing pancreatic cancer, the overall accuracy, sensitivity, and specificity were found in the ranges of 80–97.5%, 83–100%, and 50–99%, respectively [50]. Based on current data, AI-assisted EUS models have great potential as diagnostic tools for detecting pancreatic cancer.

Table 1. Studies assessing the sensitivity, specificity, and diagnostic accuracy of artificial intelligence (AI)-augmented and non-AI models for pancreatic cancer.

Study	Study Design	Artificial Intelligence Model	Patient Population	Outcomes for the Artificial Intelligence Model
Kuwahara et al. [47]	Retrospective (Japan)	Deep Learning (Convolutional Neural Networks (CNNs))	Total IPMN Patients = 50 Benign IPMN Patients = 27 Malignant IPMN Patients = 23	Recognition of Malignant IPMN: Sensitivity = 95.7% Specificity = 92.6% Accuracy = 94%
Zhang et al. [48]	Retrospective (China)	Support Vector Machine (SVM)	Total Patients = 216 Pancreatic Cancer Patients = 153 Non-Cancer Patients = 63	Recognition of Pancreatic Cancer: Sensitivity = 94.32% Specificity = 99.45% Accuracy = 97.98%
Ozkan et al. [49]	Retrospective (Turkey)	Artificial Neuronal Networks (ANNs)	Total Patients = 332 Pancreatic Cancer Patients = 202 Non-Cancer Patients = 130	Recognition of Pancreatic Cancer (All Ages): Sensitivity = 83.3% Specificity = 93.33% Accuracy = 87.5% Recognition of Pancreatic Cancer (>60 years): Sensitivity = 93.3% Specificity = 88.88% Accuracy = 91.66% Recognition of Pancreatic Cancer (40–60 years): Sensitivity = 85.7% Specificity = 91.66% Accuracy = 88.46% Recognition of Pancreatic Cancer (<40 years): Sensitivity = 87.5% Specificity = 94.11% Accuracy = 92%
Goyal et al. [50]	Systematic Review	Artificial Neural Network (ANN) Convolutional Neural Networks (CNNs) Support Vector Machine (SVM)	Total Patients = 2292 Pancreatic Cancer Patients = 1409 Non-Cancer Patients = 883	Recognition of Pancreatic Cancer: Sensitivity = 83–100% Specificity = 50–99%, Accuracy = 80–97.5%

IPMN: intraductal papillary mucinous neoplasm.

2.3. Utilization of Artificial Intelligence in Endoscopic Ultrasound to Differentiate Pancreatic Cancer from Chronic Pancreatitis

Over the last decade, imaging modalities for pancreatic lesions have improved significantly. However, differentiating between PDAC and CP is a diagnostic challenge as CP often mimics the radiological features of PDAC [51]. Cytological analysis continues to be the gold-standard test to differentiate PDAC from CP. Additionally, CP is a risk factor implicated in the development of PDAC. Hence, both clinical entities may co-exist together in the same patient [52]. In these complex cases, AI-assisted diagnostic models may help establish an accurate diagnosis. A retrospective study conducted by Das et al. for 56 patients using EUS images for digital image analysis (DIA) by an ANN noted that the AI-assisted model was highly accurate in differentiating between normal tissue, CP, and PDAC (area under the curve (AUC) of 0.93 for PDAC) [53]. Even in experienced hands, EUS imaging alone may require supplementation with FNB to differentiate malignancy from CP. Another retrospective analysis compared the accuracy of differentiation of pancreatic cancer from focal pancreatitis by an endosonographer versus a self-learning ANN model using EUS images as input data for 21 pancreatic cancer and 14 focal pancreatitis patients [54]. The authors reported that the maximal accuracy of the AI-assisted software (89%) compared favorably with the accuracy of human interpretation (85%) [54]. A cross-sectional study of 68 patients (32 PDAC, 22 normal pancreas, 11 CP, and 3 pancreatic neuroendocrine tumors) to assess the accuracy of extended neural network (ENN)-assisted real-time EUS elastography yielded an average testing performance of 95% and a high training performance of 97% in differentiating benign and malignant masses [55]. Tonozuka et al. used EUS images to develop a computer-assisted diagnosis (CAD) system using a DL model and evaluated its ability to detect PDAC using control EUS images from CP and normal pancreas patients [56]. The EUS-CAD model demonstrated excellent results (AUC 0.924 and 0.940 in the validation and test settings, respectively) in detecting PDAC [56]. Furthermore, a study by Zhu et al. utilized EUS image parameters for an SVM predictive model to differentiate pancreatic cancer and CP for 388 patients (262 pancreatic cancer and 126 CP) [57]. The authors reported the average accuracy, sensitivity, and specificity of 94.2%, 96.3%, and 93.4%, respectively, for the SVM predictive model [57].

Although numerous studies have demonstrated high diagnostic accuracy and strongly encourage the use of AI-assisted models to differentiate PDAC from other benign lesions, the main drawback is the small patient population used in each analysis, which significantly limits the input data for these AI-assisted models. Hence, multicenter studies were conducted to further validate these findings. A prospective multicenter-blinded analysis using ANN-assisted real-time EUS elastography was conducted for 258 patients at 13 tertiary academic medical centers in Europe to differentiate between pancreatic cancer and CP [58]. The authors observed that the AI-assisted model had a 91.1% training accuracy (95% CI: 89.87%–92.42%) and an 84.3% testing accuracy (95% CI, 83.09–85.44%), implying that the use of ANNs provided fast and accurate diagnoses for pancreatic malignancies [58]. Another observational prospective multicenter study that included 167 consecutive patients (112 pancreatic cancer and 55 CP) from Romania, Denmark, Germany, and Spain used parameters from the time-intensity curve (TIC) analysis of contrast EUS in an ANN model to differentiate pancreatic cancer and CP [59]. The authors reported that ANNs had high sensitivity (94.64%), specificity (94.44%), positive predictive value (97.24%), and negative predictive value (89.47%) and could be used to differentiate pancreatic cancer from CP with a high degree of accuracy [59].

In conclusion, all studies—large or small—have concluded that AI-assisted EUS models can be used in clinical practice to differentiate pancreatic cancers from CP with excellent results (Table 2).

2.4. Utilization of Artificial Intelligence in Endoscopic Ultrasound to Differentiate Pancreatic Cancer from Autoimmune Pancreatitis

AIP has been recognized as a distinct and rare fibroinflammatory subtype of chronic pancreatitis. It has characteristic features on sonographic and cross-sectional radiological imaging that mimic PDAC [60,61]. This may lead to a delayed or incorrect diagnosis. AI-assisted models can help solve this diagnostic dilemma. Mayra et al. conducted a study using a database of still images and video data from EUS examinations of 538 patients in the US to develop an EUS-based CNN model that can differentiate AIP from PDAC [62]. The authors reported that the EUS-based CNN model was 90% sensitive and 93% specific in distinguishing AIP from PDAC [62]. These findings encourage the use of AI-assisted EUS models in these subset patients for an early and accurate diagnosis. However, the data on AI-assisted EUS models to distinguish PDAC from AIP is still limited and warrant additional large multicenter prospective studies.

Table 2. Studies comparing artificial intelligence (AI)-augmented models to differentiate pancreatic cancer from other clinical entities.

Study	Study Design	Artificial Intelligence Model	Patient Population	Outcomes for the Artificial Intelligence Model
Das et al. [53]	Retrospective (United States)	Artificial Neural Network (ANN)	Normal Pancreas Patients = 22 Chronic Pancreatitis Patients = 12 Pancreatic Cancer Patients = 22	Recognition of Pancreatic Cancer: Sensitivity = 93% Specificity = 92% Recognition of Chronic Pancreatitis versus Normal Pancreas: Sensitivity = 100% Specificity = 100%
Norton et al. [54]	Retrospective (United States)	Artificial Neural Network (ANN)	Total Patients = 35 Pancreatic Cancer Patients = 21 Focal Pancreatitis Patients = 14	Recognition of Pancreatic Cancer by AI: Sensitivity = 100% Specificity = 50% Accuracy = 80% Recognition of Pancreatic Cancer by EUS: Sensitivity = 89% Specificity = 79% Accuracy = 85% Recognition of Pancreatic Cancer by Human Interpretation: Sensitivity = 73% Specificity = 100% Accuracy = 83%
Săftoiu et al. [55]	Retrospective (Europe)	Artificial Neural Network (ANN)	Total Patients = 68 Pancreatic Cancer Patients = 32 Pancreatic Neuroendocrine Tumor Patients = 3 Chronic Pancreatitis Patients = 11 Normal Pancreas Patients = 22	Recognition of Pancreatic Cancer and Pancreatic Neuroendocrine Tumors: Sensitivity = 91.4% Specificity = 87.9% Accuracy = 89.7%
Tonozuka et al. [56]	Cross-Sectional (Japan)	Convolutional Neural Networks (CNNs)	Total Patients = 139 Pancreatic Cancer Patients = 76 Chronic Pancreatitis Patients = 34 Normal Pancreas Patients = 29	Recognition of Pancreatic Cancer (Validation Set): Sensitivity = 90.2% Specificity = 74.9% Area Under the Curve = 0.924 Recognition of Pancreatic Cancer (Test Set): Sensitivity = 92.4% Specificity = 84.1% Area Under the Curve = 0.940
Zhu et al. [57]	Retrospective (China)	Support Vector Machine (SVM)	Total Patients = 388 Pancreatic Cancer Patients = 262 Chronic Pancreatitis Patients = 126	Recognition of Pancreatic Cancer: Sensitivity = 96.25% Specificity = 93.38% Accuracy = 94.2%
Săftoiu et al. [58]	Prospective Multicenter (Europe)	Artificial Neural Network (ANN)	Total Patients = 258 Pancreatic Cancer Patients = 211 Chronic Pancreatitis Patients = 47	Recognition of Pancreatic Cancer: Sensitivity = 87.59% Specificity = 82.94% Area Under the Curve = 0.94
Săftoiu et al. [59]	Prospective Multicenter Observational (Europe)	Artificial Neural Network (ANN)	Total Patients = 167 Pancreatic Cancer Patients = 112 Chronic Pancreatitis Patients = 55	Recognition of Pancreatic Cancer by AI: Sensitivity = 94.64% Specificity = 94.44% Recognition of Pancreatic Cancer by Contrast-Enhanced EUS: Sensitivity = 87.5% Specificity = 92.72%

AI: artificial intelligence. EUS: endoscopic ultrasound.

2.5. Limitations of Artificial Intelligence in Endoscopic Ultrasound for the Detection of Pancreatic Cancer

Even at the current early stage of development, AI-assisted diagnostic models provide significant value in aiding medical decision-making and planning therapeutic interventions for patients with pancreatic cancer. However, there continues to be hesitancy in their application in clinical practice by most practitioners despite promising results. In recent years, more studies reporting a higher diagnostic accuracy of AI-assisted EUS models compared to human interpretation for pancreatic cancer continued to be published. These studies are slowly changing the current landscape and building confidence in AI-assisted diagnostic models as an indispensable tool in modern medicine [50,63]. However, like any diagnostic test, AI-assisted EUS models have their own set of limitations, which will need to be addressed before they can be used as a 'go-to' diagnostic test for pancreatic cancer.

One of the most important limitations of an AI-assisted EUS model is the lack of adequate standardization of input data that are used to train the AI algorithm [63]. As per current literature, no standardized protocols for data collection, processing, and storage for the AI-assisted model have been established. Additionally, standardized principles for data analysis by the AI algorithm are also lacking. Establishing these protocols is important because if the AI-assisted EUS model trains on data that are misrepresentative of PDAC population variability, it is likely to reinforce bias, which may lead to inaccurate diagnoses, lack of generalizability, and, ultimately, adverse patient outcomes [64]. Furthermore, different types of AI-assisted EUS models may require images of the area of interest prepared in a specific manner and may not perform with a high degree of accuracy with different imaging subsets. Although universal protocols can be created for input data to increase the efficiency and accuracy of AI-assisted EUS models, it may be an extremely time and labor-expensive process [63].

Another area of concern is the quality of input data used to train the AI-assisted EUS models. Most studies in the current literature derive input data from a single institution, with only a few multicenter experiences [50,58,59,63]. This lack of diversity in the dataset leads to an information bias. For the AI-assisted EUS diagnostic models to achieve a high degree of diagnostic accuracy and generalizability to diagnose and differentiate PDAC from other etiologies, the dataset needs to be highly diverse, capturing all possible variations and variables used in the decision-making process [63]. This can be achieved by developing a quality-monitored central data collection server for EUS images from all institutions across the US, both academic and private. Furthermore, just collecting high-quality data is not sufficient. It is also imperative to ensure that the studies that utilize the data to report specific outcomes on pancreatic cancers must have high methodological quality and standards of reporting as they may influence current guidelines or help in developing future ones [65]. Poor quality studies with flawed methodologies and a lack of transparent reporting may create distrust among healthcare professionals, leading to delays in policy changes and the adoption of this newer technology in current clinical practice [65].

The AI 'Black Box' problem, particularly for ML and DL AI-assisted models, has garnered significant attention and is rapidly becoming a concern [66]. A 'Black Box' AI is an AI algorithm that allows the observer to visualize input and output data without any information on the processes and operations used to derive the output data [66,67]. Hence, the observer is unable to interpret and determine the reasoning behind how a specific variable was weighed within the AI algorithm [63,66,67]. This is concerning as gastroenterologists need to be able to visualize and understand how the information on PDAC was processed and analyzed to prevent errors that can ultimately lead to adverse patient outcomes. Therefore, for the time being, AI-assisted EUS models should be used as adjuncts to clinical experience rather than ultimate answers when recommending treatment for pancreatic cancers.

Finally, there are numerous ethical dilemmas associated with the handling and storage of sensitive patient information [68]. As the AI-assisted EUS models require a great volume of input data, appropriate de-identification of patient information is required to protect patient privacy, reduce bias, and ensure the fairness of the algorithm [68]. However, the de-identified data needs to be traceable back to the patient to aid in diagnosis and recommend treatment options. Furthermore, this information needs to be secure from cybercriminals and interested parties who may use it to exploit vulnerabilities and influence the healthcare of these individuals [68]. Figure 2 summarizes all the limitations associated with AI in EUS.

2.6. Future Directions of Artificial Intelligence in Endoscopic Ultrasound for Pancreatic Cancer

Despite its limitations, the growth and application of AI in different subspecialties of medicine, particularly GI, have increased exponentially. Collaborations between academic centers, private physicians, and industry will continue to drive the AI revolution to improve its quality, utility, ease of use in everyday clinical settings, and, most importantly, accuracy for the early detection of pancreatic cancer. We foresee the following 'near' and 'far' future applications of AI in EUS for patients with pancreatic cancer:

2.6.1. 'Near' Future Application of Artificial Intelligence in Endoscopic Ultrasound for Pancreatic Cancer

The diagnostic accuracy of AI-assisted EUS models has been compared favorably to or exceeded the diagnostic accuracy of human interpretation for pancreatic cancers [47,54]. However, it is worth noting that neither AI-assisted models nor human diagnosis has 100% diagnostic accuracy. Hence, we strongly believe that AI-assisted models should serve as a 'second set of eyes' to the endosonographer rather than a replacement (Figure 3). Furthermore, AI-assisted models can also potentially aid experienced endosonographers during biopsies while, at the same time, learning from these experts in the field. These strategies may be critical in the early detection of pancreatic cancer and differentiating them from other clinical entities. Ultimately, AI-assisted EUS models should help reduce operator variability, which has been a traditional limitation of EUS.

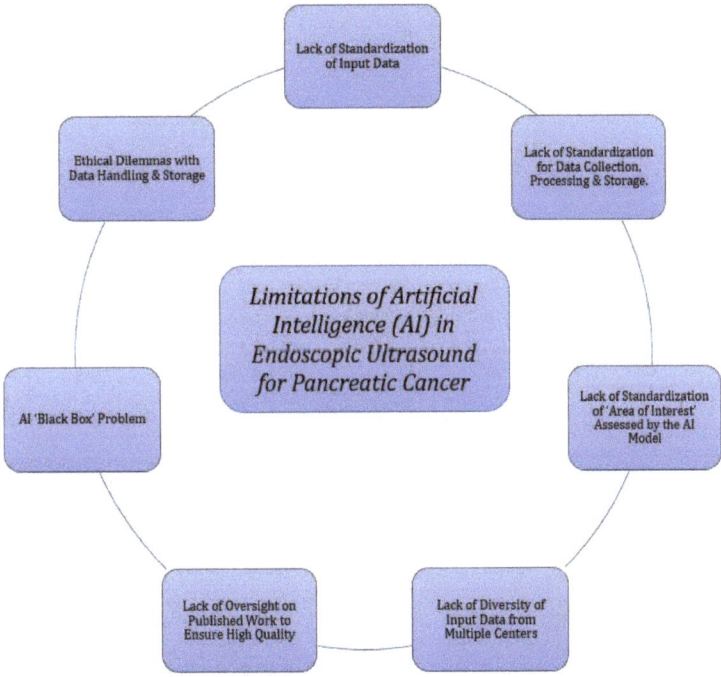

Figure 2. Limitations of artificial intelligence in endoscopic ultrasound for pancreatic cancer.

2.6.2. 'Far' Future Application of Artificial Intelligence in Endoscopic Ultrasound for Pancreatic Cancer

The application of AI technology in clinical medicine is still in the preliminary phase, with a wide scope for improvement and utilization. As AI-assisted models are ideal for the analysis of large datasets, they will have widespread utility in composite imaging, which includes the fusion of EUS and cross-sectional radiological imaging to determine vascular staging for pancreatic cancers. This information will be vital to endoscopists and other specialties (radiology, medical oncology, surgical oncology, and radiation oncology) involved in all aspects of pancreatic cancer staging. Additionally, it will help plan appropriate interventions and recommend treatment options.

AI-assisted models analyzing samples from EUS-FNA and EUS-FNB are also quickly gaining traction due to their ability to differentiate complex tissue specimens [69]. The diagnostic accuracy of MLP EUS-FNA and CNN EUS-FNB models for differentiating pancreatic cancer from other pancreatic tumors was reported to be 100% and 94.17%, respectively. However, as AI technology advances, with better AI algorithms and improved quality of EUS images/videos as input data, AI-assisted EUS models may replace traditional EUS-FNA/FNB as the gold-standard test for diagnosing pancreatic cancer due to their less invasive nature and high diagnostic accuracy.

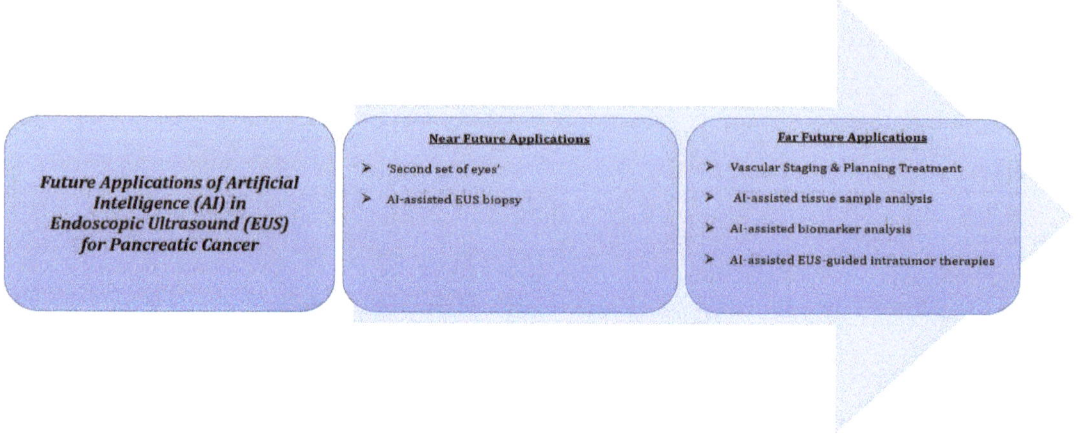

Future Applications of Artificial Intelligence (AI) in Endoscopic Ultrasound (EUS) for Pancreatic Cancer

Near Future Applications
- 'Second set of eyes'
- AI-assisted EUS biopsy

Far Future Applications
- Vascular Staging & Planning Treatment
- AI-assisted tissue sample analysis
- AI-assisted biomarker analysis
- AI-assisted EUS-guided intratumor therapies

Figure 3. Future applications of artificial intelligence in endoscopic ultrasound for pancreatic cancer.

Cancer biomarkers have widespread utility in screening, differential diagnosis, staging, risk assessment, response to treatment, monitoring disease progression, and the prognosis of any cancer [70]. However, biomarkers for pancreatic cancer currently lack sufficient sensitivity and specificity for widespread clinical application. Hence, this is an area of interest where AI-assisted models may be highly beneficial. Large sets of biomarker data from EUS-guided liquid biopsies can be analyzed using AI technology to identify pancreatic cancer at an early stage [69]. Studies investigating AI algorithms capable of analyzing biomarker data with high accuracy are an area of active research.

From an intervention perspective, AI-assisted EUS-guided fine-needle injection is another potential area of application of AI technology. Using AI-assisted real-time EUS imaging guidance, interventional endoscopists may be able to directly inject activated allogeneic lymphocyte culture or oncolytic attenuated adenovirus (ONYX-015), which are currently being studied as a potential therapy for pancreatic cancer, directly into pancreatic lesions. Traditionally, pancreatic lesions have been extremely difficult to reach by a percutaneous approach due to their depth. Hence, AI-assisted EUS-guided fine-needle injection may become the preferred approach in elderly patients or those with a high comorbidity burden, primarily due to the less invasive nature of the procedure and fewer complications. However, additional research is needed before AI-assisted EUS-guided fine-needle injection finds widespread application. Figure 3 summarizes all the potential future applications of AI in EUS for pancreatic cancer.

3. Conclusions

AI-assisted EUS models have shown promise in the early detection of pancreatic cancer, with a high degree of accuracy despite still being in the infancy of development and utilization. Compared to human interpretation, AI technology has either been compared favorably or has been noted to be far superior in identifying pancreatic cancer and differentiating it from other clinical entities that mimic pancreatic cancer on conventional radiological imaging such as CP and AIP. However, AI-assisted EUS models have a unique yet concerning set of limitations, such as the AI 'Black Box', the lack of adequate standardization and quality of data, and ethical dilemmas associated with sensitive patient information, all of which limit widespread application. Despite these limitations, AI technology may be instrumental in transforming the future of healthcare, especially for pancreatic cancer, due to its precision in analyzing and processing large datasets. AI-assisted EUS models could serve as a 'second set of eyes' to the endosonographer, improving diagnostic accuracy. AI technology could also assist in composite imaging to determine the vascular staging for pancreatic cancers and in AI-assisted EUS-guided fine-needle injection to easily treat deep pancreatic lesions. Most studies on AI are retrospective; hence, large-scale prospective clinical trials are needed to accurately evaluate the diagnostic accuracy of AI algorithms in real-world clinical settings. If successful, AI-assisted EUS models have the potential to become an indispensable tool in the management of patients with pancreatic cancer.

Author Contributions: Conceptualization, D.S.D., M.A.-H., S.C. and N.S.; methodology, D.S.D. and N.S.; software, N/A; validation, D.S.D., M.A.-H., S.C., M.K.G., M.A., B.P.M., D.R., A.C., J.B. and N.S.; formal analysis, N/A; investigation, D.S.D., M.A.-H., S.C., M.K.G., M.A., B.P.M., D.R., A.C., J.B. and N.S.; resources, D.S.D., M.A.-H., S.C. and N.S.; data curation, D.S.D., M.A.-H., S.C., M.K.G., M.A., B.P.M., D.R., A.C., J.B. and N.S.; writing—original draft preparation, D.S.D., M.A.-H., S.C., M.K.G., M.A., B.P.M., D.R., A.C., J.B. and N.S.; writing—reviewing and editing, D.S.D., M.A.-H., S.C. and N.S.; visualization, D.S.D. and N.S.; supervision, D.S.D., M.A.-H. and N.S.; project administration, D.S.D.; funding acquisition, N/A. All authors have read and agreed to the published version of the manuscript.

Funding: This research received no external funding.

Institutional Review Board Statement: Not applicable.

Informed Consent Statement: Not applicable.

Data Availability Statement: All data utilized for this narrative review is publicly available on PubMed and embedded in the reference section of the manuscript.

Conflicts of Interest: The authors declare no conflict of interest.

References

1. Sung, H.; Ferlay, J.; Siegel, R.L.; Laversanne, M.; Soerjomataram, I.; Jemal, A.; Bray, F. Global Cancer Statistics 2020: GLOBOCAN Estimates of Incidence and Mortality Worldwide for 36 Cancers in 185 Countries. *CA Cancer J. Clin.* **2021**, *71*, 209–249. [CrossRef] [PubMed]
2. Kamisawa, T.; Wood, L.D.; Itoi, T.; Takaori, K. Pancreatic cancer. *Lancet* **2016**, *388*, 73–85. [CrossRef] [PubMed]
3. Wang, S.; Zheng, Y.; Yang, F.; Zhu, L.; Zhu, X.Q.; Wang, Z.F.; Wu, X.-L.; Zhou, C.-H.; Yan, J.-Y.; Hu, B.-Y.; et al. The molecular biology of pancreatic adenocarcinoma: Translational challenges and clinical perspectives. *Signal Transduct. Target. Ther.* **2021**, *6*, 249. [CrossRef] [PubMed]
4. McGuigan, A.; Kelly, P.; Turkington, R.C.; Jones, C.; Coleman, H.G.; McCain, R.S. Pancreatic cancer: A review of clinical diagnosis, epidemiology, treatment and outcomes. *World J. Gastroenterol.* **2018**, *24*, 4846–4861. [CrossRef] [PubMed]
5. Zhao, Z.; Liu, W. Pancreatic Cancer: A Review of Risk Factors, Diagnosis, and Treatment. *Technol. Cancer Res. Treat.* **2020**, *19*, 1533033820962117. [PubMed]
6. National Cancer Institute: Surveillance Epidemiology, and End Results (SEER) Program. Cancer Stats Facts: Pancreatic Cancer: National Cancer Institute. 2022. Available online: https://seer.cancer.gov/statfacts/html/pancreas.html (accessed on 3 September 2022).
7. Kikuyama, M.; Kamisawa, T.; Kuruma, S.; Chiba, K.; Kawaguchi, S.; Terada, S.; Satoh, T. Early Diagnosis to Improve the Poor Prognosis of Pancreatic Cancer. *Cancers* **2018**, *10*, 48.
8. Iglesias-Garcia, J.; Poley, J.W.; Larghi, A.; Giovannini, M.; Petrone, M.C.; Abdulkader, I.; Monges, G.; Costamagna, G.; Arcidiacono, P.; Biermann, K.; et al. Feasibility and yield of a new EUS histology needle: Results from a multicenter, pooled, cohort study. *Gastrointest. Endosc.* **2011**, *73*, 1189–1196. [CrossRef]
9. Crinò, S.F.; Di Mitri, R.; Nguyen, N.Q.; Tarantino, I.; de Nucci, G.; Deprez, P.H.; Carrara, S.; Kitano, M.; Shami, V.M.; Fernández-Esparrach, G.; et al. Endoscopic Ultrasound-guided Fine-needle Biopsy with or Without Rapid On-site Evaluation for Diagnosis of Solid Pancreatic Lesions: A Randomized Controlled Non-Inferiority Trial. *Gastroenterology* **2021**, *161*, 899–909.e5. [CrossRef]
10. Goyal, H.; Sherazi, S.A.A.; Mann, R.; Gandhi, Z.; Perisetti, A.; Aziz, M.; Chandan, S.; Kopel, J.; Tharian, B.; Sharma, N.; et al. Scope of Artificial Intelligence in Gastrointestinal Oncology. *Cancers* **2021**, *13*, 5494. [CrossRef]
11. Cao, J.S.; Lu, Z.Y.; Chen, M.Y.; Zhang, B.; Juengpanich, S.; Hu, J.H.; Li, S.-J.; Topatana, W.; Zhou, X.-Y.; Feng, X.; et al. Artificial intelligence in gastroenterology and hepatology: Status and challenges. *World J. Gastroenterol.* **2021**, *27*, 1664–1690. [CrossRef]
12. Panch, T.; Szolovits, P.; Atun, R. Artificial intelligence, machine learning and health systems. *J. Glob. Health* **2018**, *8*, 020303. [CrossRef]
13. Gonzalo-Marin, J.; Vila, J.J.; Perez-Miranda, M. Role of endoscopic ultrasound in the diagnosis of pancreatic cancer. *World J. Gastrointest. Oncol.* **2014**, *6*, 360–368. [CrossRef]
14. Liu, E.; Bhutani, M.S.; Sun, S. Artificial intelligence: The new wave of innovation in EUS. *Endosc. Ultrasound* **2021**, *10*, 79–83.

15. Hsieh, M.H.; Sun, L.M.; Lin, C.L.; Hsieh, M.J.; Hsu, C.Y.; Kao, C.H. Development of a prediction model for pancreatic cancer in patients with type 2 diabetes using logistic regression and artificial neural network models. *Cancer Manag. Res.* **2018**, *10*, 6317–6324. [CrossRef]
16. Kenner, B.; Chari, S.T.; Kelsen, D.; Klimstra, D.S.; Pandol, S.J.; Rosenthal, M.; Rustgi, A.K.; Taylor, J.A.; Yala, A.; Abul-Husn, N.; et al. Artificial Intelligence and Early Detection of Pancreatic Cancer: 2020 Summative Review. *Pancreas* **2021**, *50*, 251–279. [CrossRef]
17. Lovejoy, C.A.; Arora, A.; Buch, V.; Dayan, I. Key considerations for the use of artificial intelligence in healthcare and clinical research. *Future Healthc. J.* **2022**, *9*, 75–78. [CrossRef]
18. Jones, L.D.; Golan, D.; Hanna, S.A.; Ramachandran, M. Artificial intelligence, machine learning and the evolution of healthcare: A bright future or cause for concern? *Bone Joint Res.* **2018**, *7*, 223–225. [CrossRef]
19. Sidey-Gibbons, J.A.M.; Sidey-Gibbons, C.J. Machine learning in medicine: A practical introduction. *BMC Med. Res. Methodol.* **2019**, *19*, 64. [CrossRef]
20. Le Berre, C.; Sandborn, W.J.; Aridhi, S.; Devignes, M.D.; Fournier, L.; Smaïl-Tabbone, M.; Danese, S.; Peyrin-Biroulet, L. Application of Artificial Intelligence to Gastroenterology and Hepatology. *Gastroenterology* **2020**, *158*, 76–94.e2. [CrossRef]
21. Cai, L.; Gao, J.; Zhao, D. A review of the application of deep learning in medical image classification and segmentation. *Ann. Transl. Med.* **2020**, *8*, 713. [CrossRef]
22. Shahid, N.; Rappon, T.; Berta, W. Applications of artificial neural networks in health care organizational decision-making: A scoping review. *PLoS ONE* **2019**, *14*, e0212356. [CrossRef] [PubMed]
23. Ahmed, Z.; Mohamed, K.; Zeeshan, S.; Dong, X. Artificial intelligence with multi-functional machine learning platform development for better healthcare and precision medicine. *Database* **2020**, *2020*, baaa010. [CrossRef] [PubMed]
24. Kinney, E.L. Medical expert systems. Who needs them? *Chest* **1987**, *91*, 3–4. [CrossRef] [PubMed]
25. Wu, L.; Zhang, J.; Zhou, W.; An, P.; Shen, L.; Liu, J.; Jiang, X.; Huang, X.; Mu, G.; Wan, X.; et al. Randomised controlled trial of WISENSE, a real-time quality improving system for monitoring blind spots during esophagogastroduodenoscopy. *Gut* **2019**, *68*, 2161. [CrossRef] [PubMed]
26. Wang, P.; Berzin, T.M.; Glissen Brown, J.R.; Bharadwaj, S.; Becq, A.; Xiao, X.; Liu, P.; Li, L.; Song, Y.; Zhang, D.; et al. Real-time automatic detection system increases colonoscopic polyp and adenoma detection rates: A prospective randomised controlled study. *Gut* **2019**, *68*, 1813–1819. [CrossRef]
27. Gohari, M.R.; Biglarian, A.; Bakhshi, E.; Pourhoseingholi, M.A. Use of an artificial neural network to determine prognostic factors in colorectal cancer patients. *Asian Pac. J. Cancer Prev.* **2011**, *12*, 1469–1472.
28. Biglarian, A.; Bakhshi, E.; Gohari, M.R.; Khodabakhshi, R. Artificial neural network for prediction of distant metastasis in colorectal cancer. *Asian Pac. J. Cancer Prev.* **2012**, *13*, 927–930. [CrossRef]
29. Nilsaz-Dezfouli, H.; Abu-Bakar, M.R.; Arasan, J.; Adam, M.B.; Pourhoseingholi, M.A. Improving Gastric Cancer Outcome Prediction Using Single Time-Point Artificial Neural Network Models. *Cancer Inform.* **2017**, *16*, 1176935116686062. [CrossRef]
30. Peng, J.H.; Fang, Y.J.; Li, C.X.; Ou, Q.J.; Jiang, W.; Lu, S.X.; Lu, Z.-H.; Li, P.-X.; Yun, J.-P.; Zhang, R.-X.; et al. A scoring system based on artificial neural network for predicting 10-year survival in stage II A colon cancer patients after radical surgery. *Oncotarget* **2016**, *7*, 22939–22947. [CrossRef]
31. Hassan, C.; Spadaccini, M.; Iannone, A.; Maselli, R.; Jovani, M.; Chandrasekar, V.T.; Antoneli, G.; Yu, H.; Areia, M.; Dinis-Ribeiro, M.; et al. Performance of artificial intelligence in colonoscopy for adenoma and polyp detection: A systematic review and meta-analysis. *Gastrointest Endosc.* **2021**, *93*, 77–85.e6. [CrossRef]
32. Bibault, J.E.; Giraud, P.; Housset, M.; Durdux, C.; Taieb, J.; Berger, A.; Coriat, R.; Chaussade, S.; Dousset, B.; Nordlinger, B.; et al. Deep Learning and Radiomics predict complete response after neo-adjuvant chemoradiation for locally advanced rectal cancer. *Sci. Rep.* **2018**, *8*, 12611. [CrossRef]
33. Lee, J.; An, J.Y.; Choi, M.G.; Park, S.H.; Kim, S.T.; Lee, J.H.; Sohn, T.S.; Bae, J.M.; Kim, S.; Lee, H.; et al. Deep Learning–Based Survival Analysis Identified Associations Between Molecular Subtype and Optimal Adjuvant Treatment of Patients with Gastric Cancer. *JCO Clin. Cancer Inform.* **2018**, *2*, 1–14. [CrossRef]
34. Pan, G.; Yan, G.; Qiu, X.; Cui, J. Bleeding detection in Wireless Capsule Endoscopy based on Probabilistic Neural Network. *J. Med. Syst.* **2011**, *35*, 1477–1484. [CrossRef]
35. Lv, G.; Yan, G.; Wang, Z. Bleeding detection in wireless capsule endoscopy images based on color invariants and spatial pyramids using support vector machines. *Annu. Int. Conf. IEEE Eng. Med. Biol. Soc.* **2011**, *2011*, 6643–6646.
36. Fu, Y.; Zhang, W.; Mandal, M.; Meng, M.Q. Computer-aided bleeding detection in WCE video. *IEEE J. Biomed. Health Inform.* **2014**, *18*, 636–642. [CrossRef]
37. Ghosh, T.; Fattah, S.A.; Shahnaz, C.; Wahid, K.A. An automatic bleeding detection scheme in wireless capsule endoscopy based on histogram of an RGB-indexed image. *Annu. Int. Conf. IEEE Eng. Med. Biol. Soc.* **2014**, *2014*, 4683–4686.
38. Sainju, S.; Bui, F.M.; Wahid, K.A. Automated bleeding detection in capsule endoscopy videos using statistical features and region growing. *J. Med. Syst.* **2014**, *38*, 25. [CrossRef]
39. Hassan, A.R.; Haque, M.A. Computer-aided gastrointestinal hemorrhage detection in wireless capsule endoscopy videos. *Comput. Methods Programs Biomed.* **2015**, *122*, 341–353. [CrossRef]
40. Jia, X.; Meng, M.Q. A deep convolutional neural network for bleeding detection in Wireless Capsule Endoscopy images. *Annu. Int. Conf. IEEE Eng. Med. Biol. Soc.* **2016**, *2016*, 639–642.

41. Usman, M.A.; Satrya, G.B.; Usman, M.R.; Shin, S.Y. Detection of small colon bleeding in wireless capsule endoscopy videos. *Comput. Med. Imaging Graph.* **2016**, *54*, 16–26. [CrossRef]
42. Liu, D.Y.; Gan, T.; Rao, N.N.; Xing, Y.W.; Zheng, J.; Li, S.; Luo, C.-S.; Zhou, Z.-J.; Wan, Y.-L. Identification of lesion images from gastrointestinal endoscope based on feature extraction of combinational methods with and without learning process. *Med. Image Anal.* **2016**, *32*, 281–294. [CrossRef]
43. Leenhardt, R.; Vasseur, P.; Li, C.; Saurin, J.C.; Rahmi, G.; Cholet, F.; Becq, A.; Marteau, P.; Histace, A.; Dray, X.; et al. A neural network algorithm for detection of GI angiectasia during small-bowel capsule endoscopy. *Gastrointest. Endosc.* **2019**, *89*, 189–194. [CrossRef]
44. Ang, T.L.; Kwek, A.B.E.; Wang, L.M. Diagnostic Endoscopic Ultrasound: Technique, Current Status and Future Directions. *Gut Liver* **2018**, *12*, 483–496. [CrossRef]
45. Harmsen, F.R.; Domagk, D.; Dietrich, C.F.; Hocke, M. Discriminating chronic pancreatitis from pancreatic cancer: Contrast-enhanced EUS and multidetector computed tomography in direct comparison. *Endosc. Ultrasound* **2018**, *7*, 395–403. [CrossRef]
46. Shahidi, N.; Ou, G.; Lam, E.; Enns, R.; Telford, J. When trainees reach competency in performing endoscopic ultrasound: A systematic review. *Endosc. Int. Open* **2017**, *5*, E239–E243. [CrossRef]
47. Kuwahara, T.; Hara, K.; Mizuno, N.; Okuno, N.; Matsumoto, S.; Obata, M.; Kurita, Y.; Koda, H.; Toriyama, K.; Onishi, S.; et al. Usefulness of Deep Learning Analysis for the Diagnosis of Malignancy in Intraductal Papillary Mucinous Neoplasms of the Pancreas. *Clin. Transl. Gastroenterol.* **2019**, *10*, 1–8. [CrossRef]
48. Zhang, M.M.; Yang, H.; Jin, Z.D.; Yu, J.G.; Cai, Z.Y.; Li, Z.S. Differential diagnosis of pancreatic cancer from normal tissue with digital imaging processing and pattern recognition based on a support vector machine of EUS images. *Gastrointest. Endosc.* **2010**, *72*, 978–985. [CrossRef]
49. Ozkan, M.; Cakiroglu, M.; Kocaman, O.; Kurt, M.; Yilmaz, B.; Can, G.; Korkmaz, U.; Dandil, E.; Eksi, Z. Age-based computer-aided diagnosis approach for pancreatic cancer on endoscopic ultrasound images. *Endosc. Ultrasound* **2016**, *5*, 101–107.
50. Goyal, H.; Sherazi, S.A.A.; Gupta, S.; Perisetti, A.; Achebe, I.; Ali, A.; Tharian, B.; Thosani, N.; Sharma, N.R. Application of artificial intelligence in diagnosis of pancreatic malignancies by endoscopic ultrasound: A systemic review. *Therap. Adv. Gastroenterol.* **2022**, *15*, 17562848221093873. [CrossRef]
51. Miura, F.; Takada, T.; Amano, H.; Yoshida, M.; Furui, S.; Takeshita, K. Diagnosis of pancreatic cancer. *HPB (Oxf.)* **2006**, *8*, 337–342. [CrossRef]
52. Wolske, K.M.; Ponnatapura, J.; Kolokythas, O.; Burke, L.M.B.; Tappouni, R.; Lalwani, N. Chronic Pancreatitis or Pancreatic Tumor? A Problem-solving Approach. *Radiographics* **2019**, *39*, 1965–1982. [CrossRef]
53. Das, A.; Nguyen, C.C.; Li, F.; Li, B. Digital image analysis of EUS images accurately differentiates pancreatic cancer from chronic pancreatitis and normal tissue. *Gastrointest. Endosc.* **2008**, *67*, 861–867. [CrossRef]
54. Norton, I.D.; Zheng, Y.; Wiersema, M.S.; Greenleaf, J.; Clain, J.E.; Dimagno, E.P. Neural network analysis of EUS images to differentiate between pancreatic malignancy and pancreatitis. *Gastrointest. Endosc.* **2001**, *54*, 625–629. [CrossRef]
55. Săftoiu, A.; Vilmann, P.; Gorunescu, F.; Gheonea, D.I.; Gorunescu, M.; Ciurea, T.; Popescu, G.L.; Iordache, A.; Hassan, H.; Iordache, S. Neural network analysis of dynamic sequences of EUS elastography used for the differential diagnosis of chronic pancreatitis and pancreatic cancer. *Gastrointest. Endosc.* **2008**, *68*, 1086–1094. [CrossRef]
56. Tonozuka, R.; Itoi, T.; Nagata, N.; Kojima, H.; Sofuni, A.; Tsuchiya, T.; Ishii, K.; Tanaka, R.; Nagakawa, Y.; Mukai, S. Deep learning analysis for the detection of pancreatic cancer on endosonographic images: A pilot study. *J. Hepatobiliary Pancreat. Sci.* **2021**, *28*, 95–104. [CrossRef]
57. Zhu, M.; Xu, C.; Yu, J.; Wu, Y.; Li, C.; Zhang, M.; Jin, Z.; Li, Z. Differentiation of pancreatic cancer and chronic pancreatitis using computer-aided diagnosis of endoscopic ultrasound (EUS) images: A diagnostic test. *PLoS ONE* **2013**, *8*, e63820. [CrossRef]
58. Săftoiu, A.; Vilmann, P.; Gorunescu, F.; Janssen, J.; Hocke, M.; Larsen, M.; Iglesias–Garcia, J.; Arcidiacono, P.; Will, U.; Giovannini, M.; et al. Efficacy of an artificial neural network-based approach to endoscopic ultrasound elastography in diagnosis of focal pancreatic masses. *Clin. Gastroenterol. Hepatol.* **2012**, *10*, 84–90.e1. [CrossRef]
59. Săftoiu, A.; Vilmann, P.; Dietrich, C.F.; Iglesias-Garcia, J.; Hocke, M.; Seicean, A.; Ignee, A.; Hassan, H.; Streba, C.T.; Ioncică, A.M.; et al. Quantitative contrast-enhanced harmonic EUS in differential diagnosis of focal pancreatic masses (with videos). *Gastrointest. Endosc.* **2015**, *82*, 59–69. [CrossRef]
60. Yoshida, K.; Toki, F.; Takeuchi, T.; Watanabe, S.; Shiratori, K.; Hayashi, N. Chronic pancreatitis caused by an autoimmune abnormality. Proposal of the concept of autoimmune pancreatitis. *Dig. Dis. Sci.* **1995**, *40*, 1561–1568. [CrossRef]
61. Sureka, B.; Rastogi, A. Autoimmune Pancreatitis. *Pol. J. Radiol.* **2017**, *82*, 233–239. [CrossRef]
62. Marya, N.B.; Powers, P.D.; Chari, S.T.; Gleeson, F.C.; Leggett, C.L.; Abu Dayyeh, B.K.; Chandrasekhara, V.; Iyer, P.G.; Majumder, S.; Pearson, R.K.; et al. Utilisation of artificial intelligence for the development of an EUS-convolutional neural network model trained to enhance the diagnosis of autoimmune pancreatitis. *Gut* **2021**, *70*, 1335. [CrossRef] [PubMed]
63. Mendoza Ladd, A.; Diehl, D.L. Artificial intelligence for early detection of pancreatic adenocarcinoma: The future is promising. *World J. Gastroenterol.* **2021**, *27*, 1283–1295. [CrossRef]
64. Norori, N.; Hu, Q.; Aellen, F.M.; Faraci, F.D.; Tzovara, A. Addressing bias in big data and AI for health care: A call for open science. *Patterns (N. Y.)* **2021**, *2*, 100347. [CrossRef]

65. Jayakumar, S.; Sounderajah, V.; Normahani, P.; Harling, L.; Markar, S.R.; Ashrafian, H.; Darzi, A. Quality assessment standards in artificial intelligence diagnostic accuracy systematic reviews: A meta-research study. *NPJ Digit. Med.* **2022**, *5*, 11. [CrossRef] [PubMed]
66. Price, W.N. Big data and black-box medical algorithms. *Sci. Transl. Med.* **2018**, *10*, eaao5333. [CrossRef]
67. Taub, S.; Pianykh, O.S. An alternative to the black box: Strategy learning. *PLoS ONE* **2022**, *17*, e0264485. [CrossRef]
68. Gerke, S.; Minssen, T.; Cohen, G. Ethical and Legal Challenges of Artificial Intelligence-Driven Healthcare. In *Artificial Intelligence in Healthcare*; Elsevier Inc.: Amsterdam, The Netherlands, 2020; pp. 295–336.
69. Huang, B.; Huang, H.; Zhang, S.; Zhang, D.; Shi, Q.; Liu, J.; Guo, J. Artificial intelligence in pancreatic cancer. *Theranostics* **2022**, *12*, 6931–6954. [CrossRef]
70. Henry, N.L.; Hayes, D.F. Cancer biomarkers. *Mol. Oncol.* **2012**, *6*, 140–146. [CrossRef]

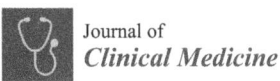

Review

Techniques and Outcomes of Endoscopic Ultrasound Guided—Pancreatic Duct Drainage (EUS- PDD)

Jun Liang Teh [1,2] and Anthony Yuen Bun Teoh [2,*]

1. Department of Surgery, Jurong health Campus, National University Health System, Singapore 609606, Singapore
2. Department of Surgery, Prince of Wales Hospital, The Chinese University of Hong Kong, Hong Kong
* Correspondence: anthonyteoh@surgery.cuhk.edu.hk; Tel.: +852-3505-2627; Fax: +852-3505-7974

Abstract: Endoscopic ultrasound guided—pancreatic duct drainage (EUS- PDD) is one of the most technically challenging procedures for the interventional endoscopist. The most common indications for EUS- PDD are patients with main pancreatic duct obstruction who have failed conventional endoscopic retrograde pancreatography (ERP) drainage or those with surgically altered anatomy. EUS- PDD can be performed via two approaches: the EUS-rendezvous (EUS- RV) or the EUS-transmural drainage (TMD) techniques. The purpose of this review is to provide an updated review of the techniques and equipment available for EUS- PDD and the outcomes of EUS- PDD reported in the literature. Recent developments and future directions surrounding the procedure will also be discussed.

Keywords: EUS-guided pancreatic duct drainage; surgically altered anatomy; transmural drainage; EUS-rendezvous ERCP

1. Introduction

Endoscopic ultrasound (EUS) pancreatic duct drainage (EUS- PDD) was first described by Bataille et al. [1] in 2002 when they reported EUS-guided main pancreatic duct (MPD) puncture for trans-duodenal rendezvous endoscopic retrograde pancreatography (ERP). Francois et al. went on to report a series of four patients who underwent EUS-guided pancreaticogastrostomy (EUS- PG) of which three out of four patients achieved satisfactory relief of pain at 1-year follow-up [2]. Currently, EUS- PDD remains a challenging yet infrequently performed procedure for the advanced interventional endoscopist. EUS- PDD serves as a rescue procedure to access the pancreatic duct when standard transpapillary ERP has failed or is not possible due to altered anatomy. Retrospective series have demonstrated that the frequency of EUS- PDD is uncommon even in specialized tertiary referral centers for pancreatic diseases, ranging between two and four cases per center per year [3–5]. Through this review, we aim to provide the reader with an update on the indications, accessories required, and techniques employed as well as a summary of the literature surrounding EUS- PDD outcomes.

2. Indications for EUS- PDD

EUS- PDD is indicated for patients with symptomatic obstruction of the MPD that is not amenable to conventional ERP drainage. The main indications and contraindications for EUS- PDD are summarized in Table 1. MPD obstruction may occur because of multiple etiologies, including fibrosis and inflammation in chronic pancreatitis, obstructing pancreatic duct stones, or malignant obstruction. Pancreatic outflow obstruction resulting in ductal hypertension is more commonly seen in benign pancreatic obstruction, and less in infiltrative malignant disease, where the need for pancreatic duct decompression is rare. EUS- PDD is also helpful for pancreatic duct drainage for pancreatico-jejunostomy anastomotic strictures (PJAS) after pancreatoduodenectomy. EUS- PDD is also indicated

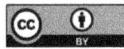

Citation: Teh, J.L.; Teoh, A.Y.B. Techniques and Outcomes of Endoscopic Ultrasound Guided—Pancreatic Duct Drainage (EUS- PDD). *J. Clin. Med.* **2023**, *12*, 1626. https://doi.org/10.3390/jcm12041626

Academic Editor: Manol Jovani

Received: 24 December 2022
Revised: 2 February 2023
Accepted: 9 February 2023
Published: 17 February 2023

Copyright: © 2023 by the authors. Licensee MDPI, Basel, Switzerland. This article is an open access article distributed under the terms and conditions of the Creative Commons Attribution (CC BY) license (https://creativecommons.org/licenses/by/4.0/).

for the management of symptomatic pancreatic duct (PD) stones and disconnected PD syndrome (DPDS). Recently, the use of EUS- PDD to manage intractable post-operative pancreatic fistula has been described [6]. EUS- PDD is a valuable technique to gain access to the pancreatic duct when the endoscopist is unable to cannulate the PD or when the PD is inaccessible due to altered post-surgical anatomy [7]. In a recent review of 2205 cases of pancreaticobiliary ductal access and drainage, Garcia- Alonso et al. reported that 107 endoscopic procedures were performed for pancreatic indications. A total of 10% eventually (n = 11) required EUS- PDD (eight transmural stenting and three EUS- RV) [8]. Four of these procedures were undertaken directly either due to anticipated failure or altered surgical anatomy and seven were undertaken after failed ERCP or performed as a combination procedure with ERCP [8]. In the management of DPDS, EUS-guided PDD aims to drain the viable upstream pancreas with a plastic stent. When direct puncture of the pancreatic duct is difficult, Ghandour et al. described two cases where the patients underwent a modified approach, with EUS-guided drainage of the fluid collection in communication with the disrupted MPD, resulting in successful symptom resolution with no recurrence of acute pancreatitis on short term follow up [9]. Although rarely indicated, EUS-guided PDD has also been described following obstructive pancreatitis in a patient with ampullary adenocarcinoma where transpapillary PD drainage was not successful [10].

Table 1. Indications and contraindications of EUS- PDD drainage.

Indications
Native Anatomy (usually after failed ERP)
Chronic pancreatitis and main pancreatic duct (MPD) obstruction
Symptomatic pancreatic stones
Disconnected Pancreatic Duct Syndrome
Surgically Altered Anatomy/Inaccessible PD
Pancreatico-jejunostomy anastomosis stricture post Whipple operation
Standard ERP indications with history of previous billroth II/Roux-en-Y Gastrectomy
Inaccessible papilla due to malignant/benign duodenal strictures
Contraindications
Technical Factors
Inability to locate the MPD on EUS
Insufficient dilatation of MPD (MPD size < 4 mm)
Intervening vessels at the puncture site
Long distance between bowel and pancreatic duct
Multi-level strictures
Patient factors
Hemodynamic instability
Uncorrected coagulopathy, thrombocytopenia

3. Contraindications for EUS- PDD

Contraindications for EUS- PDD include patient factors such as hemodynamic instability and bleeding risk due to severe coagulopathy or severe thrombocytopenia. Technical contraindications include the inability to localize the MPD on EUS or when the PD is insufficiently dilated (<4 mm), the presence of intervening vessels prohibiting safe puncture of the MPD, and the presence of multi-level strictures. There are no published data on the minimum size of PD dilatation for a successful puncture, but most series quote a median PD diameter between 4 and 6 mm [11–13]. Technical failure for PD puncture has been reported in cases of non-dilated PD measuring 2 mm [11]. In a meta-analysis consisting of 22 studies involving 714 patients, the mean MPD diameter was between 3.5 and 8.1 mm [14]. Based on these results, main PD dilatation of at least 4 mm will likely increase the chance of successful PD puncture. EUS- PDD is also contraindicated where standard ERP techniques to access the PD have not been exhausted as EUS- PDD is more invasive and may be associated with greater risk of adverse outcomes compared to standard ERP techniques [8,15].

It should be emphasized EUS- PDD is a challenging procedure and should only be attempted by interventional endoscopists skilled in both ERCP and EUS. EUS- PDD is challenging for the following reasons [3]:

a. difficult puncture with standard needles due to the small caliber of the dilated PD embedded within a fibrotic pancreas;
b. unstable scope position and consequent poor force transmission to the puncturing needle;
c. difficult wire manipulation through the needle (due to PD stricture, unfavorable needle to duct angle, preferential passage into a dilated side branch [7]), and risk of wire shearing during manipulation;
d. difficulty passing devices such as balloons or cystotomes into the PD for tract dilatation;
e. fragility of the pancreas and associated adverse events after aggressive manipulation.

In a Spanish national survey of 19 centers with limited experience in EUS-guided cholangiopancreatography, technical success rates of pancreatic EUS-guided cholangiopancreatography (ESCP) was lower than biliary ESCP (57.9% vs. 68.9%) with higher complication rates (26.3% vs. 22.6%) [15]. The main reason for technical failure was failed manipulation of the guidewire inside the pancreatic or biliary duct [15].

4. Technique of EUS- PDD

4.1. Patient Preparation

We perform EUS- PDD with the patient in a prone position under general anesthesia or monitored anesthetic care [7]. Positioning the patient in the supine position for EUS- PDD has also been described [16]. Prophylactic antibiotics are administered [7,16] prior to the start of the procedure. Anticoagulation should be corrected, and anti-thrombotic medications withheld as outlined by published guidelines [17].

4.2. Approaches and Equipment

EUS- PDD comprises two approaches to drain the pancreatic duct [13] including EUS-assisted rendezvous (EUS- RV) ERP and EUS-transmural drainage (EUS- TMD) [18]. In scenarios where the papilla is accessible with a standard therapeutic duodenoscope but cannulation of the pancreatic duct by ERP has failed previously, EUS- RV is the procedure of choice due to higher success rates, lower adverse events, and avoidance of an extra-anatomical stent [16,19,20]. Stenting performed by EUS- TMD can be either antegrade or retrograde or transpapillary/trans-anastomotic [18]. The puncture site for the pancreatic duct is usually from the stomach (EUS-pancreaticogastrostomy, EUS- PGS) or the duodenum (EUS-pancreaticoduodenostomy, EUS- PDS). Typically, to access the pancreatic duct at the body and tail, EUS- PGS is more favorable whereas EUS- PDS is more suitable for drainage of the pancreatic head. The choice of technique will depend on the accessibility of the native papilla, the ability to pass the guidewire into the PD and maneuver it across the stricture as well as the desired direction of stent drainage. These considerations are summarized in Figure 1.

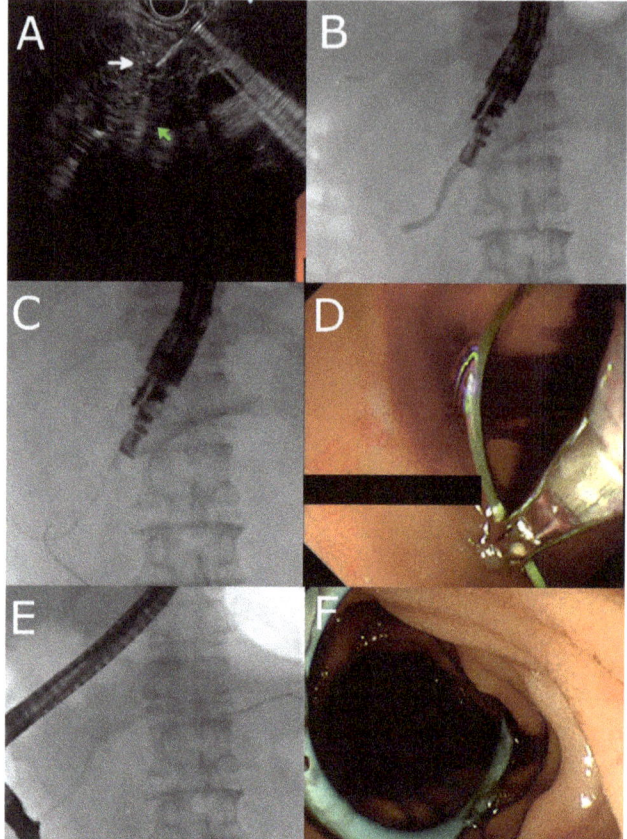

Figure 1. EUS-guided rendezvous ERP in a patient with pancreatic divisum and failed minor papilla cannulation. (**A**) EUS-guided puncture of the pancreatic duct (indicated by white arrow). (**B**) Contrast injection showing pancreatogram. (**C**) Passage of guidewire into the duodenum. (**D**) Grabbing the guidewire from the duodenal lumen after changing to a duodenoscope with micro-forceps. (**E**) Main pancreatic duct recannulated with a guidewire. (**F**) Insertion of a pancreatic duct stent after minor papillotomy.

4.3. Pancreatic Duct Access

The steps common to all approaches of EUS- PDD are first pancreatic duct puncture under EUS guidance, followed by contrast injection and guidewire placement. To gain access to the pancreatic duct, a curvilinear array echoendoscope is inserted into either the stomach or duodenal bulb and EUS performed to identify the dilated pancreatic duct. Factors affecting the choice of puncture site will include the distance between the visceral lumen and PD, the presence of intervening vessels, and the stability of scope position which facilitates subsequent tract dilatation and stent deployment [7]. The most common puncture site for PD access is the stomach. It is recommended that the pancreatic duct is punctured at an oblique angle rather than perpendicularly as the latter will result in a difficult insertion of the guidewire and subsequent device insertion into the pancreatic duct [18].

Using a 19G needle (EZ Shot 3 plus, Olympus Medical Systems, Tokyo, Japan), the PD is punctured and a diagnostic pancreatogram is performed. A 0.035-inch or 0.025-inch (VisiGlide2; Olympus Medical Systems) guidewire is inserted into the pancreatic duct, directed either toward the head of the pancreas or the tail depending on the subsequent plan. In cases where the MPD is minimally dilated or the pancreatic parenchyma is fibrotic, a 22 G needle and a corresponding 0.018-inch or 0.021-inch guidewire can be used [21]. However, 0.018 in wires lack stability for over-the-wire exchange of accessories and these wires will need to be exchanged for larger caliber guidewires after initial manipulation. Guidewire shearing has been reported during guidewire manipulation in EUS- PDD; tips to avoid guidewire shearing will include gentle manipulation of the guidewire, avoiding withdrawal of guidewire back into the needle tip, as well as retraction of the needle tip into the sheath or the echoendoscope during guidewire manipulation [18]. Allowing excess length of the guidewire in the distal pancreatic duct or forming loops in the duodenum prevents loss of access to the PD. When wire manipulation into the duodenum is unsuccessful, injection of diluted methylene blue (1–3 cc of methylene blue, diluted with 15 cc saline or contrast) via the FNA needle into the duct may help to endoscopically identify an obscured ampullary orifice to aid cannulation by the duodenoscope during EUS- RV [22,23].

4.4. EUS- RV ERP

EUS- RV ERP is indicated when the papilla is still anatomically accessible by the duodenoscope, but initial cannulation of PD by conventional ERP has failed (Figure 1). Following pancreatic duct puncture, the guidewire is introduced antegrade towards the head of the pancreas into the duodenum and allowed to form loops in the duodenum. The linear echoendoscope is removed, leaving the guidewire in situ. The therapeutic duodenoscope is then inserted in the usual fashion into the second part of the duodenum and the end of the previously inserted guidewire is grasped into the working channel of the duodenoscope using forceps or a snare and withdrawn through the accessory channel. From here, the PD can either be cannulated over the wire or alongside the wire. In patients with pancreatic divisum, the guidewire may be introduced through the pancreatic duct and directed into the duodenum via the minor papilla [24]. This allows for papillotomy of the minor papilla and insertion of a 5 cm 10 Fr plastic stent for drainage of the pancreatic duct.

4.5. Transmural Approaches with Transpapillary or Trans-Anastomotic Stenting

Transmural techniques are employed for either EUS- PGS or EUS- PDS or transpapillary/ trans-anastomotic stenting (Figure 2). Transmural EUS- PDD is performed when the papilla is inaccessible or when EUS RV is not successful l [21]. The MPD is accessed in a similar fashion as described above. The steps after initial access include dilatation of the EUS- PDS or PGS fistula track followed by deployment of the stent. Dilatation of the puncture site can be performed either with cautery or non-cautery devices [19]. Non-cautery dilatators will include either mechanical dilators or balloon dilators (Hurricane RX Biliary Dilatation Balloon, Boston Scientific, Malborough, MA, USA). Options for cautery dilators include the use of either a 6 Fr cystotome (Cysto Gastro Set; Endo-flex, GmbH, Voerde, Germany) or triple lumen needle knife (Microknife; Boston Scientific) [21]. Tract dilatation is a difficult step in EUS- PD; the endoscopist may encounter difficulty penetrating the fibrotic pancreatic parenchyma when a mechanical dilator or balloon dilator is employed for track dilatation without cautery. Conversely, several groups advocate the use of mechanical dilatators [25,26] before using cautery-assisted devices due to the risk of bleeding associated with cautery devices [27]. Recently, devices have become available. A new ultra-tapered mechanical dilator (ES dilator DC7R180S; Zeon Medical Co., Ltd., Tokyo, Japan) developed for EUS- PDD demonstrated decreased bleeding risk (0% vs. 18.2%, $p = 0.04$) with similar rates of dilatation success (93.3% vs. 95.0%, $p < 0.05$) when compared to a 6Fr cautery dilator [28]. Nakai et al. described a double-wire technique in 2019 to help stabilize the echoendoscope position when performing EUS-guided pancreatic stent placement for a patient with PJ stenosis [29]. With 0.025 in guidewire in place, fistula track dilatation with 6 Fr cystotome was performed. A double-lumen catheter (double-lumen cannula; Piolax, Kanagawa, Japan) was inserted, and an additional 0.035 in guidewire inserted (Renowave Ultrahard; Piolax) through the PJ stricture into the jejunum [29]. The introduction of the additional guidewire reduces the angulation between the puncture site and the PD which facilitates the insertion of the stent device and other accessories. Two plastic stents were then placed separately over the two guidewires. On the other hand, a plastic stent can also be deployed across the papilla or PJ anastomosis, with the distal end of the stent in the jejunum and the proximal end of the stent in the gastric lumen (i.e., "ring drainage" or gastro-pancreatico-jejunostomy) [5,30]. Ring drains facilitate future stent exchanges by keeping the pancreatico-gastric fistula track patent and reduces the risk of stent migration risk [30].

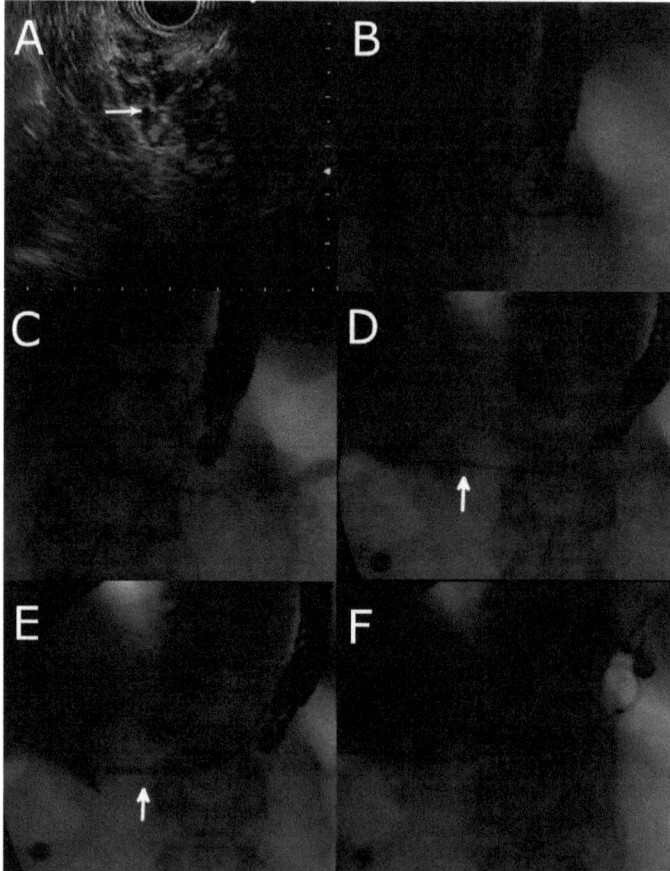

Figure 2. EUS-guided drainage of a pancreatico-jejunal anastomotic stricture after Whipple operation. (**A**) EUS-guided puncture of the pancreatic duct (arrow indicates the position of the needle) (**B**) Injection of contrast through the needle showing a pancreatogram. (**C**) Passage of guidewire and cystotome into the pancreatic duct. (**D**) Passage of the guidewire across the anastomotic stricture (indicated by the arrow) with the use of the cystotome as a pivot. Contrast injection through the cystotome outlined the jejunum and also part of the bile duct. (**E**) Dilation of the stricture with a 4 mm balloon (indicated by the arrow). (**F**) Placement of a plastic stent across the PJ anastomosis into the stomach.

4.6. Transmural Stenting with Antegrade/Retrograde Stenting

Transmural antegrade or retrograde stenting is performed when there is difficulty passing the guidewire beyond the pancreatic duct stricture or PJ anastomotic stricture.

Transmural stenting can be either antegrade when the stent is placed towards the head of the pancreas or retrograde when placed towards the tail of the pancreas. Following pancreatic duct access and fistula track dilatation as described above, plastic stents (usually 5 or 7 Fr plastic stents) are deployed with the distal end in the pancreatic duct and the proximal end in the enteric lumen. When choosing plastic stents for the creation of PDS or PGS, one should choose a plastic stent without a side aperture (Tannenbaum type) to avoid pancreatic juice leakage into the peritoneum via the side hole [31]. The use of modified anti-migratory FCSEMS with proximal and distal anchoring flaps (M.I. Tech, Seoul, Korea) across the pancreatico-gastric or enteric anastomosis has also been described [32], although there is a risk of obstructive pancreatitis if side branches of the PD are blocked. Success rates and long-term outcomes following FCSEMS in patients with pancreatico-jejunostomy anastomotic strictures (PJAS) following a Whipple operation have also been described [33]. Out of 23 patients who underwent FCSEMS, 5 patients (21.7%) developed late adverse events of which only 1 (4.3%) was due to stent occlusion which resulted in symptom recurrence [33]. Uncovered SEMS is not used due to the risk of pancreatic fluid leakage between the stomach and the pancreas.

To circumvent the problem of difficult fistula track dilatation and subsequent passage of stent across the gastric wall and pancreatic parenchyma into the MPD, Hayat et al. described PGS creation using small caliber accessories. After EUS-guided puncture of the PD and pancreatogram, over 0.018 inch guidewire, a 4 Fr angiogplasty balloon (Sterling, Boston Scientific, Malborough, MA, USA) was used to dilate the pancreatico-gastrostomy fistula track. A 3 Fr single pigtail stent was used to drain the pancreatic duct with the pigtail end in the intestine lumen or proximal PD, and the proximal end in the gastric lumen [34].

4.7. Per Oral Pancreaticoscopy

Per-oral pancreaticoscopy (POPS) following the creation of pancreatico-gastrostomy (PGS) and stent insertion has been described [35]. Three months following the PGS creation, a guidewire is inserted alongside the previously inserted stent and the stent is removed. The fistula and stricture sites were dilated with a 4 mm balloon (4-mm REN; Kaneka). A digital cholangiopancreatoscope (Spy Scope DS; Boston Scientific) was used to evaluate the cause of the stricture and perform electrohydraulic lithotripsy (EHL) of any pancreatic stones. The plastic stents were then regularly exchanged every two to three months for a year.

Per-oral pancreaticoscopy was performed in 13 out of 19 patients who underwent EUS-PGS [35]. Technical success of POPS was 100% with the median length of the procedure taking 66 min. POPS resulted in mild pancreatitis in one patient (8%), and asymptomatic stent migration in another. Following POPS, two or three 7-Fr plastic stents were placed across the stricture for dilatation. At the time of data analysis, four patients with benign fibrotic pancreatic strictures who had reached 1-year follow-up had improvement in pancreatic duct strictures and were stent free.

5. Outcomes

The outcomes of patient cohorts undergoing EUS- PDD are summarized in Table 2. Kahaleh reported in 2007 a series of 13 patients who underwent EUS-guided PGS with a plastic stent, of which 7 patients had surgically altered anatomy and the rest had pancreatic duct stricture due to pancreatitis or neoplastic process [4]. A total of 10 patients had successful stent placement across the PGS fistula (76.9%). After a mean follow-up of 14 months, mean pancreatic duct size was reduced from 4.6 to 3.0 mm ($p = 0.01$) with significant improvement in pain score from 7.3 to 3.6 ($p = 0.01$) [4]. Adverse events occurred in two patients, one with bleeding and another with contained perforation. Will et al. described a series of 12 patients over a 3-year period who underwent EUS- PGS after failing standard ERP and drainage of the pancreatic duct [36]. Pancreatography was successful in all patients and drainage was achieved in 69% of patients [36]. The adverse events rate was 42.9% with post-procedural pain accounting for most events. A total of 14.3% of patients needed repeat endoscopic drainage and another 14.3% required surgical drainage of the pancreatic duct. Krafft et al. described a dual-center study of 28 patients undergoing anterograde EUS- PGS for chronic pancreatitis or PJ stenosis after Whipple surgery [11]. The technical and clinical success rates were 82% (23/28) and 77% (17/22), respectively, with an adverse event rate of 14% (4/28).

Table 2. Outcomes of EUS-guided pancreatic duct intervention.

Author	Type of Study	Patients	Indications	Technical Success, n (%)	Clinical Success, n (%)	Adverse Events, n (%)	Comments
Kahaleh et al. (2007) [4]	Prospective	13 [EUS- TMD]	SAA, strictures secondary to pancreatitis, IPMN	10/13 (77%)	NR	2/13 (15.3%) Bleeding (1), perforation (1)	Improvement in MPD diameter, pain score, and weight on long term follow up
Tessier et al. (2007) [37]	Retrospective	36 [EUS- TMD]	SAA, chronic pancreatitis, PJAS	33/36 (92%)	Pain relief: 25/36 (69%) Stent dysfunction: 20/36 (55%)	5/35 (13.8%) 2 severe, 3 mild	
Barkay et al. (2010) [38]	Retrospective	21 [EUS- RV]	Failed ERP	10/21 (48%)	NR	2/20 (10%) 1 case of pancreatitis 1 case of peripancreatic abscess)	Dilated PD was associated with greater likelihood of EUS-guided pancreatography
Ergun et al. (2011) [39]	Retrospective	20 [total]/ 24 procedures 5 [EUS- RV] 19 [EUS- TMD]	CP, PJAS	18/20 (90%) 5/5 (100%) 15/19 (79%)	Pain term pain resolution: 13/18 (72%)	2/20 (10%) including bleeding and perigatric collection. 9/18 (50%) developed stent dysfunction	Significant decrease in pain scores and MPD size after long-term follow-up.
Shah et al. (2012) [40]	Retrospective	24 [total]/30 procedures 16 [EUS- RV] 14 [EUS- TMD]	CP, pancreatic duct leak, PJAS	19/30 (63%) 9/16 (56%) 10/14 (71%)	NR	4/ 22 (18%)	
Kurihara et al. (2013) [20]	Retrospective	14 [total]/17 procedures 11 [EUS- RV] 5 [EUS- TMD]	PJAS, CP	14/17 (82.3%) 11/17 (64.7%) 3/5 (60%)	NR	1/17 (5.8%) 1 case developed pancreatic pseudocyst with aneurysm	Patients underwent EUS-PD after failed EUS- RV.
Fujii et al. (2013) [12]	Retrospective	45 [total]	SAA, failed ERP	32/43 (74%) 14 [EUS- RV] 18 [EUS- TMD]	Long-term symptom resolution: 24/29 (83%)	3/45 (6.6%) with severe complications 16/35 (35.5%) developed abdominal pain	EUS- RV significantly longer than EUS-TMD (130 vs. 125 min, $p = 0.05$)
Will et al. (2015) [41]	Retrospective	94 [total]/111 procedures	CP, pancreatic divisum, DPDS, POPF	47/83 (56.6%) 21 [EUS- RV] 26 [EUS- TMD]	68/83 (81.9%)	24/111 (21.6%) (2 severe, 20 intermediate, 2 minor AEs)	
Chen et al. (2017) [42]	Retrospective	40 [Total] 37 [EUS- TMD] 3 [EUS- RV]	Pancreatic intervention post-Whipple operation	37/40 (92.5%) 34/ 37 (91.8%) 3/3 (100%)	32/40 (87.5%) 29/37 (78.3%) 3/3 (100%)	14/40 (35.0%)	
Tyberg et al. (2018) [5]	Retrospective	80 [total] 66 [EUS- RV] 14 [EUS- TMD]	Malignancy, chronic pancreatitis	71/ 80 (89%)	65/80 (81%)	Immediate 16/80 (20%); Delayed 9/80 (11%)	Comparative study of EUS-PDD and e-ERP. EUS- PDD had higher clinical and technical success.
Uchida et al. (2018) [25]	Retrospective	15 [total] 2 [EUS- RV] 13 [EUS- TMD]	Pancreatic strictures (8 benign, 7 malignant)	13/15 (86%) Benign 75% (6/8) malignant 100% (7/7)	12/13 (92.3%) Benign 100% (6/6), malignant 87.5% (6/7)	4/15 (26.7%)–peritonitis, stent migration, bleeding	

Table 2. Cont.

Author	Type of Study	Patients	Indications	Technical Success, n (%)	Clinical Success, n (%)	Adverse Events, n (%)	Comments
Tellez-Avina et al. (2018) [43]	Retrospective	21 [EUS- TMD]	DPDS	21/21 (100%)	17/21 (80.9%)	5/21 (23.8%)	
Matsunami et al. (2019) [44]	Retrospective	30 [EUS- TMD]	Acute recurrent pancreatitis with stricture	30/30 (100%)	23/30 (76%)	7/30 (23%): mild abdominal pain/bleeding/pancreatitis 6/25 (24%): stent dislodgement	
Oh et al. (2019) [33]	Retrospective	23 [total] 3 patients underwent plastic stenting 20 patients underwent FCSEMS	PJAS	23/23 (100%)	23/23 (100%)	Early adverse events: 4/23 (17.4%) Late adverse events: 5/23 (21.7%)	Utilized FCSEMS.
Krafft et al. (2020) [11]	Retrospective	28 [EUS- TMD]	CP, PJS	23/28 (82%)	21/28 (75%)	4/28 (14.2%)	Long-term outcomes: 52% developed DM, 14.2% developed exocrine insufficiency, 83% had stents in situ after 12 months
Dalal et al. (2020) [16]	Retrospective	44 [total] 23/44 [EUS- RV] 21/44 [EUS- TMD]	Failed ERP, SAA	39/44 (88.6%) 22/23 (95.6%) 17/21 (80.9%)	35/44 (79.5%) 19/23 (82.6%) 16/21 (76.1%)	10/44 (22.7%)	2/28 patients underwent gastropancreaticoenterostomy "ring drainage"

Legend: SAA–surgically altered anatomy, IPMN–intraductal papillary mucinous neoplasm, MPD–main pancreatic duct, PJAS–pancreatico-jejunal anastomotic strictures, ERP–endoscopic retrograde pancreatography, CP chronic pancreatitis, DPDS–disconnected pancreatic duct syndrome, POPF–post-operative pancreatic fistula, EUS- RV–EUS rendezvous, EUS- TMD–EUS-transmural stenting, FCSEMs–fully covered self-expanding metal stents.

5.1. Long-Term Outcomes

Fujii et al. [12] published long-term follow-up of 29 patients who successfully underwent EUS- PDD. Of 23 patients who successfully underwent EUS- PDD and had > 1-year follow-up, 16 patients (69.6%) had complete symptom resolution. Stents were removed after a median of 4 months in 23 patients, and symptom recurrence was seen in 13.1 % (n = 4) of patients after a median of 14 months follow-up (range 2–45 months). No further surgical or endoscopic intervention was required for these patients who had symptom recurrence or incomplete symptom resolution. Tellez et al. reported long-term results of permanent indwelling transmural stents for patients with disconnected pancreatic duct syndrome [43]. Technical success was 100% with clinical success of 80.9% (17/21 patients). A total of 25.3% of the cohort developed adverse events, most of which were stent migration.

An international multi-center prospective study reported the outcomes of 80 patients who underwent EUS- PDD [5]. A total of 83% (n = 66) of this cohort had malignant disease and 45% (n = 36) had surgically altered anatomy. Technical success was achieved in 89% (n = 71) and clinical success in 81% of patients (n = 65). The immediate adverse event rate was 20% (n = 16). A total of 12 out of 16 immediate adverse events were classified as major and included post-ERCP pancreatitis, pancreatic fluid collection, pancreatic duct leakage, and bowel perforation. The method of approach (either antegrade or retrograde) did not predict technical success or clinical success [5]. Uchida et al. compared outcomes of EUS- PGS for patients with benign strictures compared to malignant obstructions. Technical success (75% vs. 100%) and clinical success (100% vs. 85.7%) were similar for EUS- PGS performed for benign and malignant indications respectively with a non-significant difference in adverse event rates [25].

Recently, Sakai et al. described the endoscopic outcomes following endoscopic transpapillary pancreatic drainage (ETPD) and EUS- PDD in patients with benign pancreatic duct obstruction [45]. Eight out of ten patients who failed ETPD underwent EUS-PDD together with two patients undergoing EUS- PDD as a primary procedure. When added to ETPD, EUS- PDD improved the technical success rates of endoscopic intervention from 82% to 91% for chronic pancreatitis and 0 % to 80% in patients with pancreaticojejunostomy stricture [45]. The overall clinical success rate of endoscopic interventions was 97%. Post-procedural pancreatitis in the EUS- PDD group was 30% (n = 3). Sakai's study demonstrated that EUS- PDD was more likely to achieve technical success than ETPD for PJ stenosis; when added to ETPD as a salvage procedure, decreased the number of patients who would otherwise require surgical drainage for pancreatic obstruction [45].

5.2. Post-Operative Pancreatic Fistula

In a study of 24 patients undergoing POPF drainage after pancreatic resection, the POPF could be visualized on EUS from the gastric position in five patients and hence underwent EUS- transmural drainage (TMD). The remaining 19 patients underwent percutaneous drainage. Both EUS- TMD and percutaneous drainage achieved a technical success of 100%. The short- and long-term clinical success rates of EUS- TMD were both 100%, compared to 61.1% and 83% for percutaneous drainage. The time until clinical success for EUS- TD was markedly shorter (5.8 days vs. 30.4 days, $p = 0.0013$) in patients undergoing EUS- TMD [46].

5.3. Comparison between e-ERP vs. EUS- PDD

Chen et al. compared the efficacy of EUS- PDD compared to enteroscopy-assisted ERP (e-ERP) in an international multi-center comparative retrospective study. A total of 75 procedures (40 EUS- PDD and 35 e-ERP) were performed in 66 patients. Technical (92.5% vs. 20%, $p < 0.001$) and clinical success (87.5% vs. 23.1%, $p < 0.001$) were significantly superior in the EUS- PDD group compared to e-ERP but resulted in more adverse events (35.0% vs. 2.9%, OR 18.3, $p < 0.01$) [42]. The lower technical success in the e-ERP group was due to failed cannulation in 42.9%, failed identification of PJ anastomosis (35.7%), and inability to reach the PJ in 21.4% [42]. Kogure et al. reported the outcomes of pancreatic interventions performed via double-balloon enteroscopy (DBE- assisted) ERP compared to EUS- PDD [47]. EUS- PDD was utilized as a salvage procedure when DBE -ERP failed and vice versa. The technical success of DB-ERP was 70.7% compared to 100% for EUS- PDD ($p = 0.092$). The clinical success of DB- ERP was similar to EUS- PDD (68.3% vs. 66.7%) and overall clinical success improved to 85.0% by combining both DB-ERP and EUS- PD [47].

5.4. Comparison between EUS- RV and EUS- TMD

Dalal et al. compared the outcomes of patients undergoing EUS-guided rendezvous technique compared to those who underwent antegrade stenting. Technical success for EUS- RV was 95.6% (22/23 patients) compared to 77.8% (14/18) in EUS- PGS ($p = 0.08$). Clinical success was also similar between the two techniques (RV 86.9% vs. PGS 72.2%). The rendezvous technique had a non-significant reduction in adverse events compared to EUS-guided PGS (17.4% vs. 33.3 %, $p > 0.05$) [16].

5.5. Overall Outcomes from Meta-Analyses and Systemic Reviews

Published reports currently estimate the technical success of EUS- PDD to be around 80% with an adverse event rate of 20% [14,18,48]. Imoto et al. summarized in a review the outcomes of 401 patients who underwent EUS-guided transmural stenting. The overall technical and clinical success rates were 85% (339/401 patients) and 88% (328/372 patients) respectively [19]. Adverse outcomes occurred in 25% (102/401 patients), of which 5% (20/401) were classified as severe adverse events. Bhurwal et al. summarized the outcomes of EUS-guided pancreatic duct decompression in a recent meta-analysis [48]. In this meta-analysis comprising 503 patients, the technical success rate was 81.4%, clinical success was 84.6% with an overall adverse event rate of 21.3% (mostly post-procedural pain), and pooled event rate of 5% for EUS- PD pancreatitis. Results from an earlier meta-analysis [14] were similar with a pooled technical success rate of 84.8% (95% CI 79.1–89.2) and clinical success of 89.2% (95% CI 82.1–93.7). Pooled adverse event rates were 18.1% (95% CI 14.2–22.9) and 6.6% (95% CI 4.5–9.4) for acute pancreatitis, 4.1% (95% CI 2.7–6.2) for bleeding, 3.1% (95% CI 1.9–5) for perforation and 2.3% (95% CI 1.4–4) for pancreatic leakage.

In a systemic review comparing pancreatic duct cannulation outcomes of patients who underwent ERP guided vs. EUS-guided pancreatic access for pancreatico-jejunostomy (PJ) stenosis, an EUS-guided approach resulted in higher pancreatic duct opacification (87% vs. 30%, $p <0.001$), cannulation success (79% vs. 26%, $p < 0.001$), and stent placement (72% vs. 20%, $p< 0.001$) [49]. Clinical success was also higher in the EUS group compared to the ERP group (79% vs. 19%, $p < 0.001$) [49] even though the definition of clinical success was not standardized.

6. EUS- PDD Training

Tyberg et al. reported the learning curve of EUS- PDD for a single expert ERCP / EUS operator from a retrospective registry [50]. In a series comprising 56 patients, the median procedural time was found to be 80 min (range 49–159 min). CUSUM analysis showed a progressive reduction in procedural time with a procedural time of 80 min achieved on the 27th procedure, indicating procedural efficiency. Procedural duration further reduced until the 40th procedure before reaching a plateau indicating proficiency. These results suggest that even for the experienced interventional endoscopist, 40 cases are required prior to mastery of the procedure [50]. Technical success was achieved in 84% of patients and the overall adverse event rate was 24% in this series [50].

7. Future Directions

Over the last two decades, EUS- PDD has evolved significantly and now plays an important role in the management of pancreatic duct obstruction, especially in patients with altered surgical anatomy and failed drainage by traditional ERP techniques. Case series regarding EUS- PDD have mostly been retrospective in nature involving small cohorts of patients. Consequently, guidelines surrounding EUS- PDD have only provided guiding statements backed up by low-quality evidence [51,52]. There is a need for larger prospective and long-term comparative studies in the field of EUS- PDD. Several studies consist of mixed cohorts of EUS- PDD patients who have undergone EUS- RV and transmural stenting and outcomes are not reported separately [4,5,36]; future studies should report the outcomes of EUS- RV and transmural stenting independently as these procedures have varying technical considerations as well as varying technical success. Furthermore, definitions for technical and clinical success in EUS- PDD have not been standardized. Technical success in EUS- PDD varies and has been defined as a successful pancreatogram, successful negotiation of the guidewire past the obstruction, as well as stent placement into the MPD in different studies. The lack of standardization makes the comparison of results difficult, and this is evident in the results of a meta-analysis in EUS- PDD where heterogeneity has been noted [14,48]. EUS- PDD is a challenging procedure due to several technical factors as previously discussed, as well as the lack of dedicated accessories and limited training opportunities due to the rare indications for the procedure. The development of dedicated accessories such as small caliber accessories [34] may improve the technical success of EUS- PDD but direct head-to-head comparisons with standard accessories have not been performed. Adverse events still occur in about 20% of EUS- PDD cases and guidelines have suggested that experience in other EUS-guided drainage procedures may improve the success rates and reduce the risk of adverse events [52]. Given that the learning curve of EUS- PDD has recently been described to be around 40 cases [50], it is imperative to research how the EUS- PDD learning curve can be surmounted in fewer cases through better standardized training and the provision of better accessories to improve the success rates and safety of the procedure.

The advent of per-oral pancreatoscopy is an exciting development in EUS-guided pancreatic duct access. Currently, there are few case series proving the efficacy and safety of POPS [35]; per oral cholecystoscopy after EUS- gallbladder drainage opened a whole new paradigm into the treatment of gallbladder-related diseases, such as cholecystoscopy-guided target biopsy of gallbladder neoplasm and lithotripsy of gallbladder stones [53]. Similarly, POPS can expand the indications for EUS-guided PD access and allow the development of a new tool for luminal diagnosis and management of pancreatic diseases.

8. Conclusions

EUS- PDD is a valuable skill in the interventional endoscopist's armamentarium of skills to deal with main pancreatic duct obstruction when traditional ERP techniques have failed. It is especially valuable in cases with altered surgical anatomy, such as in PJAS after the Whipple operation. In skilled hands, EUS- PDD is associated with high technical and clinical success rates, although one in five patients who undergo EUS- PDD may still experience adverse events. Standardization of EUS- PDD techniques, the introduction of dedicated accessories, and the provision of structured training in high-volume centers will improve the outcomes of patients who undergo EUS- PDD who might otherwise require surgical management which is associated with high morbidity and mortality.

Author Contributions: J.L.T. was involved in the literature review, formulation, and revision of the manuscript. A.Y.B.T. was involved in the study conception, formulation, critical revision, and final approval of the manuscript. All authors have read and agreed to the published version of the manuscript.

Funding: This research received no external funding.

Conflicts of Interest: A.Y.B.T. is a consultant for Boston Scientific, Cook, Taewoong, Microtech, and MI Tech Medical Corporations. J.L.T. has no conflicts of interest to disclose.

References

1. Bataille, L.; Deprez, P. A new application for therapeutic EUS: Main pancreatic duct drainage with a "pancreatic rendezvous technique". *Gastrointest. Endosc.* **2002**, *55*, 740–743. [CrossRef]
2. François, E.; Kahaleh, M.; Giovannini, M.; Matos, C.; Devière, J. EUS-guided pancreaticogastrostomy. *Gastrointest. Endosc.* **2002**, *56*, 128–133. [CrossRef]
3. Devière, J. EUS-guided pancreatic duct drainage: A rare indication in need of prospective evidence. *Gastrointest. Endosc.* **2017**, *85*, 178–180. [CrossRef]
4. Kahaleh, M.; Hernandez, A.J.; Tokar, J.; Adams, R.B.; Shami, V.M.; Yeaton, P. EUS-guided pancreaticogastrostomy: Analysis of its efficacy to drain inaccessible pancreatic ducts. *Gastrointest. Endosc.* **2007**, *65*, 224–230. [CrossRef]
5. Tyberg, A.; Sharaiha, R.Z.; Kedia, P.; Kumta, N.; Gaidhane, M.; Artifon, E.; Giovannini, M.; Kahaleh, M. EUS-guided pancreatic drainage for pancreatic strictures after failed ERCP: A multicenter international collaborative study. *Gastrointest. Endosc.* **2017**, *85*, 164–169. [CrossRef]
6. Toshima, T.; Fujimori, N.; Yoshizumi, T.; Itoh, S.; Nagao, Y.; Harada, N.; Oono, T.; Mori, M. A Novel Strategy of Endoscopic Ultrasonography-Guided Pancreatic Duct Drainage for Pancreatic Fistula After Pancreaticoduodenectomy. *Pancreas* **2021**, *50*, e21–e22. [CrossRef]
7. Chapman, C.G.; Waxman, I.; Siddiqui, U.D. Endoscopic Ultrasound (EUS)-Guided Pancreatic Duct Drainage: The Basics of When and How to Perform EUS-Guided Pancreatic Duct Interventions. *Clin. Endosc.* **2016**, *49*, 161–167. [CrossRef]
8. García-Alonso, F.J.; Peñas-Herrero, I.; Sanchez-Ocana, R.; Villarroel, M.; Cimavilla, M.; Bazaga, S.; De Benito Sanz, M.; Gil-Simon, P.; de la Serna-Higuera, C.; Perez-Miranda, M. The role of endoscopic ultrasound guidance for biliary and pancreatic duct access and drainage to overcome the limitations of ERCP: A retrospective evaluation. *Endoscopy* **2021**, *53*, 691–699. [CrossRef]
9. Ghandour, B.; Akshintala, V.S.; Bejjani, M.; Szvarca, D.; Khashab, M.A. A modified approach for endoscopic ultrasound-guided management of disconnected pancreatic duct syndrome via drainage of a communicating collection. *Endoscopy* **2022**, *54*, 917–919. [CrossRef]
10. Miyata, T.; Kamata, K.; Takenaka, M. Endoscopic ultrasonography-guided transenteric pancreatic duct drainage without cautery for obstructive pancreatitis as a result of ampullary carcinoma. *Dig. Endosc.* **2018**, *30*, 403–404. [CrossRef]
11. Krafft, M.R.; Croglio, M.P.; James, T.W.; Baron, T.H.; Nasr, J.Y. Endoscopic endgame for obstructive pancreatopathy: Outcomes of anterograde EUS-guided pancreatic duct drainage. A dual-center study. *Gastrointest. Endosc.* **2020**, *92*, 1055–1066. [CrossRef]

12. Fujii, L.L.; Topazian, M.D.; Abu Dayyeh, B.K.; Baron, T.H.; Chari, S.T.; Farnell, M.B.; Gleeson, F.C.; Gostout, C.J.; Kendrick, M.L.; Pearson, R.K.; et al. EUS-guided pancreatic duct intervention: Outcomes of a single tertiary-care referral center experience. *Gastrointest. Endosc.* **2013**, *78*, 854–864.e1. [CrossRef] [PubMed]
13. Chen, Y.I.; Saxena, P.; Ngamruengphong, S.; Haito-Chavez, Y.; Bukhari, M.; Artifon, E.; Khashab, M.A. Endoscopic ultrasound-guided pancreatic duct drainage: Technical approaches to a challenging procedure. *Endoscopy* **2016**, *48* (Suppl. 1), E192–E193. [CrossRef] [PubMed]
14. Chandan, S.; Mohan, B.P.; Khan, S.R.; Kassab, L.L.; Ponnada, S.; Ofosu, A.; Bhat, I.; Singh, S.; Adler, D.G. Efficacy and safety of endoscopic ultrasound-guided pancreatic duct drainage (EUS-PDD): A systematic review and meta-analysis of 714 patients. *Endosc. Int. Open* **2020**, *8*, E1664–E1672. [CrossRef]
15. Vila, J.J.; Pérez-Miranda, M.; Vazquez-Sequeiros, E.; Abadia, M.A.; Pérez-Millán, A.; González-Huix, F.; Gornals, J.; Iglesias-Garcia, J.; De la Serna, C.; Aparicio, J.R.; et al. Initial experience with EUS-guided cholangiopancreatography for biliary and pancreatic duct drainage: A Spanish national survey. *Gastrointest. Endosc.* **2012**, *76*, 1133–1141. [CrossRef] [PubMed]
16. Dalal, A.; Patil, G.; Maydeo, A. Six-year retrospective analysis of endoscopic ultrasonography-guided pancreatic ductal interventions at a tertiary referral center. *Dig. Endosc.* **2020**, *32*, 409–416. [CrossRef] [PubMed]
17. Veitch, A.M.; Radaelli, F.; Alikhan, R.; Dumonceau, J.M.; Eaton, D.; Jerrome, J.; Lester, W.; Nylander, D.; Thoufeeq, M.; Vanbiervliet, G.; et al. Endoscopy in patients on antiplatelet or anticoagulant therapy: British Society of Gastroenterology (BSG) and European Society of Gastrointestinal Endoscopy (ESGE) guideline update. *Gut* **2021**, *70*, 1611–1628. [CrossRef]
18. Nakai, Y.; Kogure, H.; Isayama, H.; Koike, K. Endoscopic ultrasound-guided pancreatic duct drainage. *Saudi J. Gastroenterol.* **2019**, *25*, 210–217. [CrossRef]
19. Imoto, A.; Ogura, T.; Higuchi, K. Endoscopic Ultrasound-Guided Pancreatic Duct Drainage: Techniques and Literature Review of Transmural Stenting. *Clin. Endosc.* **2020**, *53*, 525–534. [CrossRef]
20. Kurihara, T.; Itoi, T.; Sofuni, A.; Itokawa, F.; Moriyasu, F. Endoscopic ultrasonography-guided pancreatic duct drainage after failed endoscopic retrograde cholangiopancreatography in patients with malignant and benign pancreatic duct obstructions. *Dig. Endosc.* **2013**, *25* (Suppl. 2), 109–116. [CrossRef]
21. Abdelqader, A.; Kahaleh, M. When ERCP Fails: EUS-Guided Access to Biliary and Pancreatic Ducts. *Dig. Dis. Sci.* **2022**, *67*, 1649–1659. [CrossRef] [PubMed]
22. Elmunzer, B.J.; Piraka, C.R. EUS-Guided Methylene Blue Injection to Facilitate Pancreatic Duct Access After Unsuccessful ERCP. *Gastroenterology* **2016**, *151*, 809–810. [CrossRef] [PubMed]
23. Aneese, A.M.; Ghaith, G.; Cannon, M.E.; Manuballa, V.; Cappell, M.S. EUS-guided methylene blue injection to facilitate endoscopic cannulation of an obscured pancreatic duct orifice after ampullectomy. *Am. J. Gastroenterol.* **2018**, *113*, 782–783. [CrossRef] [PubMed]
24. Will, U.; Meyer, F.; Manger, T.; Wanzar, I. Endoscopic ultrasound-assisted rendezvous maneuver to achieve pancreatic duct drainage in obstructive chronic pancreatitis. *Endoscopy* **2005**, *37*, 171–173. [CrossRef] [PubMed]
25. Uchida, D.; Kato, H.; Saragai, Y.; Takada, S.; Mizukawa, S.; Muro, S.; Akimoto, Y.; Tomoda, T.; Matsumoto, K.; Horiguchi, S.; et al. Indications for Endoscopic Ultrasound-Guided Pancreatic Drainage: For Benign or Malignant Cases? *Can. J. Gastroenterol. Hepatol.* **2018**, *2018*, 8216109. [CrossRef]
26. Itoi, T.; Yasuda, I.; Kurihara, T.; Itokawa, F.; Kasuya, K. Technique of endoscopic ultrasonography-guided pancreatic duct intervention (with videos). *J. Hepatobiliary Pancreat. Sci.* **2014**, *21*, E4–E9. [CrossRef]
27. Park, D.H.; Jang, J.W.; Lee, S.S.; Seo, D.W.; Lee, S.K.; Kim, M.H. EUS-guided biliary drainage with transluminal stenting after failed ERCP: Predictors of adverse events and long-term results. *Gastrointest. Endosc.* **2011**, *74*, 1276–1284. [CrossRef]
28. Honjo, M.; Itoi, T.; Tsuchiya, T.; Tanaka, R.; Tonozuka, R.; Mukai, S.; Sofuni, A.; Nagakawa, Y.; Iwasaki, H.; Kanai, T. Safety and efficacy of ultra-tapered mechanical dilator for EUS-guided hepaticogastrostomy and pancreatic duct drainage compared with electrocautery dilator (with video). *Endosc. Ultrasound.* **2018**, *7*, 376–382. [CrossRef]
29. Nakai, Y.; Kogure, H.; Koike, K. Double-guidewire technique for endoscopic ultrasound-guided pancreatic duct drainage. *Dig. Endosc.* **2019**, *31* (Suppl. 1), 65–66. [CrossRef]
30. Krafft, M.R.; Nasr, J.Y. Anterograde Endoscopic Ultrasound-Guided Pancreatic Duct Drainage: A Technical Review. *Dig. Dis. Sci.* **2019**, *64*, 1770–1781. [CrossRef]
31. Itoi, T.; Kasuya, K.; Sofuni, A.; Itokawa, F.; Kurihara, T.; Yasuda, I.; Nakai, Y.; Isayama, H.; Moriyasu, F. Endoscopic ultrasonography-guided pancreatic duct access: Techniques and literature review of pancreatography, transmural drainage and rendezvous techniques. *Dig. Endosc.* **2013**, *25*, 241–252. [CrossRef] [PubMed]
32. Oh, D.; Park, D.H.; Cho, M.K.; Nam, K.; Song, T.J.; Lee, S.S.; Seo, D.W.; Lee, S.K.; Kim, M.H. Feasibility and safety of a fully covered self-expandable metal stent with antimigration properties for EUS-guided pancreatic duct drainage: Early and midterm outcomes (with video). *Gastrointest. Endosc.* **2016**, *83*, 366–373.e2. [CrossRef] [PubMed]
33. Oh, D.; Park, D.H.; Song, T.J.; Lee, S.S.; Seo, D.W.; Lee, S.K.; Kim, M.H. Long-term outcome of endoscopic ultrasound-guided pancreatic duct drainage using a fully covered self-expandable metal stent for pancreaticojejunal anastomosis stricture. *J. Gastroenterol. Hepatol.* **2020**, *35*, 994–1001. [CrossRef] [PubMed]
34. Hayat, U.; Freeman, M.L.; Trikudanathan, G.; Azeem, N.; Amateau, S.K.; Mallery, J. Endoscopic ultrasound-guided pancreatic duct intervention and pancreaticogastrostomy using a novel cross-platform technique with small-caliber devices. *Endosc. Int. Open* **2020**, *8*, E196–E202. [CrossRef] [PubMed]

35. Suzuki, A.; Ishii, S.; Fujisawa, T.; Saito, H.; Takasaki, Y.; Takahashi, S.; Yamagata, W.; Ochiai, K.; Tomishima, K.; Isayama, H. Efficacy and Safety of Peroral Pancreatoscopy Through the Fistula Created by Endoscopic Ultrasound-Guided Pancreaticogastrostomy. *Pancreas* **2022**, *51*, 228–233. [CrossRef]
36. Will, U.; Fueldner, F.; Thieme, A.K.; Goldmann, B.; Gerlach, R.; Wanzar, I.; Meyer, F. Transgastric pancreatography and EUS-guided drainage of the pancreatic duct. *J. Hepatobiliary Pancreat. Surg.* **2007**, *14*, 377–382. [CrossRef]
37. Tessier, G.; Bories, E.; Arvanitakis, M.; Hittelet, A.; Pesenti, C.; Le Moine, O.; Giovannini, M.; Deviere, J. EUS-guided pancreatogastrostomy and pancreatobulbostomy for the treatment of pain in patients with pancreatic ductal dilatation inaccessible for transpapillary endoscopic therapy. *Gastrointest. Endosc.* **2007**, *65*, 233–241. [CrossRef]
38. Barkay, O.; Sherman, S.; McHenry, L.; Yoo, B.M.; Fogel, E.L.; Watkins, J.L.; DeWitt, J.; Al-Haddad, M.A.; Lehman, G.A. Therapeutic EUS-assisted endoscopic retrograde pancreatography after failed pancreatic duct cannulation at ERCP. *Gastrointest. Endosc.* **2010**, *71*, 1166–1173. [CrossRef]
39. Ergun, M.; Aouattah, T.; Gillain, C.; Gigot, J.F.; Hubert, C.; Deprez, P.H. Endoscopic ultrasound-guided transluminal drainage of pancreatic duct obstruction: Long-term outcome. *Endoscopy* **2011**, *43*, 518–525. [CrossRef]
40. Shah, J.N.; Marson, F.; Weilert, F.; Bhat, Y.M.; Nguyen-Tang, T.; Shaw, R.E.; Binmoeller, K.F. Single-operator, single-session EUS-guided anterograde cholangiopancreatography in failed ERCP or inaccessible papilla. *Gastrointest. Endosc.* **2012**, *75*, 56–64. [CrossRef]
41. Will, U.; Reichel, A.; Fueldner, F.; Meyer, F. Endoscopic ultrasonography-guided drainage for patients with symptomatic obstruction and enlargement of the pancreatic duct. *World J. Gastroenterol.* **2015**, *21*, 13140–13151. [CrossRef]
42. Chen, Y.I.; Levy, M.J.; Moreels, T.G.; Hajijeva, G.; Will, U.; Artifon, E.L.; Hara, K.; Kitano, M.; Topazian, M.; Abu Dayyeh, B.; et al. An international multicenter study comparing EUS-guided pancreatic duct drainage with enteroscopy-assisted endoscopic retrograde pancreatography after Whipple surgery. *Gastrointest. Endosc.* **2017**, *85*, 170–177. [CrossRef] [PubMed]
43. Téllez-Aviña, F.I.; Casasola-Sánchez, L.E.; Ramírez-Luna, M.; Saúl, Á.; Murcio-Pérez, E.; Chan, C.; Uscanga, L.; Duarte-Medrano, G.; Valdovinos-Andraca, F. Permanent Indwelling Transmural Stents for Endoscopic Treatment of Patients with Disconnected Pancreatic Duct Syndrome: Long-term Results. *J. Clin. Gastroenterol.* **2018**, *52*, 85–90. [CrossRef] [PubMed]
44. Matsunami, Y.; Itoi, T.; Sofuni, A.; Tsuchiya, T.; Kamada, K.; Tanaka, R.; Tonozuka, R.; Honjo, M.; Mukai, S.; Fujita, M.; et al. Evaluation of a new stent for EUS-guided pancreatic duct drainage: Long-term follow-up outcome. *Endosc. Int. Open* **2018**, *6*, E505–E512. [CrossRef] [PubMed]
45. Sakai, T.; Koshita, S.; Kanno, Y.; Ogawa, T.; Kusunose, H.; Yonamine, K.; Miyamoto, K.; Kozakai, F.; Okano, H.; Ohira, T.; et al. Early and long-term clinical outcomes of endoscopic interventions for benign pancreatic duct stricture/obstruction-the possibility of additional clinical effects of endoscopic ultrasonography-guided pancreatic drainage. *Pancreatology* **2022**, *22*, 58–66. [CrossRef] [PubMed]
46. Onodera, M.; Kawakami, H.; Kuwatani, M.; Kudo, T.; Haba, S.; Abe, Y.; Kawahata, S.; Eto, K.; Nasu, Y.; Tanaka, E.; et al. Endoscopic ultrasound-guided transmural drainage for pancreatic fistula or pancreatic duct dilation after pancreatic surgery. *Surg. Endosc.* **2012**, *26*, 1710–1717. [CrossRef]
47. Kogure, H.; Sato, T.; Nakai, Y.; Ishigaki, K.; Hakuta, R.; Saito, K.; Saito, T.; Takahara, N.; Hamada, T.; Mizuno, S.; et al. Endoscopic management of pancreatic diseases in patients with surgically altered anatomy: Clinical outcomes of combination of double-balloon endoscopy- and endoscopic ultrasound-guided interventions. *Dig. Endosc.* **2021**, *33*, 441–450. [CrossRef]
48. Bhurwal, A.; Tawadros, A.; Mutneja, H.; Gjeorgjievski, M.; Shah, I.; Bansal, V.; Patel, A.; Sarkar, A.; Bartel, M.; Brahmbhatt, B. EUS guided pancreatic duct decompression in surgically altered anatomy or failed ERCP—A systematic review, meta-analysis and meta-regression. *Pancreatology* **2021**, *21*, 990–1000. [CrossRef]
49. Basiliya, K.; Veldhuijzen, G.; Gerges, C.; Maubach, J.; Will, U.; Elmunzer, B.J.; Stommel, M.W.J.; Akkermans, R.; Siersema, P.D.; van Geenen, E.M. Endoscopic retrograde pancreatography-guided versus endoscopic ultrasound-guided technique for pancreatic duct cannulation in patients with pancreaticojejunostomy stenosis: A systematic literature review. *Endoscopy* **2021**, *53*, 266–276. [CrossRef]
50. Tyberg, A.; Bodiwala, V.; Kedia, P.; Tarnasky, P.R.; Khan, M.A.; Novikov, A.; Gaidhane, M.; Ardengh, J.C.; Kahaleh, M. EUS-guided pancreatic drainage: A steep learning curve. *Endosc. Ultrasound.* **2020**, *9*, 175–179. [CrossRef]
51. van der Merwe, S.W.; van Wanrooij, R.L.J.; Bronswijk, M.; Everett, S.; Lakhtakia, S.; Rimbas, M.; Hucl, T.; Kunda, R.; Badaoui, A.; Law, R.; et al. Therapeutic endoscopic ultrasound: European Society of Gastrointestinal Endoscopy (ESGE) Guideline. *Endoscopy* **2022**, *54*, 185–205. [CrossRef] [PubMed]
52. Teoh, A.Y.B.; Dhir, V.; Kida, M.; Yasuda, I.; Jin, Z.D.; Seo, D.W.; Almadi, M.; Ang, T.L.; Hara, K.; Hilmi, I.; et al. Consensus guidelines on the optimal management in interventional EUS procedures: Results from the Asian EUS group RAND/UCLA expert panel. *Gut* **2018**, *67*, 1209–1228. [CrossRef] [PubMed]
53. Yoo, H.W.; Moon, J.H.; Lee, Y.N.; Song, Y.H.; Yang, J.K.; Lee, T.H.; Cha, S.W.; Cho, Y.D.; Park, S.H. Peroral cholecystoscopy using a multibending ultraslim endoscope through a lumen-apposing metal stent for endoscopic ultrasound-guided gallbladder drainage: A feasibility study. *Endoscopy* **2022**, *54*, 384–388. [CrossRef] [PubMed]

Disclaimer/Publisher's Note: The statements, opinions and data contained in all publications are solely those of the individual author(s) and contributor(s) and not of MDPI and/or the editor(s). MDPI and/or the editor(s) disclaim responsibility for any injury to people or property resulting from any ideas, methods, instructions or products referred to in the content.

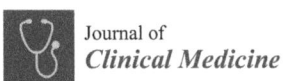

Review

EUS-Guided Vascular Interventions

Michelle Baliss [1], Devan Patel [2], Mahmoud Y. Madi [1] and Ahmad Najdat Bazarbashi [2,*]

[1] Division of Gastroenterology, Saint Louis University Hospital, St. Louis, MO 63104, USA
[2] Division of Gastroenterology, Washington University in St. Louis, St. Louis, MO 63130, USA
* Correspondence: bazarbashi@wustl.edu

Abstract: Endoscopic ultrasound (EUS) has numerous advanced applications as a diagnostic and therapeutic modality in contemporary medicine. Through intraluminal placement, EUS offers a real-time Doppler-guided endoscopic visualization and access to intra-abdominal vasculature, which were previously inaccessible using historical methods. We aim to provide a comprehensive review of key studies on both current and future EUS-guided vascular applications. This review details EUS-based vascular diagnostic techniques of portal pressure measurements in the prognostication of liver disease and portal venous sampling for obtaining circulating tumor cells in the diagnosis of cancer. From an interventional perspective, we describe effective EUS-guided treatments via coiling and cyanoacrylate injections of gastric varices and visceral artery pseudoaneurysms. Specific attention is given to clinical studies on efficacy and procedural techniques described by investigators for each EUS-based application. We explore novel and future emerging EUS-based interventions, such as liver tumor ablation and intrahepatic portosystemic shunt placement.

Keywords: endoscopic ultrasound; vascular; gastric varices; portal pressure gradient; pseudoaneurysms; portal venous sampling

Citation: Baliss, M.; Patel, D.; Madi, M.Y.; Bazarbashi, A.N. EUS-Guided Vascular Interventions. *J. Clin. Med.* 2023, 12, 2165. https://doi.org/10.3390/jcm12062165

Academic Editor: Takuji Iwashita

Received: 18 January 2023
Revised: 18 February 2023
Accepted: 21 February 2023
Published: 10 March 2023

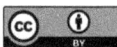

Copyright: © 2023 by the authors. Licensee MDPI, Basel, Switzerland. This article is an open access article distributed under the terms and conditions of the Creative Commons Attribution (CC BY) license (https://creativecommons.org/licenses/by/4.0/).

1. Introduction

Since the introduction of endoscopic ultrasound (EUS) as a diagnostic modality in the 1980s, advances in EUS over the years have expanded its applications to an interventional platform by adopting conventional radiological and minimally invasive surgical techniques [1]. While diagnostic EUS interventions have been premised on solid and cystic non-vascular pathology in the foregut, their diagnostic and therapeutic repertoire have recently expanded to vascular pathology. The proximity of the gastrointestinal (GI) tract to major blood vessels in the mediastinum and abdomen and the capability of EUS to provide a real-time Doppler-guided endoscopic visualization of extraluminal structures make EUS uniquely suited for guiding vascular access and therapeutic maneuvers [2]. From a vascular standpoint, EUS guidance can be used to understand vascular anatomy, to determine the presence or absence of vascular flow through a Doppler and waveform analysis, and to intervene with precision at targeted vascular sites that may be less accessible using conventional methods. The ability to visualize and access the portal vein with EUS guidance allows for direct portal pressure measurements, portal venous sampling, and the ablation of liver pathology. EUS-guided vascular coiling offers a minimally invasive alternative to interventional radiology techniques for the management of gastric varices (GVs) and visceral pseudoaneurysmal bleeding. With a shift towards less invasive approaches to the diagnosis and management of GI pathology, the applications of EUS-guided vascular interventions will continue to evolve. Here, we provide a comprehensive review of these promising diagnostic and therapeutic modalities and shed light on possible future applications, including EUS-guided intrahepatic portosystemic shunt placement and EUS-guided cardiopulmonary interventions (Table 1).

Table 1. General overview of current and future EUS-guided diagnostic and therapeutic techniques.

EUS-Guided Vascular Interventions	
Category	Intervention
Diagnostic	Portal pressure measurement
	Portal venous sampling
Therapeutic	Gastric variceal coiling
	Arterial pseudoaneurysm coiling
Future directions	Liver tumor ablation
	Intrahepatic portosystemic shunt placement

2. EUS-Guided Vascular Interventions

2.1. Diagnostic Applications

2.1.1. EUS-Guided Portal Pressure Measurement

Portal hypertension (PH), most commonly seen as a consequence of cirrhosis, results from complex intrahepatic and extrahepatic pathophysiological alterations that cause an increase in intrahepatic vascular resistance [3]. Identifying the presence and severity of PH in cirrhosis has become an important clinical prognostic tool that can be used to guide management [4]. For example, more severe portal hypertension predicts the presence and risk of bleeding from esophagogastric varices. Currently, the standard method of evaluating clinically significant PH consists of measuring the hepatic venous pressure gradient (HVPG), performed by interventional radiologists. HVPG serves as a surrogate for portal venous pressure (PVP) but is not a direct measurement of the portal pressure gradient (PPG). It is measured by inserting a catheter percutaneously into the hepatic vein and calculating the difference between the free hepatic vein pressure and the wedged hepatic vein pressure (WHVP). In addition to being an indirect measurement of PVP, HVPG is invasive, requires radiation exposure and the use of intravenous contrast, and has been shown to poorly correlate with directly measured portal pressures in patients with non-cirrhotic and presinusoidal causes of PH [5].

The largest barrier to a direct portal pressure measurement is its limited accessibility. Historically, a portal pressure measurement was performed through direct surgical access into the portal vein, which was considered invasive. With the advancement of EUS, we have almost turned full circle, returning our focus on direct portal access for pressure measurements at a less invasive cost. An EUS-guided portal pressure gradient (EUS-PPG) measurement is an alternative novel method of directly measuring the PPG by taking advantage of the proximity of the portal vein to the tip of the echoendoscope in the stomach (Figure 1). With the patient in the supine position under general or monitored anesthesia care, the middle hepatic vein waveform is identified using Doppler flow. A transgastric transhepatic approach is used to introduce a heparin-flushed 25G FNA needle into the hepatic vein. This needle is attached to a manometer, which provides a real-time pressure measurement. A total of three separate hepatic vein pressure recordings are documented, and the average of the three is recorded as the mean hepatic venous pressure (HVP). The FNA needle is then withdrawn, and the same process is repeated with the umbilical portion of the left portal vein, which can be easily identified on EUS and confirmed with a Doppler and waveform analysis (Figure 1). To calculate the PPG, the mean PVP is subtracted from the mean HVP. The concept of a gradient eliminates the potential error associated with using an external zero reference point and with the false elevations in PVP or WHVP caused by factors such as ascites and increased intra-abdominal pressure [6]. While still novel and in its early phases, various animal and human pilot studies conducted over the years have demonstrated the safety and feasibility of EUS-PPG measurements with a high degree of technical success and correlation with HVPG [7–10]. In a prospective study by Zhang et al., the feasibility and safety of EUS-PPG and the consistency between EUS-PPG and HVPG were explored in 12 patients. EUS-PPG measurements were technically successful in 91.7% of patients, with a high degree of safety and accuracy [7].

The current literature demonstrates high technical success rates. In the largest study of 83 patients, Choi et al. reported a 100% technical success rate. In a more recent study from Zhang et al., the technical success rate was 92%. In both studies, no early- or late-onset adverse events were reported. While these studies reported high technical success rates without significant adverse events, we would like to highlight the potential risks and adverse events of this technique, which include but are not limited to bleeding from the needle puncture (intrahepatic or extrahepatic), bile leak, infection, and peritonitis [7,11]. While EUS-PPG measurements remain similarly invasive to HVPG, the possibility of using EUS as a one-stop shop for PPG measurements, liver biopsy, elastography, and variceal assessment during the same procedure is an attractive option that may ultimately emerge as the standard approach for select patients. Future studies are needed to fully evaluate this modality and compare its outcomes and clinical significance to the current gold-standard HVPG and to non-invasive testing for portal hypertension.

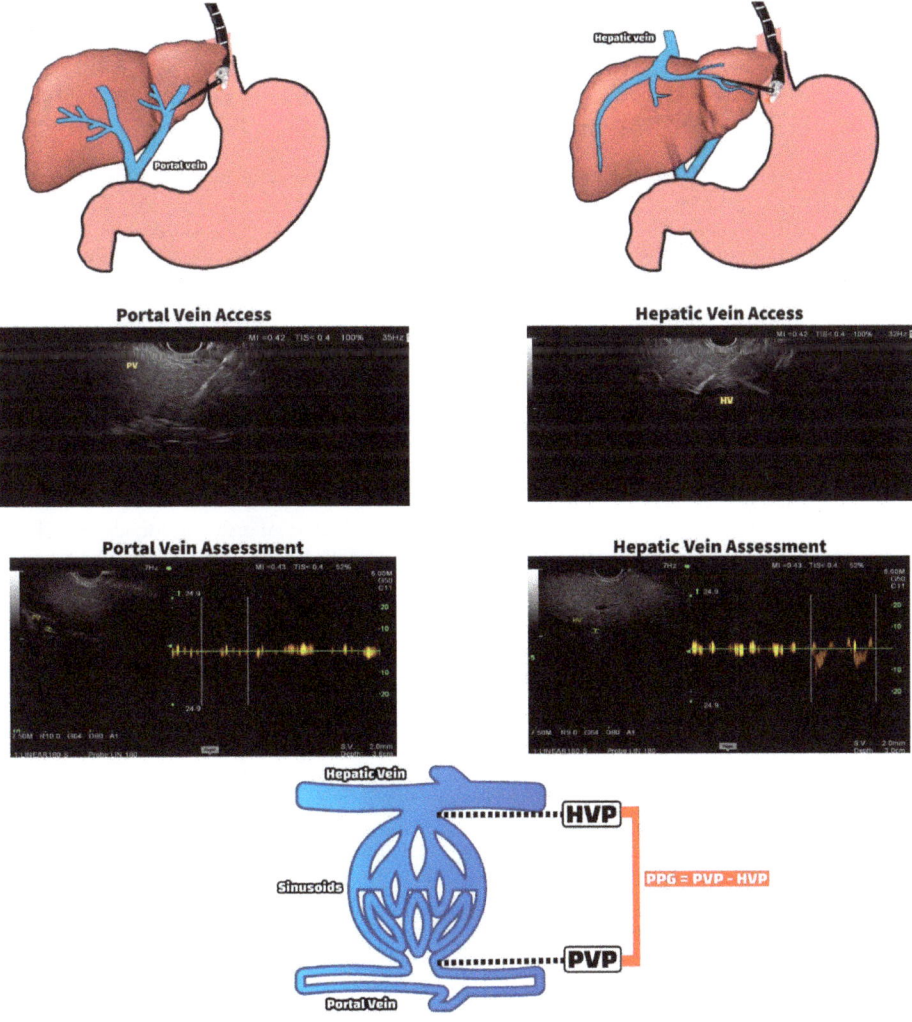

Figure 1. EUS-guided portal pressure gradient measurement.

2.1.2. EUS-Guided Portal Venous Sampling

Pancreatic cancer remains one of the most aggressive GI malignancies with a poor prognosis due to a lack of early symptoms and disease biomarkers. The criteria for curative surgical resection in patients with pancreatic cancer are in part dependent on the radiological evaluation of metastatic disease. While the currently available imaging modalities can provide information on the macroscopic evidence of metastasis, they are limited in terms of their ability to identify early micrometastatic disease. This, in turn, could affect the adequacy of prognostication and the prediction of postoperative recurrence risk.

Circulating tumor cells (CTCs) are cells that shed from primary tumors and travel through the systemic circulation to secondary sites where they deposit and act as early seeds for distant metastasis. There is increasing evidence to support the role of CTCs in the early diagnosis of pancreatic cancer and in predicting the risk of metastatic disease [12]. The acquisition of CTCs from vessels proximal to the primary tumor can increase the possibility of detecting enough CTCs to predict the risk of metastatic disease. In the case of pancreatic cancer, which commonly metastasizes to the liver, pancreatic venous drainage into the portal circulation makes the portal vein a potential target for CTC detection.

The utility of CTC acquisition from the mesenteric and portal circulation compared to peripheral blood for prognostication and guidance on the use of adjuvant chemotherapy was initially explored in the surgical setting. In a 2012 study of patients undergoing the surgical resection of colorectal cancer, CTCs were found at a higher rate and count in the mesenteric circulation compared to peripheral blood, and the presence of CTCs was associated with a higher rate of liver metastases at the 3-year follow-up interval [13]. Subsequently, in 2016, the intraoperative acquisition of portal venous blood for CTC enumeration was explored in patients with periampullary and pancreatic adenocarcinoma, and it similarly demonstrated a higher CTC count and detection rate than peripheral venous sampling and a higher rate of liver metastases at the 6-month follow up interval in CTC-positive patients [14].

The surgical collection of CTCs is limited by infrequent patient eligibility for surgery and is prone to inaccuracy due to the potential release of CTCs from intraoperative pancreatic manipulation. Additionally, intraoperative access to the portal vein to collect CTCs in many of these patients is invasive. EUS provides a minimally invasive approach to access the portal vein with precision and to isolate CTCs for risk stratification preoperatively. The portal vein can easily be seen and accessed by a needle from a transduodenal view. In a 2015 single-center cohort study, Catenacci et al. demonstrated the safety and feasibility of EUS-guided portal venous sampling of isolated CTCs in patients with pancreaticobiliary malignancies with a higher yield than peripheral blood samples [15]. These findings were further supported by a prospective study of 40 patients with suspected pancreaticobiliary cancer conducted by Zhang et al. in 2021 [16].

EUS-guided portal venous sampling should be preceded by standard EUS staging and diagnostic confirmation with EUS-FNA (Figure 2). Cross-sectional imaging should be studied to evaluate for aberrant anatomy or possible contraindications to needle access. For blood sample acquisition, Chapman et al. recommend the use of a 19G EUS-FNA needle for improved blood flow, which reduces clotting and the time spent within the vessel. Before introducing the needle into the portal vein, a Doppler-guided assessment of vessel anatomy and a confirmation of vessel patency and flow should be performed. Special care should be taken to avoid needle contact with any metastatic lesions or lymph nodes. Negative suction should be used during aspiration once the portal vein is accessed. Once the sample is acquired, the needle is slowly withdrawn with close attention to the intrahepatic needle track and puncture site using Doppler visualization to identify sites at high risk of persistent bleeding.

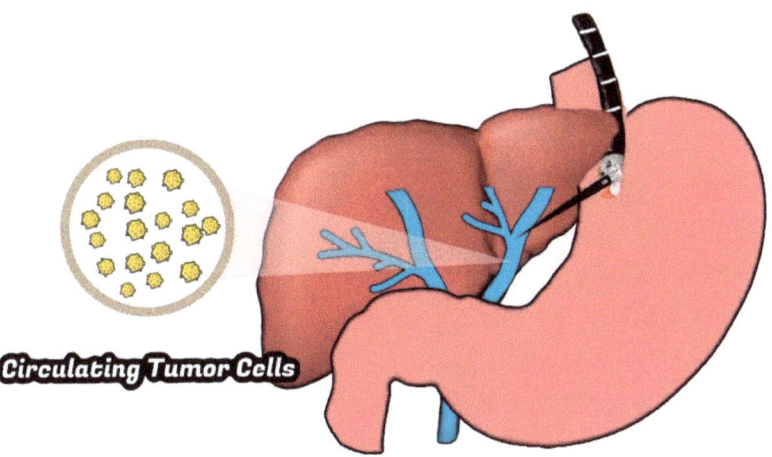

Figure 2. EUS-guided portal venous sampling for circulating tumor cells.

2.2. Therapeutic Applications

2.2.1. EUS-Guided Gastric Variceal Coiling

Gastroesophageal varices (GVs) are dilated portosystemic collateral veins that can cause significant gastrointestinal bleeding in patients with cirrhosis and portal hypertension. Although GVs represent 20% of variceal bleeding, they are associated with poorer outcomes, including more severe bleeding at index presentation, higher transfusion requirements, and an increased risk of rebleeding compared to esophageal varices (EVs) [17,18]. Despite having worse outcomes, there exist sparse evidenced-based guidelines for the management of GVs (actively bleeding and prophylactic GVs), especially when compared to EV management.

While various GV classification systems exist, the Sarin classification has been the most used, particularly when it comes to management decisions (Figure 3) [19]. GOV-1 is treated similarly to EV, such as with endoscopic band ligation. Meanwhile, GOV-2, IGV-2, and IGV-2 can be treated with direct endoscopic injection therapies, transjugular intrahepatic portosystemic shunts (TIPSs), or balloon retrograde transvenous obliteration (BRTO). However, these treatments have significant limitations, such as recurrent bleeding, systemic embolization, limited feasibility in GVs associated with splenic vein thrombosis, and occasionally limited resources to these modalities [18]. More recently, EUS-guided GV management has emerged as an alternative intervention, with promising clinical success and low risks of complications and recurrent bleeding [20–24].

EUS can assist in the identification of GVs and reveal important characteristics, such as varix size and flow, which can provide information to guide optimal management at the point of care [17]. Flow information is especially useful for EUS-guided cyanoacrylate (CYA) glue injections to ensure that an optimal amount of CYA is delivered for obturation and the risk reduction of CYA-related embolization. EUS GV coiling was later introduced in 2010 as a promising therapy and has recently been adopted as the more common EUS-guided technique for GV management, including for actively bleeding GVs and for prophylaxis [17]. EUS-guided coil therapy may include the deployment of coils alone or coils alongside injectate, such as acrylate polymers (cyanoacrylate) or an absorbable gelatin sponge [25].

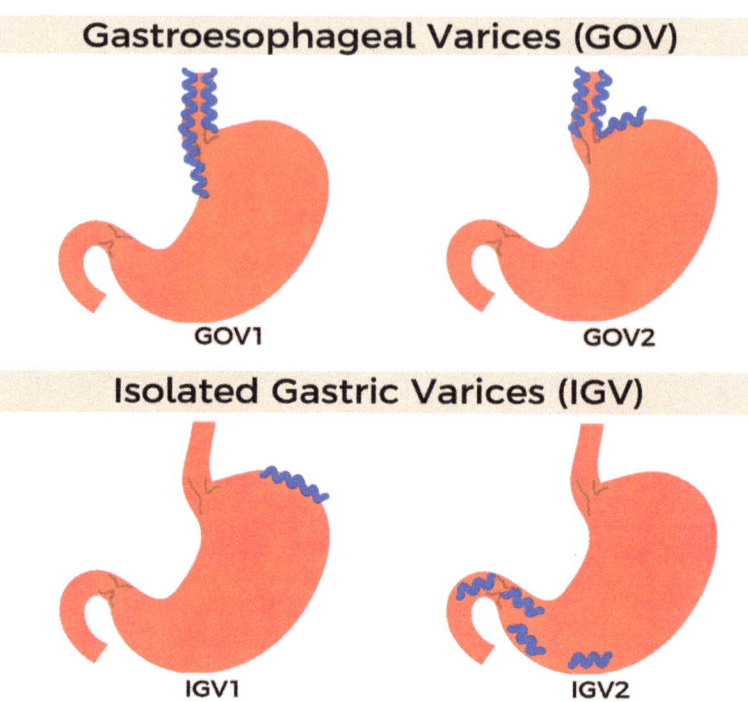

Figure 3. Sarin classification of gastric varices.

While no standardized technique for EUS-guided coiling exists, many institutions have adopted common steps to ensure a safe deployment, high clinical success, and a minimal risk of adverse events. Patients are in the left lateral position and often sedated with general anesthesia. An upper endoscopy is performed to evaluate the location and size of the gastric varices and to obtain information on concurrent esophageal varices. Antibiotics are often administered for prophylaxis. Next, a linear echoendoscope is advanced to the distal esophagus or gastric fundus to assess the anatomy of the GV and feeding vessels along with flow patterns. Water is infused in the fundus to assist with the better delineation of the GV to enhance acoustics and improve ultrasound image quality. Coils of various lengths and diameters are delivered through a 19G or 22G needle into the varix and/or feeder vessel under EUS guidance. The coils are advanced into the varix with the assistance of a stylet, under endosonographic and sometimes fluoroscopic guidance. The number of coils deployed is often operator-dependent and relies on evidence of a diminished or abrupt cessation of Doppler flow. An iodinated contrast agent can be injected into varices after coil deployment to ensure that there is no evidence of a persistent shunt. Cyanoacrylate can then be injected as adjunctive therapy [17,18,25] (Figure 4).

While cyanoacrylate has been proven to be an effective therapy for the treatment of GVs, with or without coil use, it does carry certain limitations, such as the risk of damaging endoscopes and causing adverse events, including rebleeding and systemic embolization. Additionally, cyanoacrylate can polymerize early and lead to the deroofing of the varix when the needle is pulled back. Lipiodol can assist in preventing early polymerization. More recently, an absorbable gelatin sponge has been used as an alternative to cyanoacrylate, as it does not carry similar risks. Bazarbashi et al. recently evaluated the use of absorbable gelatin sponges (such as Gelfoam or Surgiflo) as adjunctive therapy with coils (instead of cyanoacrylate). An absorbable gelatin sponge has been used for intravascular thrombolysis with IR and carries low risks of embolization. In their matched cohort study, Bazarbashi et al. demonstrated the superiority of AGS to cyanoacrylate for the treatment of GVs [25].

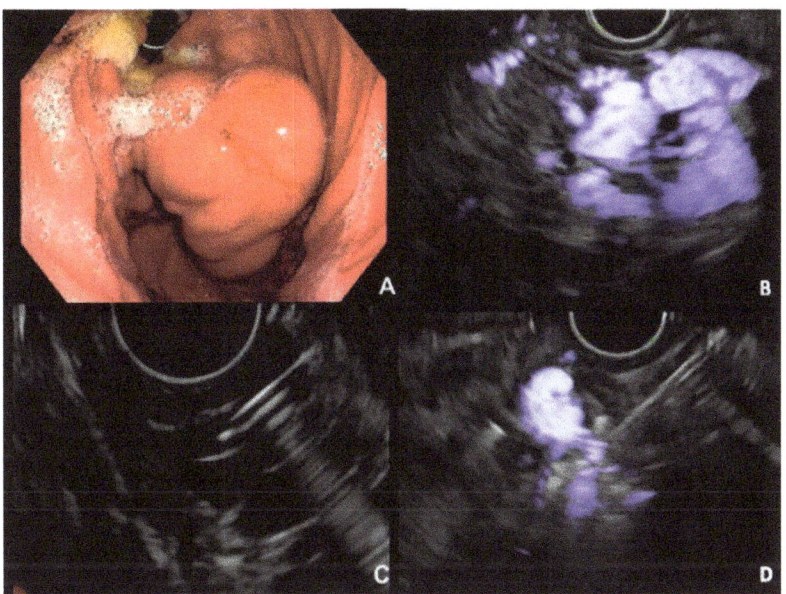

Figure 4. (**A**) Endoscopic examination of large GV on retroflexion. (**B**) EUS confirming Doppler flow within large varices. (**C**) Needle access into GV under endosonographic guidance with coil deployment. (**D**) Diminished Doppler flow on EUS after coil injection.

Surveillance EUS to monitor GVs after coil therapy is typically carried out at 1, 6, and 12 months. Repeat EUS-guided coil and gel injections may be needed depending on the response after index endoscopy and the size of the varices and ongoing Doppler flow. The complications of EUS-guided coils and therapy include the systemic gel embolization of concurrent injectate (cyanoacrylate embolization), transient abdominal pain, minor bleeding from the needle site puncture, and benign coil tip extrusion [17,25]. To date, based on the literature and to the best of our knowledge, there is no evidence of coil migration after EUS-guided coil therapy for GVs.

EUS-guided coil therapy is limited by the availability of expertise and EUS equipment and a lack of evidence on coil size and the requisite number for optimal outcomes. Despite these limitations, EUS-guided coiling has been demonstrated in multiple studies to obturate gastric varices with excellent outcomes, including low rates of rebleeding and adverse events [17,18].

2.2.2. EUS-Guided Arterial Pseudoaneurysm Coiling

Visceral arterial pseudoaneurysms (VAPAs) are rare, abnormally dilated arteries associated with significant morbidity and mortality. Intra-abdominal organ pathologies, such as surgery and pancreatitis, can lead to the development of VAPAs. The commonly involved arteries include the splenic, hepatic, superior mesenteric, and pancreaticoduodenal arteries. Unlike true aneurysms, VAPAs represent ballooned blood vessels with thin walls, resulting in a higher risk of rupture and significant bleeding. In chronic pancreatitis, studies demonstrate a risk of rupture up to 50% and a mortality post-rupture between 15 and 40% [25].

Interventional radiology procedures and surgery have been historically utilized to treat these lesions. However, these procedures can be technically challenging, especially in cases of small pseudoaneurysms not detected by imaging and in anatomically difficult locations in which endovascular methods may not be feasible. EUS may overcome such barriers by providing an improved visualization and access to previously inaccessible abdominal pseudoaneurysmal lesions. In turn, VAPAs can be directly injected with EUS-guided devices, such as coils, thrombin, and glue, in a minimally invasive manner, resulting in an effective and safe therapy [26].

EUS-guided pseudoaneurysm coiling follows a similar technique to that of EUS-guided coil therapy for GVs (Figure 5). An echoendoscope is introduced into the stomach. The Doppler technique is used to detect the VAPA, including a waveform analysis, and to accurately measure the pseudoaneurysm to guide coil placement (the diameter of the coil and the number of coils). A 19G fine-needle aspiration needle is inserted directly into the VAPA. Once secure, the needle stylet is removed, and embolization coils are loaded via the FNA needle into the VAPA and can subsequently be injected for further treatment. Further coils are injected until VAPA obliteration occurs, which can be confirmed using Doppler technique.

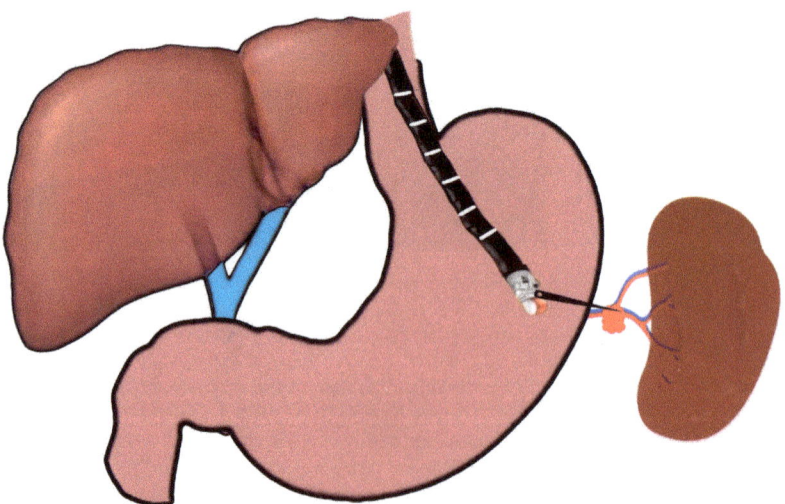

Figure 5. EUS-guided splenic artery embolization.

In 2018, Rai et al. described a standard EUS-guided coiling approach in splenic artery pseudoaneurysm treatment [27]. Coils were deployed under EUS guidance followed by an injection of N-butyl-2-cyanoacrylate glue. All patients achieved both technical and clinical success, as defined by VAPA obliteration on a 12-week follow-up EUS and no evidence of blood loss. Patients required one–two treatment sessions with one–three coils inserted. They reported no procedure-related adverse events or deaths [27]. Comparable results of a high technical success have been reported in EUS-guided thrombin injections and EUS-guided salvage therapy in previously treated splenic artery pseudoaneurysms via an endovascular approach, reflecting the effective nature of the EUS-guided treatment of VAPAs [26,28,29].

However, EUS-guided techniques may be limited by echoendoscopic detection, the possible need for repeat therapies to achieve obliteration, and lesion accessibility [30]. The complications of EUS-guided therapies have been reported to be post-procedural pain; rebleeding, especially in incompletely obliterated VAPAs; coil migration and erosion (as can be seen in IR-guided coil therapy); infection; and thrombosis [26]. Coil erosion can be particularly devastating. After a patient presented with a complicated coil migration into his stomach via a gastrosplenic artery fistula, he underwent a partial gastrectomy, distal pancreatectomy, and splenic artery pseudoaneurysm resection as treatment [31].

EUS-guided coil embolization represents a promising effective application of endoscopic ultrasound in the treatment of highly morbid intra-abdominal vascular pseudoaneurysms that should be added to the armamentarium of VAPA management, particularly when standard IR-guided therapies are limited or contraindicated.

2.3. Future Directions

Future applications of EUS-guided vascular interventions are expected to emerge with further advances in endoscopic technology and the availability of longer-term data. Some applications currently being explored, include EUS-guided liver tumor ablation, EUS-guided intrahepatic portosystemic shunt placement, EUS-guided cardiac interventions, and EUS-guided thrombolysis of pulmonary arterial thrombosis [32,33].

2.3.1. EUS-Guided Liver Tumor Ablation

Various innovative ablative techniques are routinely utilized in the treatment of primary and metastatic liver tumors. Whether for cure or for palliation, the percutaneous ablation of liver tumors under ultrasound, computed tomography, or magnetic resonance guidance aims to detrimentally impact a pathologic lesion whilst sparing the surrounding tissues. In certain instances, the application of percutaneous ablative techniques is limited by difficult anatomical locations, such as the caudate and left lobe of the liver. EUS-guided liver tumor ablation, though primarily experimental and in its early stages, is a promising addition to the therapeutic repertoire with an enticing potential for advancement in the coming years. This allows for a safe, effective, and readily available intervention for tumors in difficult locations when alternative methods may not be feasible [34].

EUS-guided liver tumor ablation can be accomplished using different techniques [35] (Figure 6). An EUS fine-needle injection (FNI) entails the injection of sclerosing agents, such as ethanol gels or antitumor agents, directly into the tumor cells or the portal circulation. Ethanol gel, the most commonly used sclerosing agent, not only has a destructive effect on tumor cells but also induces local vasculitis leading to a reduction in recurrence rates. EUS thermal ablation is another option with radiofrequency ablation (RFA), cryotherapy, and interstitial laser coagulation (ILC), where energy is applied directly to liver tumors. With RFA, the goal is to generate and sustain 50–100 °C in the target lesion to achieve adequate ablation. Nd:YAG is the predominantly used type of laser in ILC, with small enough fibers allowing passage into the EUS scope and through FNA needles. Cryotherapy is a technique that primarily damages tissues by freezing followed by thawing. This technique is of futuristic interest, as it has not yet been used to ablate liver tumors. Other techniques that may theoretically be of value include EUS-brachytherapy with radioactive seeds or gel and EUS-guided photodynamic therapy. EUS portal vein embolization allows for access to the left (supplying segments 5, 6, 7, and 8) and right portal veins (supplying segments 2, 3, and 4) given its clear visibility on transduodenal views. From a transgastric view, the umbilical portion of the left portal vein can be accessed. While this will allow for multi-segment embolization, the feasibility for single-liver-segment EUS-guided embolization, by accessing the sub-branches of the left and right portal veins is not known. This would be prudent for oncological planning and may pose a limitation to EUS-guided ablation [36].

Despite the promising nature of EUS-guided liver tumor ablation, the limitations must be acknowledged at this time. These include the current experimental nature of the majority of the methods described in our review and the lack of the current primary role of interventions, such as EUS-FNI, in liver tumor ablation, in addition to the smaller yet present risk of malignant seeding when compared to percutaneous techniques [37].

As our technologies continue to rapidly advance, the production and development of EUS-specific needle ablative systems while maintaining flexibility and limiting the diameter are required. Accurate mapping methods are also in demand to allow for precise therapy. More importantly, further research with comparative studies and randomized controlled clinical trials must be conducted to ensure the effectiveness, safety, and applicability of EUS-guided liver tumor ablation.

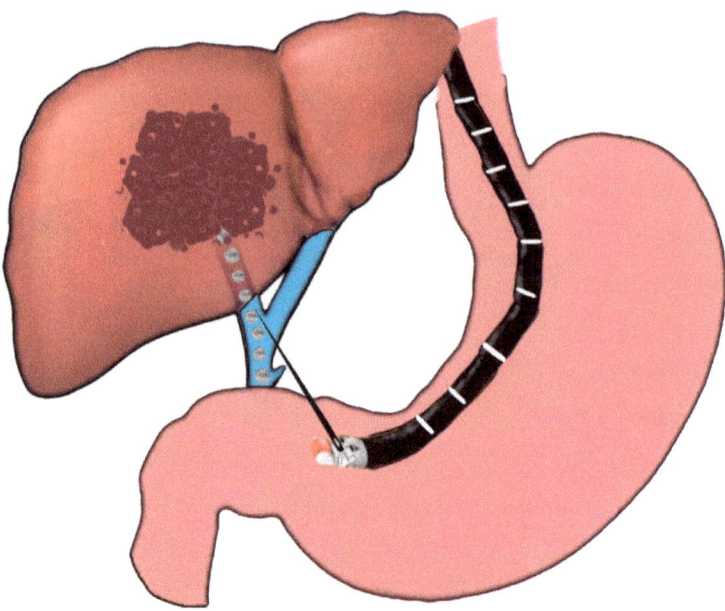

Figure 6. EUS-guided liver tumor ablation.

2.3.2. EUS-Guided Intrahepatic Portosystemic Shunt Placement

Transjugular intrahepatic portosystemic shunt (TIPS) placement remains the most frequently performed procedure to alleviate portal hypertension (PH) and its consequences, with high technical success and efficacy and a low risk of adverse events compared to surgical shunting techniques [38,39]. PH drives the major complications in cirrhosis leading to increased readmissions and mortality. With TIPS, an angiographic technique involving transjugular access and the advancement of a catheter and a guidewire through the right heart to the inferior vena cava is employed to create an artificial low-resistance channel between the portal and hepatic veins, thereby directing blood flow to the systemic circulation to alleviate PH and reduce its risk of complications.

While TIPS is largely safe and effective, adverse events can occur due to the route of access. These complications, while rare, include inadvertent arterial, tracheal, and biliary injuries and cardiac conduction and rhythm events [40].

Advances in EUS have led to experimental and animal model work evaluating the possible role of an EUS-guided portosystemic shunt (EIPS). While in its infancy with much work to be carried out, EIPS may have a potential role in the future management of patients with PH, particularly when vascular access with TIPS carries a high risk of complications. EIPS does not require entrance into the right heart or inferior vena cava; does not involve radiation exposure; and can be combined with EUS-guided interventions, such as direct portal pressure measurements or GV management in a one-stop shop fashion. Other major technical differences of EIPS from conventional TIPS include transluminal access to the hepatic vein from the upper gastrointestinal tract instead of transvascular catheterization, an EUS-guided puncture instead of a radiologic and percutaneous US-guided puncture, and stent type.

The technique of EIPS was first described by Buscaglia et al. in 2009 in a liver porcine model using a self-expandable tubular metal stent [41]. In this study, the fully expanded stent did not adequately cover the area between the PV and HV in some animals, and a second stent was deployed as a bridge. No major complications were noted, and a 2-week survival period was reported. Subsequently, in 2011, Binmoeller et al. reported a similar

EIPS technique for the successful novel transgastric deployment of a lumen-apposing metal stent (LAMS) in a non-survival porcine model [42].

In 2017, Schulman et al. conducted an animal survival study model in which the high technical feasibility of EIPS (with a technical success rate of 100%) combined with a simultaneous direct digital PVP measurement was demonstrated [43]. A lumen-apposing metal stent was also used in this non-cirrhotic animal model study, and while this did confirm its feasibility, this technique remains primitive with many parameters that require further investigation in humans, particularly in those with cirrhosis in whom the risks of coagulopathy and infection are high. Some complications seen in this study included the development of liver abscesses in two of the animals; however, prophylactic antibiotics were not utilized. In-stent thrombosis was also seen in several animals; thus, stent modifications for the purpose of intravascular use may be needed.

2.3.3. EUS-Guided Cardiac Interventions and Thrombolysis

The location of the heart and pulmonary vessels in proximity to the esophagus has prompted the early exploration of EUS-guided transesophageal cardiopulmonary interventions. In 2007, Fritscher-Ravens et al. described the use of EUS in porcine models to guide a puncture of the heart and ultimately performed radiofrequency ablative therapy, pericardial fluid aspiration, cardiac tumor puncture, and pacing wire insertion. No arrhythmias were noted during the procedure, and no cardiac abnormalities resulted [44]. Subsequently, the successful EUS-guided drainage of a pericardial cyst was reported by Larghi et al. in 2009 [45]. In 2019, Romero-Castro et al. reported the use of an EUS-guided biopsy to confirm the diagnosis of a right atrial lymphoma and right atrial myxoma [32]. More recently, an EUS-guided biopsy of an intraventricular fibroadipose mass was reported by Mehta et al. in 2022 [46].

The use of EUS to direct vascular thrombolysis was explored by Sharma et al. in 2017 in the case of an acute portal venous thrombus [47]. EUS was used to guide a puncture into the superior mesenteric vein followed by the placement of a cannula into the vein. The cannula was routed through the nose and used to infuse a thrombolytic agent continuously. Although there was a reported radiological improvement, subsequent bleeding was reported from the site of injection, which was treated by inflating a G-EYE balloon after failure to achieve hemostasis with epinephrine and hemostatic clip placement. Sharma et al. later reported seven cases of EUS-guided thrombolysis for acute portal vein thrombosis in 2019 with a 100% technical success rate [48]. In five cases, the EUS-guided puncture allowed access to the portal venous system, and continuous catheter thrombolysis was administered for 72 h to 10 days via a cannula, which was routed through the nares. In the remaining three cases, bolus injections were administered. For the bolus injections, the splenic vein was accessed through a puncture of the body of the stomach, the portal vein was accessed through a duodenal bulb puncture, and the superior mesenteric vein was accessed through the pancreas. Among the seven cases, one patient experienced catheter site bleeding with the catheter in situ, one patient experienced mild oozing following catheter removal, and one patient developed a splenic infarct on day 7. In 2019, Somani et al. similarly used EUS-guided thrombolysis in a patient with superior mesenteric vein and pulmonary artery thrombosis in whom systemic anticoagulation was contraindicated in light of a recent hemorrhagic stroke. This resulted in a substantial reduction in thrombus size without reported complications [33].

EUS-guided cardiac interventions and vascular thrombolysis are experimental interventions seen in animal model studies and isolated human case reports. While unlikely to be common approaches given the less invasive and more well-established access that currently exists, EUS can provide rare diagnostic and therapeutic benefits for cardiac pathology and for vascular thrombolysis.

2.4. Limitations and Complications

While studies have shown promising results for the safety and technical success of EUS-guided vascular interventions, it is important to note that this field remains in its infancy, and much of the data available are limited to case series and retrospective single-center studies. Therefore, it is prudent that we highlight the potential pitfalls and limitations of EUS-guided vascular therapies. First and foremost, EUS-guided vascular interventions, when compared to gold-standard therapies, are compared to IR-guided vascular interventions. IR-guided vascular interventions have proven to be extremely successful, with high clinical and technical success rates. IR-guided interventions allow for safe access to various splanchnic and visceral vessels through the percutaneous route. We envision the role of EUS-guided vascular therapy to be supplemental, rather than a substitute, to IR-guided vascular interventions. Another limitation includes the limited knowledge on the vascular anatomy of the GI tract when applied to EUS. This is an evolving field, but much work is needed to better delineate the vascular anatomy of the GI tract to ensure safe and effective access and subsequent therapies. The third limitation is that many of the tools and techniques available for EUS are not specifically designed for vascular interventions and that many of the tools used for EUS vascular access and treatment are adopted from those used in interventional radiology (for example, GV coiling).

In terms of complications, we want to highlight that, while these are rare, they can be significant. The risks and complications that need to be highlighted include bleeding (from the target vessel or puncture site); infection, including peritonitis and liver abscess formation; systemic embolization; and visceral perforation.

3. Conclusions

The applications of EUS-guided vascular interventions continue to evolve, affording multiple therapeutic avenues for various conditions. The unique location of the GI tract in proximity to major vascular structures allows for the use of EUS to guide these vascular interventions and offers potential alternatives to standard diagnostic and treatment modalities performed by interventional radiology. Although smaller-scale studies have shown promising safety results, clinical efficacy, and technical success rates, future larger-scale studies are needed to demonstrate how these parameters compare with the currently available approaches for the management of these conditions. A better understanding of vascular anatomy, improved EUS resolution and acoustics with a vascular assisted analysis, and the development of vascular-friendly EUS-deployed stents and coils will hopefully assist with the advancement of this promising field.

Author Contributions: Conceptualization, methodology, drafting, review and supervision, A.N.B. Writing, original draft preparation, and re-view, M.B., D.P. and M.Y.M. All authors have read and agreed to the published version of the manuscript.

Funding: This research received no external funding.

Data Availability Statement: Research data available from publicly archived datasets available online.

Conflicts of Interest: The authors declare no conflict of interest.

References

1. DiMagno, E.P.; DiMagno, M.J. Endoscopic Ultrasonography: From the Origins to Routine EUS. *Dig. Dis. Sci.* **2015**, *61*, 342–353. [CrossRef]
2. Burmester, E.; Tiede, U. Longitudinal Endoscopic Ultrasound–Anatomical Guiding Structures in the Upper Abdomen (Cranial–Right). *Video J. Encycl. GI Endosc.* **2013**, *1*, 501–504. [CrossRef]
3. Iwakiri, Y.; Trebicka, J. Portal hypertension in cirrhosis: Pathophysiological mechanisms and therapy. *JHEP Rep.* **2021**, *3*, 100316. [CrossRef] [PubMed]
4. Bosch, J.; Abraldes, J.G.; Berzigotti, A.; García-Pagan, J.C. The clinical use of HVPG measurements in chronic liver disease. *Nat. Rev. Gastroenterol. Hepatol.* **2009**, *6*, 573–582. [CrossRef] [PubMed]
5. Pomier-Layrargues, G.M.D.; Kusielewicz, D.; Willems, B.; Villeneuve, J.; Marleau, D.; Côté, J.; Huet, P. Presinusoidal portal hypertension in non-alcoholic cirrhosis. *Hepatology* **1985**, *5*, 415–418. [CrossRef] [PubMed]

6. Bazarbashi, A.N.; Ryou, M. Portal pressure measurement: Have we come full circle? *Gastrointest. Endosc.* **2021**, *93*, 573–576. [CrossRef]
7. Zhang, W.; Peng, C.; Zhang, S.; Huang, S.; Shen, S.; Xu, G.; Zhang, F.; Xiao, J.; Zhang, M.; Zhuge, Y.; et al. EUS-guided portal pressure gradient measurement in patients with acute or subacute portal hypertension. *Gastrointest. Endosc.* **2020**, *93*, 565–572. [CrossRef]
8. Huang, J.Y.; Samarasena, J.B.; Tsujino, T.; Chang, K.J. EUS-guided portal pressure gradient measurement with a novel 25-gauge needle device versus standard transjugular approach: A comparison animal study. *Gastrointest. Endosc.* **2016**, *84*, 358–362. [CrossRef]
9. Huang, J.Y.; Samarasena, J.B.; Tsujino, T.; Lee, J.; Hu, K.-Q.; McLaren, C.E.; Chen, W.-P.; Chang, K.J. EUS-guided portal pressure gradient measurement with a simple novel device: A human pilot study. *Gastrointest. Endosc.* **2016**, *85*, 996–1001. [CrossRef]
10. Samarasena, J.B.; Huang, J.Y.; Tsujino, T.; Thieu, D.; Yu, A.; Hu, K.Q.; Lee, J.; Chang, K.J. EUS-guided portal pressure gradient measurement with a simple novel device: A human pilot study. *VideoGIE* **2018**, *3*, 361–363. [CrossRef]
11. Choi, A.Y.; Kolb, J.; Shah, S.; Chahine, A.; Hashimoto, R.; Patel, A.; Tsujino, T.; Huang, J.; Hu, K.; Chang, K.; et al. Endoscopic ultrasound-guided portal pressure gradient with liver biopsy: 6 years of endo-hepatology in practice. *J. Gastroenterol. Hepatol.* **2022**, *37*, 1373–1379. [CrossRef]
12. Yeo, D.; Bastian, A.; Strauss, H.; Saxena, P.; Grimison, P.; Rasko, J.E.J. Exploring the Clinical Utility of Pancreatic Cancer Circulating Tumor Cells. *Int. J. Mol. Sci.* **2022**, *23*, 1671. [CrossRef]
13. Bissolati, M.; Sandri, M.T.; Burtulo, G.; Zorzino, L.; Balzano, G.; Braga, M. Portal vein-circulating tumor cells predict liver metastases in patients with resectable pancreatic cancer. *Tumor Biol.* **2015**, *36*, 991–996. [CrossRef]
14. Tien, Y.W.; Kuo, H.C.; Ho, B.I.; Chang, M.C.; Chang, Y.T.; Cheng, M.F.; Chen, H.L.; Liang, T.Y.; Wang, C.F.; Huang, C.Y. A High Circulating Tumor Cell Count in Portal Vein Predicts Liver Metastasis from Periampullary or Pancreatic Cancer: A High Portal Venous CTC Count Predicts Liver Metastases. *Medicine* **2016**, *95*, e3407. [CrossRef]
15. Catenacci, D.V.; Chapman, C.G.; Xu, P.; Koons, A.; Konda, V.J.; Siddiqui, U.D.; Waxman, I. Acquisition of Portal Venous Circulating Tumor Cells from Patients with Pancreaticobiliary Cancers by Endoscopic Ultrasound. *Gastroenterology* **2015**, *149*, 1794–1803.e4. [CrossRef]
16. Zhang, Y.; Su, H.; Wang, H.; Xu, C.; Zhou, S.; Zhao, J.; Shen, S.; Xu, G.; Wang, L.; Zou, X.; et al. Endoscopic Ultrasound-Guided Acquisition of Portal Venous Circulating Tumor Cells as a Potential Diagnostic and Prognostic Tool for Pancreatic Cancer. *Cancer Manag. Res.* **2021**, *13*, 7649–7661. [CrossRef]
17. Thiruvengadam, S.S.; Sedarat, A. The Role of Endoscopic Ultrasound (EUS) in the Management of Gastric Varices. *Curr. Gastroenterol. Rep.* **2021**, *23*, 1–10. [CrossRef]
18. Bazarbashi, A.N.; Ryou, M. Gastric variceal bleeding. *Curr. Opin. Gastroenterol.* **2019**, *35*, 524–534. [CrossRef]
19. Sarin, S.K.; Kumar, A. Gastric varices: Profile, classification, and management. *Am. J. Gastroenterol.* **1989**, *84*, 1244–1249.
20. Iwase, H.; Maeda, O.; Shimada, M.; Tsuzuki, T.; Peek, R.M., Jr.; Nishio, Y.; Ando, T.; Ina, K.; Kusugami, K. Endoscopic ablation with cyanoacrylate glue for isolated gastric variceal bleeding. *Gastrointest. Endosc.* **2001**, *53*, 585–592. [CrossRef]
21. Cheng, L.-F.; Wang, Z.-Q.; Li, C.-Z.; Cai, F.-C.; Huang, Q.-Y.; Linghu, E.-Q.; Li, W.; Chai, G.-J.; Sun, G.-H.; Mao, Y.-P.; et al. Treatment of gastric varices by endoscopic sclerotherapy using butyl cyanoacrylate: 10 years' experience of 635 cases. *Chin. Med. J.* **2007**, *120*, 2081–2085. [CrossRef] [PubMed]
22. Fry, L.C.; Neumann, H.; Olano, C.; Malfertheiner, P.; Mönkemüller, K. Efficacy, complications and clinical outcomes of endoscopic sclerotherapy with N-butyl-2-cyanoacrylate for bleeding gastric varices. *Dig. Dis.* **2008**, *26*, 300–303. [CrossRef] [PubMed]
23. Robles-Medranda, C.; Valero, M.; Nebel, J.A.; de Britto, S.R., Jr.; Puga-Tejada, M.; Ospina, J.; Muñoz-Jurado, G.; Pitanga-Lukashok, H. Endoscopic-ultrasound-guided coil and cyanoacrylate embolization for gastric varices and the roles of endoscopic Doppler and endosonographic varicealography in vascular targeting. *Dig. Endosc.* **2019**, *31*, 283–290. [CrossRef] [PubMed]
24. Bhat, Y.M.; Weilert, F.; Fredrick, R.T.; Kane, S.D.; Shah, J.N.; Hamerski, C.M.; Binmoeller, K.F. EUS-guided treatment of gastric fundal varices with combined injection of coils and cyanoacrylate glue: A large U.S. experience over 6 years (with video). *Gastrointest. Endosc.* **2016**, *83*, 1164–1172. [CrossRef]
25. Bazarbashi, A.N.; Wang, T.J.; Jirapinyo, P.; Thompson, C.C.; Ryou, M. Endoscopic Ultrasound-Guided Coil Embolization with Absorbable Gelatin Sponge Appears Superior to Traditional Cyanoacrylate Injection for the Treatment of Gastric Varices. *Clin. Transl. Gastroenterol.* **2020**, *11*, e00175. [CrossRef]
26. Maharshi, S.; Sharma, S.S.; Sharma, D.; Sapra, B.; Nijhawan, S. Endoscopic ultrasound-guided thrombin injection, a management approach for visceral artery pseudoaneurysms. *Endosc. Int. Open* **2020**, *8*, E407–E412. [CrossRef]
27. Bokun, T.; Grgurevic, I.; Kujundzic, M.; Banic, M. EUS-Guided Vascular Procedures: A Literature Review. *Gastroenterol. Res. Pract.* **2013**, *2013*, 865945. [CrossRef]
28. Rai, P.; Kc, H.; Goel, A.; Aggarwal, R.; Sharma, M. Endoscopic ultrasound-guided coil and glue for treatment of splenic artery pseudo-aneurysm: New kid on the block! *Endosc. Int. Open* **2018**, *6*, E821–E825. [CrossRef]
29. Gamanagatti, S.; Thingujam, U.; Garg, P.; Nongthombam, S.; Dash, N.R. Endoscopic ultrasound guided thrombin injection of angiographically occult pancreatitis associated visceral artery pseudoaneurysms: Case series. *World J. Gastrointest. Endosc.* **2015**, *7*, 1107–1113. [CrossRef]
30. Villa, E.; Melitas, C.; Ibrahim Naga, Y.M.; Pandhi, M.; Shah, K.; Boulay, B. Endoscopic ultrasound-guided embolization of refractory splenic pseudoaneurysm. *VideoGIE* **2022**, *7*, 331–333. [CrossRef]

31. Sharma, M.; Jindal, S.; Somani, P.; Basnet, B.K.; Bansal, R. EUS-guided coiling of hepatic artery pseudoaneurysm in 2 stages. *Videogie* **2017**, *2*, 262–263. [CrossRef]
32. Romero-Castro, R.; Rios-Martin, J.J.; Jimenez-Garcia, V.A.; Pellicer-Bautista, F.; Hergueta-Delgado, P. EUS-FNA of 2 right atrial masses. *Videogie* **2019**, *4*, 323–324. [CrossRef]
33. Somani, P.; Talele, R.; Sharma, M. Endoscopic Ultrasound-Guided Thrombolysis of Pulmonary Artery Thrombus and Mesenteric Vein Thrombus. *Am. J. Gastroenterol.* **2019**, *114*, 379. [CrossRef]
34. Tekola, B.D.; Arner, D.M.; Behm, B.W. Coil Migration after Transarterial Coil Embolization of a Splenic Artery Pseudoaneurysm. *Case Rep. Gastroenterol.* **2013**, *7*, 487–491. [CrossRef]
35. Wallace, M.B.; Sabbagh, L.C. EUS 2008 Working Group document: Evaluation of EUS-guided tumor ablation. *Gastrointest. Endosc.* **2009**, *69*, S59–S63. [CrossRef]
36. Okasha, H.H.; Farouk, M.; El Hendawy, R.I.; Mahmoud, R.M.; El-Meligui, A.; Atalla, H.; Hashim, A.M.; Pawlak, K.M. Practical approach to linear EUS examination of the liver. *Endosc. Ultrasound* **2021**, *10*, 161–167. [CrossRef]
37. Chua, T.; Faigel, D.O. Endoscopic Ultrasound-Guided Ablation of Liver Tumors. *Gastrointest. Endosc. Clin. N. Am.* **2019**, *29*, 369–379. [CrossRef]
38. Chang, K.J.; Irisawa, A. EUS 2008 Working Group document: Evaluation of EUS-guided injection therapy for tumors. *Gastrointest. Endosc.* **2009**, *69*, S54–S58. [CrossRef]
39. Boyer, T.D.; Haskal, Z.J.; American Association for the Study of Liver Diseases. The role of transjugular intrahepatic portosystemic shunt in the management of portal hypertension. *Hepatology* **2005**, *41*, 386–400. [CrossRef]
40. Colombato, L. The Role of Transjugular Intrahepatic Portosystemic Shunt (TIPS) in the Management of Portal Hypertension. *J. Clin. Gastroenterol.* **2007**, *41*, S344–S351. [CrossRef]
41. Buscaglia, J.M.; Dray, X.; Shin, E.J.; Magno, P.; Chmura, K.M.; Surti, V.C.; Dillon, T.E.; Ducharme, R.W.; Donatelli, G.; Thuluvath, P.J.; et al. A new alternative for a transjugular intrahepatic portosystemic shunt: EUS-guided creation of an intrahepatic portosystemic shunt (with video). *Gastrointest. Endosc.* **2009**, *69*, 941–947. [CrossRef] [PubMed]
42. Binmoeller, K.F.; Shah, J.N. Sa1428 EUS-Guided Transgastric Intrahepatic Portosystemic Shunt Using the Axios Stent. *Gastrointest. Endosc.* **2011**, *73*, AB167. [CrossRef]
43. Schulman, A.R.; Ryou, M.; Aihara, H.; Abidi, W.; Chiang, A.; Jirapinyo, P.; Sakr, A.; Ajeje, E.; Ryan, M.B.; Thompson, C.C. EUS-guided intrahepatic portosystemic shunt with direct portal pressure measurements: A novel alternative to transjugular intrahepatic portosystemic shunting. *Gastrointest. Endosc.* **2017**, *85*, 243–247. [CrossRef] [PubMed]
44. Fritscher-Ravens, A.; Ganbari, A.; Mosse, C.A.; Swain, P.; Koehler, P.; Patel, K. Transesophageal endoscopic ultra-sound-guided access to the heart. *Endoscopy* **2007**, *39*, 385–389. [CrossRef] [PubMed]
45. Larghi, A.; Stobinski, M.; Galasso, D.; Amato, A.; Familiari, P.; Costamagna, G. EUS-guided drainage of a pericardial cyst: Closer to the heart (with video). *Gastrointest. Endosc.* **2009**, *70*, 1273–1274. [CrossRef]
46. Mehta, N.; Joseph, A.; Harb, S.; Kapadia, S.; Bhatt, A. EUS–guided biopsy of an intraventricular mass in a patient with ventricular tachycardia. *Videogie* **2022**, *7*, 322–323. [CrossRef]
47. Sharma, M.; Somani, P.; Jindal, S. EUS-Guided Continuous Catheter Thrombolysis of Portal Venous System: 1614. *Am. J. Gastroenterol.* **2017**, *112*, S877–S879. [CrossRef]
48. Sharma, M.; Somani, P.; Jindal, S. EUS-Guided Continuous Catheter Thrombolysis of Portal Venous System. *Am. J. Gastroenterol.* **2019**, *89*, AB605. [CrossRef]

Disclaimer/Publisher's Note: The statements, opinions and data contained in all publications are solely those of the individual author(s) and contributor(s) and not of MDPI and/or the editor(s). MDPI and/or the editor(s) disclaim responsibility for any injury to people or property resulting from any ideas, methods, instructions or products referred to in the content.

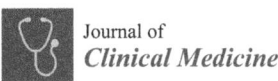

Review

Endoscopic Ultrasound-Guided Biliary Drainage

John B. Doyle and Amrita Sethi *

Division of Digestive and Liver Diseases, Columbia University Irving Medical Center, New York-Presbyterian Hospital, New York, NY 10032, USA
* Correspondence: as3614@cumc.columbia.edu

Abstract: Endoscopic retrograde cholangiopancreatography (ERCP) and percutaneous transhepatic biliary drainage (PTBD) are currently first- and second-line therapeutic options, respectively, for the relief of biliary obstruction. In recent years, however, endoscopic ultrasound-guided biliary drainage (EUS-BD) has become an established alternative therapy for biliary obstruction. There are multiple different techniques for EUS-BD, which can be distinguished based on the access point within the biliary tree (intrahepatic versus extrahepatic) and the location of stent placement (transenteric versus transpapillary). The clinical and technical success rates of biliary drainage for EUS-BD are similar to both ERCP and PTBD, and complication rates are favorable for EUS-BD relative to PTBD. As EUS-BD becomes more widely practiced and endoscopic tools continue to advance, the outcomes will likely improve, and the breadth of indications for EUS-BD will continue to expand.

Keywords: endoscopic ultrasound; biliary obstruction; choledochoduodenostomy; hepaticogastrostomy

1. Introduction

Endoscopic retrograde cholangiopancreatography (ERCP) is currently the first-line therapeutic option for the relief of benign and malignant biliary obstruction [1]. During ERCP, a side-viewing duodenoscope is used to cannulate the ampulla of Vater, through which the biliary tree and pancreatic duct can be accessed for dilation or stent placement. However, ERCP is unsuccessful in relieving biliary obstruction in 5–10% of cases [2,3]. This is often due to anatomical abnormalities or post-surgical changes that render cannulating the ampulla either difficult or impossible.

For decades, the second-line therapeutic intervention for biliary drainage following a failed ERCP has been percutaneous transhepatic biliary drainage (PTBD). In PTBD, the biliary system is accessed via a cutaneous incision, and biliary obstruction is relieved by an external biliary drain [4]. PTBD can have notable complications, including bacteremia, hemobilia, and the dislodgement, occlusion, or leakage of the external biliary drain [5–7]. Relative to internal enteric biliary drainage, the presence of an external biliary catheter that is required in PTBD can also lead to frequent bag exchanges, skin irritation, and reduced quality of life [8–10].

In recent years, endoscopic ultrasound-guided biliary drainage (EUS-BD) has been recognized as an appealing alternative to PTBD to relieve biliary obstruction after failed ERCP. In this review, we highlight the current indications, techniques, and outcomes of EUS-BD. We also discuss its potential as a primary option for biliary drainage as new endoscopic tools can improve the feasibility and accessibility of EUS-BD.

2. EUS-BD: Indications and Technique

EUS-BD was first described in 2001 by Giovannini et al., who reported the successful drainage of the common bile duct with a transduodenal plastic stent [11]. In the two decades since, techniques have been refined and expanded, and EUS-BD has become an essential endoscopic therapy for patients with biliary obstruction.

Citation: Doyle, J.B.; Sethi, A. Endoscopic Ultrasound-Guided Biliary Drainage. *J. Clin. Med.* **2023**, *12*, 2736. https://doi.org/10.3390/jcm12072736

Academic Editor: Antonio M Caballero-Mateos

Received: 6 March 2023
Revised: 3 April 2023
Accepted: 5 April 2023
Published: 6 April 2023

Copyright: © 2023 by the authors. Licensee MDPI, Basel, Switzerland. This article is an open access article distributed under the terms and conditions of the Creative Commons Attribution (CC BY) license (https://creativecommons.org/licenses/by/4.0/).

At present, EUS-BD is most commonly indicated for patients with malignant obstruction of the distal biliary tree when ERCP is unsuccessful or not feasible. This is often due to anatomical pathology, which makes it difficult or impossible to cannulate the papilla with a side-viewing duodenoscope, including gastric outlet obstruction, duodenal stenosis, ampullary tumor, or periampullary diverticulum. In addition, EUS-BD is useful for patients with surgically-altered anatomy, particularly following surgeries such as Roux-en-Y gastric bypass, Roux-en-Y hepaticojejunostomy, pancreaticoduodenectomy, or partial gastrectomy, in which access to the ampulla is technically cumbersome [12,13]. EUS-BD has also been used in patients with existing gastroduodenal stents that obstruct ampullary access [14].

There are multiple different techniques for EUS-BD, which have been distinguished based on their access point within the biliary tree (intrahepatic vs. extrahepatic) and the location of stent placement (transenteric vs. transpapillary). The choice of technique is based largely on patient anatomy and operator expertise [15,16].

2.1. EUS-Guided Hepaticogastrostomy (EUS-HGS)

In this technique, an echoendoscope is positioned in the gastric body to provide the ultrasound visualization of the left intrahepatic bile ducts [16–19]. Under this ultrasound visualization, a needle is used to access the intrahepatic biliary ducts, and a color doppler is used to identify and avoid any intervening vasculature. After needle access is obtained, a cholangiogram is performed to confirm biliary access and delineate biliary anatomy. A guidewire is then advanced through the needle and into the intrahepatic duct and biliary tree. After dilation, a stent can be deployed over the guidewire to create a hepaticogastrostomy and allow bile drainage directly into the stomach lumen.

EUS-HGS is particularly useful for patients with a gastroduodenal obstruction or post-surgical anatomy, including patients with prior pancreaticoduodenectomy or Roux-en-Y hepaticojejunostomy [16]. Given that EUS-HGS techniques typically involve access to the dilated left intrahepatic biliary ducts, the utility of EUS-HGS may be more limited in patients without intrahepatic ductal dilation or with only a right-sided intrahepatic biliary obstruction [18]. Relative contraindications include coagulopathy, massive ascites, and stomach wall pathology, such as a tumor or ulceration [16]. The most common complications of EUS-HGS include infection (including cholangitis, pancreatitis, and biliary peritonitis), bleeding, and bile leaks.

2.2. EUS-Guided Choledochoduodenostomy (EUS-CDS)

In EUS-CDS, an echoendoscope is positioned in the duodenal bulb, and a needle is placed into the extrahepatic biliary tree under direct ultrasound guidance. In a similar fashion to the EUS-HGS technique, a contrast is then injected to obtain a cholangiogram, and a guidewire is inserted into the common hepatic duct or the common biliary duct. A fistulous tract is created with cautery or dilation, and a stent is deployed [17–19]. The result is a transduodenal stent draining the extrahepatic biliary tree, as opposed to EUS-HGS, which results in a transgastric stent draining the intrahepatic biliary tree.

EUS-CDS can be a useful technique for biliary drainage in patients with distal malignant biliary obstruction due to periampullary malignancy and mass or papillary stenosis. It has similar complications and contraindications to EUS-HGS. If performed in the setting of a pending or existing duodenal obstruction, then adequate bile drainage needs to be established, either with a duodenal stent or a gastrojejunostomy, which can be performed endoscopically at the time of EUS-CDS. In recent years, lumen-apposing metal stents (LAMS) have been increasingly used in EUS-CDS, which can improve anastomotic creation and anchoring between the enteric lumen and the biliary tree [12,20,21]. Electrocautery-enhanced LAMS, in particular, allows for a single-stage biliary puncture and stent placement and, thus, has the potential to decrease the procedure difficulty and complication risk [21,22].

2.3. EUS-Guided Antegrade Stent Placement

While EUS-HGS and EUS-CDS both involve transenteric stenting and biliary drainage, EUS-guided antegrade stent placement is a technique that can achieve transpapillary biliary stenting. In this technique, either intrahepatic or extrahepatic access is created via the gastric or duodenal lumen under ultrasound guidance, as described above. Once the biliary tree is accessed, a guidewire can be used to traverse the biliary obstruction and the ampulla [16,17]. Contrast can be injected to confirm extravasation into the small bowel to ensure proper placement, and if confirmed, a transpapillary stent can be placed in the antegrade fashion. This technique requires that a guidewire is able to pass distally to the obstructed biliary tree.

EUS-guided antegrade stent placement has a theoretical advantage over EUS-HGS or EUS-CDS in that it can avoid the creation of a new anastomosis at the biliary access site and any consequent adverse events [12]. EUS-guided antegrade stent placement can be especially useful in patients with surgically-altered anatomies, such as the Roux-en-Y gastric bypass, and who have preserved ampullary anatomy and physiology. With a transpapillary stent, however, there is a higher risk of pancreatitis or cholangitis that is relative to EUS-HGS or EUS-CG [12]. In patients with suitable anatomy, EUS-guided antegrade stent placement can also be combined with EUS-HGS; relative to EUS-HGS alone, this combined technique has the potential advantages of decreased adverse events (such as bile peritonitis) and prolonged stent patency [23].

2.4. EUS-Guided Rendezvous Technique

In the EUS-guided rendezvous technique, extrahepatic or intrahepatic access can be obtained using the echoendoscope and the methods described above. Similar to EUS-guided antegrade stent placement, once biliary access is obtained and a guidewire is placed across the biliary obstructions, across the ampulla, and into the small bowel. The guidewire is then left in place, and a duodenoscope is maneuvered to the second portion of the duodenum; the wire is used to facilitate ampullary cannulation, and a conventional ERCP can then be performed.

As with the EUS-guided antegrade stent placement, this achieves transpapillary drainage without transluminal anastomosis at the biliary access site [12,18,19]. This rendezvous technique can be useful when the second portion of the duodenum is accessible, but the conventional cannulation of the papilla is technically difficult [12,17,19].

3. Outcomes of EUS-BD

3.1. Efficacy and Adverse Events of EUS-BD

EUS-BD has a high technical and clinical success rate in relieving biliary obstruction, along with a favorable adverse event rate profile that is relative to alternative interventions. Much of the current literature has explored the role of EUS-BD after failed ERCP in the relief of MBO in particular. Systematic reviews and meta-analyses have demonstrated the technical and clinical success rates of EUS-BD to be 90–95% in this setting, respectively [8,18,24]. Meta-analyses have demonstrated procedure-related adverse event rates to be between 15 and 24%, with the most common complications being infection (including cholangitis, pancreatitis, and biliary peritonitis), bleeding, pneumoperitoneum, and bile leaks [8,18,24,25]. In EUS-HGS, a transesophageal puncture has also been reported, which can result in pneumothorax or mediastinitis [25].

The optimal technique for EUS-BD remains unclear, as it is difficult to compare different biliary access sites or the direction of stent placement, given the heterogeneity of patient populations and the relative rarity of each technique. Two randomized controlled trials (n = 49 and 47, respectively) have compared EUS-HGS to EUS-CDS for distal MBO after failed ERCP, and neither found significant differences in terms of technical or clinical success, adverse event rates, or morbidity [26,27]. One recent multicenter retrospective review (n = 182) found that choledochoduodenostomy was associated with longer stent patency than hepaticogastrostomy but otherwise noted a similar efficacy between the two approaches [28]. Other retrospective reviews and meta-analyses have demonstrated similar or conflicting results [12,24,29]. An ongoing randomized, multicenter clinical comparison between EUS-HGS and EUS-guided antegrade stent placement may shed light on the differences between these approaches [30]. Currently, however, the literature comparing different EUS-BD techniques is limited, so the optimal approach at many centers remains dependent upon patient anatomy and endoscopist expertise.

3.2. EUS-BD vs. PTBD

Given that PTBD remains the conventional therapeutic intervention for biliary obstruction following failed ERCP, investigators have compared the outcomes between PTBD and EUS-BD [8,9,31–34]. Recent randomized controlled trials have found that EUS-BD and PTBD were equivalent in terms of the technical and clinical success of relieving biliary obstruction [31,34], and multiple retrospective studies and meta-analyses have demonstrated similar findings [8,9,32,33,35]. In one large meta-analysis, Moole et al. found the pooled odds ratio for successful biliary drainage in EUS-BD vs. PTBD to be 3.1 (95% CI 1.1–8.4), suggesting that EUS-BD may be even more efficacious than PTBD in patients with malignant biliary strictures [8].

The current literature also suggests that EUS-BD is associated with lower adverse events and complications than PTBD. One randomized trial found that the procedure-related adverse event rate for EUS-BD (8.8%) was significantly lower than that for PTBD (31.2%) [31]; a second found a lower rate of re-intervention for EUS-BD [34]. Retrospective studies and meta-analyses have found similar results, with EUS-BD demonstrating lower infectious complications [8], fewer repeat interventions [9,35], and less post-procedural pain [35]. Other postulated advantages of EUS-BD over PTBD include improved patient quality of life (given the lack of an external catheter) and the ability to perform EUS-BD in the same session as a failed ERCP [8,10]. A multicenter, randomized trial comparison between EUS-BD and PTBD after failed ERCP for distal MBO is underway to more definitively answer these questions, which will be the largest prospective trial to date [36].

3.3. EUS-BD vs. ERCP as First-Line Intervention for Malignant Biliary Obstruction

Although EUS-BD is currently considered a second-line therapy after failed ERCP, several studies in recent years have compared EUS-BD to ERCP as the first-line intervention for biliary obstruction. The theoretical advantages of transenteric stenting (via EUS-HGS or EUS-CDS) relative to transpapillary stenting via ERCP include: the minimization of papillary manipulation leading to pancreatitis; the avoidance of stent tumor ingrowth which can occur when the stent is placed through a distal malignant biliary stricture; and the ability to access biliary ducts despite surgically-altered anatomy or gastroduodenal stents.

Meta-analyses have found that EUS-BD and ERCP have similarly high rates of technical success and clinical success when used as the primary option for biliary obstruction [25]. EUS-BD and ERCP also have similar rates of adverse events; while bile peritonitis remains a concern in EUS-BD (occurring in up to 2.4% of cases), EUS-BD has significantly lower rates of post-procedure pancreatitis and stent patency relative to ERCP. This was demonstrated in a randomized, controlled multicenter trial (n = 125) which found that EUS-BD was non-inferior to ERCP as a primary option for MBO; the study also found lower rates of overall adverse events for EUS-BD relative to ERCP (6.3% vs. 19.7%, respectively), including post-procedure pancreatitis (0 vs. 14.8%) and reintervention (15.6% vs. 42.6%), as well as a higher rate of stent patency (85.1% vs. 48.9%) with EUS-BD [37]. EUS-BD (specifically EUS-HGS and EUS-CG) may also have superior technical success to ERCP in patients with indwelling gastroduodenal stents who develop a subsequent biliary obstruction [14].

4. Limitations and Future Directions in EUS-BD

A major barrier to the widespread adoption of EUS-BD is operator expertise relative to PTBD, which is more widely practiced in most parts of the world [18,25]. Relative to ERCP or PTBD, EUS-BD is a relatively new therapeutic intervention that is practiced mainly at tertiary care centers. As such, EUS-BD is associated with a notable learning curve for endoscopists. For instance, in one cohort of 101 patients undergoing EUS-BD in a single center between 2006 and 2013, there were six procedure-related deaths; five of these deaths were among the first 50 patients in which the procedure was performed, and only one death was among the last 51 patients [29]. This may be true on a population level as well: one meta-analysis on different EUS-BD approaches found that studies published after 2013 had a higher technical success rate than those published prior to 2013 [24]. It seems likely that EUS-BD outcomes will continue to improve as endoscopist experience increases and adoption expands.

New endoscopic devices are likely to improve operability and clinical success rates for EUS-BD. While early studies have lacked the tools specific to EUS-BD and have instead relied on devices borrowed from other procedures, new endoscopic stents, and dilators have already changed how EUS-BD is performed. EUS-BD originally relied on traditional plastic stents; for instance, newly designed plastic stents with a tapered tip and four flanges with pigtail anchors have been developed specifically for EUS-HGS and have demonstrated good technical and clinical success [38]. Similarly, the adoption of newer covered self-expanding metal stents (CSEMS) has been associated with significantly lower adverse events in EUS-BD over time [24]. As noted previously, electrocautery-enhanced LAMS delivery systems have been increasingly used in EUS-CDS, which allow for single-step biliary access and stent placement with high technical success rates and acceptable adverse event rates [12,20,21]. Data from a recent large nationwide analysis of EUS-CDS with LAMS demonstrated reproducible efficacy and safety across different centers with a range of endoscopist expertise, suggesting that technological advancements such as LAMS have the potential to democratize the utilization of EUS-BD techniques beyond tertiary medical centers [21]. Other technological advancements—such as stent anti-migratory systems [39] and drill dilators, which are specific for intrahepatic bile ducts [40]—are expected to continue to shape the way EUS-BD is performed.

Ultimately, as endoscopic tools for EUS-BD continue to advance and EUS-BD becomes more widely practiced, the utilization and indications for EUS-BD are likely to expand. As noted above, research trials are already underway to determine which patients would benefit from EUS-BD rather than ERCP as the first-line option for biliary obstruction. Other areas that are being explored include using EUS-BD as a preferred method for gallbladder drainage in patients who are not surgical candidates [41–43]. EUS-BD also has the potential to become the preferred pre-operative management for MBO in patients ultimately undergoing surgery [44]. Taken together, EUS-BD and related techniques have the potential to transform the current paradigms that define how patients with hepatobiliary diseases are treated.

Author Contributions: J.B.D. and A.S. conceptualization, writing, editing. All authors have read and agreed to the published version of the manuscript.

Funding: This research received no external funding.

Institutional Review Board Statement: Not applicable.

Informed Consent Statement: Not applicable.

Data Availability Statement: Not applicable.

Conflicts of Interest: J.B.D.: no disclosures. A.S.: Consulting for Boston Scientific, Interscope, Olympus, and Medtronic; Research for Boston Scientific, Fujifilm; Advisory board for Endosound.

References

1. Early, D.S.; Ben-Menachem, T.; Decker, G.A.; Evans, J.A.; Fanelli, R.D.; Fisher, D.A.; Fukami, N.; Hwang, J.H.; Jain, R.; Jue, T.L.; et al. Appropriate use of GI endoscopy. *Gastrointest. Endosc.* **2012**, *75*, 1127–1131. [CrossRef]
2. Enochsson, L.; Swahn, F.; Arnelo, U.; Nilsson, M.; Löhr, M.; Persson, G. Nationwide, population-based data from 11,074 ERCP procedures from the Swedish Registry for Gallstone Surgery and ERCP. *Gastrointest. Endosc.* **2010**, *72*, 1175–1184.e1-3. [CrossRef]
3. Dumonceau, J.M.; Tringali, A.; Papanikolaou, I.S.; Blero, D.; Mangiavillano, B.; Schmidt, A.; Vanbiervliet, G.; Costamagna, G.; Devière, J.; García-Cano, J.; et al. Endoscopic biliary stenting: Indications, choice of stents, and results: European Society of Gastrointestinal Endoscopy (ESGE) Clinical Guideline–Updated October 2017. *Endoscopy* **2018**, *50*, 910–930. [CrossRef] [PubMed]
4. Kavanagh, P.V.; van Sonnenberg, E.; Wittich, G.R.; Goodacre, B.W.; Walser, E.M. Interventional Radiology of the Biliary Tract. *Endoscopy* **1997**, *29*, 570–576. [CrossRef]
5. Oh, H.-C.; Lee, S.; Lee, T.; Kwon, S.; Lee, S.S.; Seo, D.-W.; Kim, M.-H. Analysis of percutaneous transhepatic cholangioscopy-related complications and the risk factors for those complications. *Endoscopy* **2007**, *39*, 731–736. [CrossRef] [PubMed]
6. Ginat, D.; Saad, W.E.A.; Davies, M.G.; Saad, N.E.; Waldman, D.L.; Kitanosono, T. Incidence of Cholangitis and Sepsis Associated With Percutaneous Transhepatic Biliary Drain Cholangiography and Exchange: A Comparison Between Liver Transplant and Native Liver Patients. *AJR Am. J. Roentgenol.* **2011**, *196*, W73–W77. [CrossRef]
7. Molina, H.; Chan, M.M.; Lewandowski, R.J.; Gabr, A.; Riaz, A. Complications of Percutaneous Biliary Procedures. *Semin. Interv. Radiol.* **2021**, *38*, 364–372. [CrossRef]
8. Moole, H.; Bechtold, M.L.; Forcione, D.; Puli, S.R. A meta-analysis and systematic review: Success of endoscopic ultrasound guided biliary stenting in patients with inoperable malignant biliary strictures and a failed ERCP. *Medicine* **2017**, *96*, e5154. [CrossRef] [PubMed]
9. Khashab, M.A.; El Zein, M.H.; Sharzehi, K.; Marson, F.P.; Haluszka, O.; Small, A.J.; Nakai, Y.; Park, D.H.; Kunda, R.; Teoh, A.Y.; et al. EUS-guided biliary drainage or enteroscopy-assisted ERCP in patients with surgical anatomy and biliary obstruction: An international comparative study. *Endosc. Int. Open* **2016**, *04*, E1322–E1327. [CrossRef]
10. Park, D.H.; Nam, K.; Kim, D.U.; Lee, T.H.; Iwashita, T.; Nakai, Y.; Bolkhir, A.; Castro, L.A.; Vazquez-Sequeiros, E.; De La Serna, C.; et al. Patient perception and preference of EUS-guided drainage over percutaneous drainage when endoscopic transpapillary biliary drainage fails: An international multicenter survey. *Endosc. Ultrasound* **2018**, *7*, 48–55. [CrossRef]
11. Giovannini, M.; Moutardier, V.; Pesenti, C.; Bories, E.; Lelong, B.; Delpero, J.R. Endoscopic Ultrasound-Guided Bilioduodenal Anastomosis: A New Technique for Biliary Drainage. *Endoscopy* **2001**, *33*, 898–900. [CrossRef]
12. Canakis, A.; Baron, T.H. Relief of biliary obstruction: Choosing between endoscopic ultrasound and endoscopic retrograde cholangiopancreatography. *BMJ Open Gastroenterol.* **2020**, *7*, e000428. [CrossRef]
13. Elfert, K.; Zeid, E.; Duarte-Chavez, R.; Kahaleh, M. Endoscopic ultrasound guided access procedures following surgery. *Best Pr. Res. Clin. Gastroenterol.* **2022**, *60–61*, 101812. [CrossRef]
14. Yamao, K.; Kitano, M.; Takenaka, M.; Minaga, K.; Sakurai, T.; Watanabe, T.; Kayahara, T.; Yoshikawa, T.; Yamashita, Y.; Asada, M.; et al. Outcomes of endoscopic biliary drainage in pancreatic cancer patients with an indwelling gastroduodenal stent: A multicenter cohort study in West Japan. *Gastrointest. Endosc.* **2018**, *88*, 66–75.e2. [CrossRef]
15. Tyberg, A.; Desai, A.P.; Kumta, N.A.; Brown, E.; Gaidhane, M.; Sharaiha, R.Z.; Kahaleh, M. EUS-guided biliary drainage after failed ERCP: A novel algorithm individualized based on patient anatomy. *Gastrointest. Endosc.* **2016**, *84*, 941–946. [CrossRef] [PubMed]
16. Boulay, B.R.; Lo, S.K. Endoscopic Ultrasound–Guided Biliary Drainage. *Gastrointest. Endosc. Clin. N. Am.* **2018**, *28*, 171–185. [CrossRef] [PubMed]
17. Mishra, A.; Tyberg, A. Endoscopic ultrasound guided biliary drainage: A comprehensive review. *Transl. Gastroenterol. Hepatol.* **2019**, *4*, 10. [CrossRef] [PubMed]
18. Nussbaum, J.S.; Kumta, N.A. Endoscopic Ultrasound-Guided Biliary Drainage. *Gastrointest. Endosc. Clin. N. Am.* **2019**, *29*, 277–291. [CrossRef] [PubMed]
19. Dietrich, C.; Braden, B.; Burmeister, S.; Aabakken, L.; Arciadacono, P.; Bhutani, M.; Götzberger, M.; Healey, A.; Hocke, M.; Hollerbach, S.; et al. How to perform EUS-guided biliary drainage. *Endosc. Ultrasound* **2022**, *11*, 342. [CrossRef]
20. Krishnamoorthi, R.; Dasari, C.S.; Chandrasekar, V.T.; Priyan, H.; Jayaraj, M.; Law, J.; Larsen, M.; Kozarek, R.; Ross, A.; Irani, S. Effectiveness and safety of EUS-guided choledochoduodenostomy using lumen-apposing metal stents (LAMS): A systematic review and meta-analysis. *Surg. Endosc.* **2020**, *34*, 2866–2877. [CrossRef]
21. Fugazza, A.; Fabbri, C.; Di Mitri, R.; Petrone, M.C.; Colombo, M.; Cugia, L.; Amato, A.; Forti, E.; Binda, C.; Maida, M.; et al. EUS-guided choledochoduodenostomy for malignant distal biliary obstruction after failed ERCP: A retrospective nationwide analysis. *Gastrointest. Endosc.* **2022**, *95*, 896–904.e1. [CrossRef]
22. Yi, H.; Liu, Q.; He, S.; Zhong, L.; Wu, S.-H.; Guo, X.-D.; Ning, B. Current uses of electro-cautery lumen apposing metal stents in endoscopic ultrasound guided interventions. *Front. Med.* **2022**, *9*, 1002031. [CrossRef] [PubMed]
23. Ogura, T.; Kitano, M.; Takenaka, M.; Okuda, A.; Minaga, K.; Yamao, K.; Yamashita, Y.; Hatamaru, K.; Noguchi, C.; Gotoh, Y.; et al. Multicenter prospective evaluation study of endoscopic ultrasound-guided hepaticogastrostomy combined with antegrade stenting (with video). *Dig. Endosc.* **2018**, *30*, 252–259. [CrossRef]

24. Wang, K.; Zhu, J.; Xing, L.; Wang, Y.; Jin, Z.; Li, Z. Assessment of efficacy and safety of EUS-guided biliary drainage: A systematic review. *Gastrointest. Endosc.* **2016**, *83*, 1218–1227. [CrossRef] [PubMed]
25. Jin, Z.; Wei, Y.; Lin, H.; Yang, J.; Jin, H.; Shen, S.; Zhang, X. Endoscopic ultrasound-guided versus endoscopic retrograde cholangiopancreatography-guided biliary drainage for primary treatment of distal malignant biliary obstruction: A systematic review and meta-analysis. *Dig. Endosc.* **2020**, *32*, 16–26. [CrossRef]
26. Artifon, E.L.; Marson, F.P.; Gaidhane, M.; Kahaleh, M.; Otoch, J.P. Hepaticogastrostomy or choledochoduodenostomy for distal malignant biliary obstruction after failed ERCP: Is there any difference? *Gastrointest. Endosc.* **2015**, *81*, 950–959. [CrossRef] [PubMed]
27. Minaga, K.; Ogura, T.; Shiomi, H.; Imai, H.; Hoki, N.; Takenaka, M.; Nishikiori, H.; Yamashita, Y.; Hisa, T.; Kato, H.; et al. Comparison of the efficacy and safety of endoscopic ultrasound-guided choledochoduodenostomy and hepaticogastrostomy for malignant distal biliary obstruction: Multicenter, randomized, clinical trial. *Dig. Endosc.* **2019**, *31*, 575–582. [CrossRef]
28. Kahaleh, M.; Tyberg, A.; Napoleon, B.; Robles-Medranda, C.; Shah, J.; Bories, E.; Kumta, N.; Yague, A.; Vazquez-Sequeiros, E.; Lakhtakia, S.; et al. Hepaticogastrostomy versus choledochoduodenostomy: An international multicenter study on their long-term patency. *Endosc. Ultrasound* **2022**, *11*, 38. [CrossRef] [PubMed]
29. Poincloux, L.; Rouquette, O.; Buc, E.; Privat, J.; Pezet, D.; Dapoigny, M.; Bommelaer, G.; Abergel, A. Endoscopic ultrasound-guided biliary drainage after failed ERCP: Cumulative experience of 101 procedures at a single center. *Endoscopy* **2015**, *47*, 794–801. [CrossRef] [PubMed]
30. Liao, Y.; Giovannini, M.; Zhong, N.; Xiao, T.; Sheng, S.; Wu, Y.; Zhang, J.; Wang, S.; Liu, X.; Sun, S.; et al. Comparison of endoscopic ultrasound-guided hepaticogastrostomy and the antegrade technique in the management of unresectable malignant biliary obstruction: Study protocol for a prospective, multicentre, randomised controlled trial. *Trials* **2020**, *21*, 1–7. [CrossRef]
31. Lee, T.H.; Choi, J.-H.; Park, D.H.; Song, T.J.; Kim, D.U.; Paik, W.H.; Hwangbo, Y.; Lee, S.S.; Seo, D.W.; Lee, S.K.; et al. Similar Efficacies of Endoscopic Ultrasound–guided Transmural and Percutaneous Drainage for Malignant Distal Biliary Obstruction. *Clin. Gastroenterol. Hepatol.* **2016**, *14*, 1011–1019.e3. [CrossRef]
32. Sharaiha, R.Z.; Khan, M.A.; Kamal, F.; Tyberg, A.; Tombazzi, C.R.; Ali, B.; Tombazzi, C.; Kahaleh, M. Efficacy and safety of EUS-guided biliary drainage in comparison with percutaneous biliary drainage when ERCP fails: A systematic review and meta-analysis. *Gastrointest. Endosc.* **2017**, *85*, 904–914. [CrossRef]
33. Baniya, R.; Upadhaya, S.; Madala, S.; Subedi, S.C.; Mohammed, T.S.; Bachuwa, G. Endoscopic ultrasound-guided biliary drainage versus percutaneous transhepatic biliary drainage after failed endoscopic retrograde cholangiopancreatography: A meta-analysis. *Clin. Exp. Gastroenterol.* **2017**, *10*, 67–74. [CrossRef]
34. Marx, M.; Caillol, F.; Autret, A.; Ratone, J.-P.; Zemmour, C.; Boher, J.M.; Pesenti, C.; Bories, E.; Barthet, M.; Napoléon, B.; et al. EUS-guided hepaticogastrostomy in patients with obstructive jaundice after failed or impossible endoscopic retrograde drainage: A multicenter, randomized phase II Study. *Endosc. Ultrasound* **2022**, *11*, 495. [CrossRef] [PubMed]
35. Hassan, Z.; Gadour, E. Systematic review of endoscopic ultrasound-guided biliary drainage versus percutaneous transhepatic biliary drainage. *Clin. Med.* **2022**, *22*, 14. [CrossRef]
36. Schmitz, D.; Valiente, C.T.; Dollhopf, M.; Perez-Miranda, M.; Küllmer, A.; Gornals, J.; Vila, J.; Weigt, J.; Voigtländer, T.; Redondo-Cerezo, E.; et al. Percutaneous transhepatic or endoscopic ultrasound-guided biliary drainage in malignant distal bile duct obstruction using a self-expanding metal stent: Study protocol for a prospective European multicenter trial (PUMa trial). *PLoS ONE* **2022**, *17*, e0275029. [CrossRef] [PubMed]
37. Paik, W.H.; Lee, T.H.; Park, D.H.; Choi, J.-H.; Kim, S.-O.; Jang, S.; Kim, D.U.; Shim, J.H.; Song, T.J.; Lee, S.S.; et al. EUS-Guided Biliary Drainage Versus ERCP for the Primary Palliation of Malignant Biliary Obstruction: A Multicenter Randomized Clinical Trial. *Am. J. Gastroenterol.* **2018**, *113*, 987–997. [CrossRef] [PubMed]
38. Umeda, J.; Itoi, T.; Tsuchiya, T.; Sofuni, A.; Itokawa, F.; Ishii, K.; Tsuji, S.; Ikeuchi, N.; Kamada, K.; Tanaka, R.; et al. A newly designed plastic stent for EUS-guided hepaticogastrostomy: A prospective preliminary feasibility study (with videos). *Gastrointest. Endosc.* **2015**, *82*, 390–396.e2. [CrossRef]
39. Anderloni, A.; Fugazza, A.; Spadaccini, M.; Colombo, M.; Capogreco, A.; Carrara, S.; Maselli, R.; Ferrara, E.; Galtieri, P.; Pellegatta, G.; et al. Feasibility and safety of a new dedicated biliary stent for EUS-guided hepaticogastrostomy: The FIT study (with video). *Endosc. Ultrasound* **2023**, *12*, 59. [CrossRef]
40. Ogura, T.; Uba, Y.; Yamamura, M.; Kawai, J.; Nishikawa, H. Successful endoscopic ultrasound-guided hepaticogastrostomy with use of a novel drill dilator for challenging tract dilation. *Endoscopy* **2023**, *55*, E149–E150. [CrossRef]
41. Adler, D.; Kamal, F.; Khan, M.; Lee-Smith, W.; Sharma, S.; Acharya, A.; Farooq, U.; Aziz, M.; Kouanda, A.; Dai, S.-C.; et al. Efficacy and safety of EUS-guided gallbladder drainage for rescue treatment of malignant biliary obstruction: A systematic review and meta-analysis. *Endosc. Ultrasound* **2022**, *12*, 8. [CrossRef] [PubMed]
42. Robles-Medranda, C.; Oleas, R.; Puga-Tejada, M.; Alcivar-Vasquez, J.; Del Valle, R.; Olmos, J.; Arevalo-Mora, M.; Egas-Izquierdo, M.; Tabacelia, D.; Baquerizo-Burgos, J.; et al. Prophylactic EUS-guided gallbladder drainage prevents acute cholecystitis in patients with malignant biliary obstruction and cystic duct orifice involvement: A randomized trial (with video). *Gastrointest. Endosc.* **2023**, *97*, 445–453. [CrossRef]

43. Hemerly, M.C.; de Moura, D.T.H.; Junior, E.S.D.M.; Proença, I.M.; Ribeiro, I.B.; Yvamoto, E.Y.; Ribas, P.H.B.V.; Sánchez-Luna, S.A.; Bernardo, W.M.; de Moura, E.G.H. Endoscopic ultrasound (EUS)-guided cholecystostomy versus percutaneous cholecystostomy (PTC) in the management of acute cholecystitis in patients unfit for surgery: A systematic review and meta-analysis. *Surg. Endosc.* **2022**. [CrossRef] [PubMed]
44. Mukai, S.; Itoi, T.; Tsuchiya, T.; Ishii, K.; Tonozuka, R.; Nagakawa, Y.; Kozono, S.; Takishita, C.; Osakabe, H.; Sofuni, A. Clinical feasibility of endoscopic ultrasound-guided biliary drainage for preoperative management of malignant biliary obstruction (with videos). *J. Hepato-Biliary-Pancreatic Sci.* **2022**. [CrossRef] [PubMed]

Disclaimer/Publisher's Note: The statements, opinions and data contained in all publications are solely those of the individual author(s) and contributor(s) and not of MDPI and/or the editor(s). MDPI and/or the editor(s) disclaim responsibility for any injury to people or property resulting from any ideas, methods, instructions or products referred to in the content.

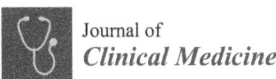

Review

Endoscopic Ultrasound-Guided Local Ablative Therapies for the Treatment of Pancreatic Neuroendocrine Tumors and Cystic Lesions: A Review of the Current Literature

Alexander M. Prete [1] and Tamas A. Gonda [2,*]

1. Department of Medicine, New York University (NYU) Grossman School of Medicine, New York, NY 10016, USA
2. Division of Gastroenterology and Hepatology, New York University (NYU) Langone Health, New York, NY 10016, USA
* Correspondence: tamas.gonda@nyulangone.org

Abstract: Since its emergence as a diagnostic modality in the 1980s, endoscopic ultrasound (EUS) has provided the clinician profound access to gastrointestinal organs to aid in the direct visualization, sampling, and subsequent identification of pancreatic pathology. In recent years, advancements in EUS as an interventional technique have promoted the use of local ablative therapies as a minimally invasive alternative to the surgical management of pancreatic neuroendocrine tumors (pNETs) and pancreatic cystic neoplasms (PCNs), especially for those deemed to be poor operative candidates. EUS-guided local therapies have demonstrated promising efficacy in addressing a spectrum of pancreatic neoplasms, while also balancing local adverse effects on healthy parenchyma. This article serves as a review of the current literature detailing the mechanisms, outcomes, complications, and limitations of EUS-guided local ablative therapies such as chemical ablation and radiofrequency ablation (RFA) for the treatment of pNETs and PCNs, as well as a discussion of future applications of EUS-guided techniques to address a broader scope of pancreatic pathology.

Keywords: EUS-guided local therapies; interventional EUS; radiofrequency ablation; ethanol ablation; chemical ablation; intratumoral drug delivery; pancreatic neuroendocrine tumors; pancreatic cystic neoplasms; pancreatobiliary disease

1. Introduction

Endoscopic ultrasound (EUS) emerged as a diagnostic modality approximately five decades ago and has since grown significantly in its utilization to aid in the identification of gastrointestinal (GI) pathology [1–3]. Given the proximity of the pancreas to the hollow organs of the GI tract, EUS offers excellent resolution of the pancreatic parenchyma, main duct, and its adjacent structures, including the common bile duct, portal and splenic veins, and mesenteric lymph nodes [1]. Therefore, EUS has become a reliable technique for the evaluation of pancreatobiliary disorders, demonstrating higher sensitivity in detecting early pancreatic tumors when compared to non-invasive imaging techniques such as positron-emission tomography (PET), computed tomography (CT), or transabdominal ultrasound [4]. Within the past decade, EUS has evolved from a purely diagnostic modality to an interventional technique, with new EUS-guided procedures showing great promise in addressing structural pathology of the pancreas.

Starting with the first human pilot study of EUS-guided ethanol ablation to treat pancreatic cystic neoplasms (PCNs) in 2005 [5], the field of EUS-guided local ablative therapy for pancreatic disease has shown subsequent expansion in both technique and therapeutic application. To date, ablative techniques are numerous and in various stages of clinical application, including chemical ablation (such as ethanol lavage and intratumoral chemotherapy delivery [6,7]), radiofrequency ablation, laser ablation, microwave ablation,

and cryoablation therapy [8]. Though diverse in their mechanisms, these methods are unified in their minimally invasive approach, involving the use of ultrasound guidance to advance an electrode or needle tip into a target lesion while avoiding vascular or ductal structures [8]. These ablative techniques generate local necrosis of the target lesion while balancing potential adverse effects on healthy parenchyma (i.e., pancreatitis and pancreatic necrosis) and surrounding structures (i.e., portal venous thrombosis) [9].

EUS-guided ablative techniques have been applied to an ever-growing spectrum of pancreatic pathologies, chief among them neoplastic lesions. This includes both solid neoplasms, such as pancreatic neuroendocrine tumors (pNETs) and pancreatic ductal adenocarcinoma (PDAC), as well as cystic lesions. Traditionally, surgical management has been the definitive therapy of choice for neoplastic lesions that are symptomatic [9], malignant [10], or harboring malignant potential [11]. However, these procedures carry significant morbidity and mortality; depending on the malignant potential and individual risk, surgery may carry an unacceptable risk-to-benefit ratio [12]. EUS-guided local ablation has offered a minimally invasive therapeutic alternative to surgery [13]. Adding to its advantages, EUS-guided local ablative therapy has the potential to be conducted on an outpatient basis, resulting in reduced post-operative morbidity when compared to surgery [8].

Despite its growing appeal, the efficacy and safety of EUS-guided ablative therapies has been reported in the literature through a limited number of case reports and observational studies. To date, these therapies have yet to be compared vis-à-vis surgical management through a randomized controlled trial. While many ablative techniques remain in the experimental or pre-clinical phases of application, radiofrequency ablation (RFA) and chemical ablation with ethanol (EA) or chemotherapeutic substrate have been broadly reported in the literature, especially in the management of pNETs and PCNs. Thus, this article will serve as a review of selected studies reporting the use of EUS-guided RFA and chemical ablation in the treatment of pNETs and PCNs, providing an overview of therapeutic rationale, mechanisms, efficacy, safety, and pitfalls. Additionally, this article will briefly touch upon the future applications of EUS-guided local ablative therapy, including new ablative techniques and the growing pathologic scope of this exciting intervention.

2. Clinical Definitions and Classification of Pancreatic Lesions

2.1. Definitons and Classification of PCNs

PCNs are a common lesion, with an estimated prevalence of CT detectable asymptomatic cysts reported in the literature as 2.2% of the general population [14]. However, despite their frequency, cystic lesions of the pancreas constitute a heterogenous group of tumors that are classified according to their histopathologic features [15]. Broadly, the main groups of PCNs include serous cystic neoplasms (SCNs), mucinous cystic neoplasms (MCNs), and intraductal papillary mucinous neoplasms (IPMNs), with the latter two harboring the potential for malignant transformation [11]. Given this, current consensus guidelines suggest surveillance of MCNs and IPMNs with progression to surgical resection should high-risk or worrisome features develop [16]. However, the absence of widely accepted evidence-based guidelines for PCN management has posed the clinical challenge of weighing the risks of unnecessary surgery with the potential for untreated malignant evolution.

2.2. Definitons and Classification of pNETs

pNETs constitute a small percentage of all pancreatic tumors, comprising only 1.3% of all cancers that originate in the pancreas [17]. These tumors are generally classified as either functional or non-functional, depending on whether they are capable of releasing hormones that may produce symptoms in the afflicted individual. While 60–90% of pNETs are non-functional, functional pNETs produce hormones such as insulin, gastrin, glucagon, somatostatin, and vasoactive intestinal peptide, generating hallmark symptoms that usually lead to earlier clinical detection and subsequent management [18]. Insulinomas are the most common functional pNET and result from neoplastic growth of beta cells in the islets of Langerhans [18].

3. Clinical Rationale for EUS-Guided Local Ablative Therapy

3.1. Clinical Rationale for EUS-Guided Local Ablative Therapy of PCNs

Due to recent technologic advances in modern imaging modalities, the detection rate of PCNs has only increased, many of which constitute incidental findings [15]. In fact, it has been reported that incidental pancreatic cysts now make up nearly one-third of resected lesions seen in surgical practice [19]. EUS has become a potent tool to aid in pre-operative diagnosis and classification of either symptomatic or incidentally detected cystic lesions of the pancreas. International guidelines have distinguished features of potentially malignant cystic lesions (including cyst size, location, internal and capsular structure, and association with changes in the size or caliber of the main pancreatic duct (MPD) [20]), all of which can be detected using EUS. Additionally, EUS-guided fine needle aspiration (FNA) allows the clinician to sample intra-cystic fluid in real-time, with subsequent fluid cytology and analysis of carcinoembryonic antigen (CEA) levels to aid in the diagnosis of a mucinous neoplasm [21].

Should the diagnostic features of a mucinous PCN reveal high-risk for malignancy or high-grade dysplasia (HGD), definitive surgical management is deemed the gold standard therapy [22]. Unfortunately, in many instances, histologic diagnosis of HGD or carcinoma cannot be achieved preoperatively, and the clinician must make a management decision based on the radiographic and biochemical surrogate markers detailed above [23]. Thus, there is a growing clinical interest in exploring an effective, minimally invasive technique to treat pre-malignant lesions prior to their transformation to invasive carcinoma while also avoiding the significant perioperative morbidity and mortality of invasive surgery [24]. In patients with unilocular or oligolocular mucinous cysts without definite pancreatic mass who are poor operative candidates, ablation can be considered as a therapeutic option that avoids the safety concerns of invasive surgery while allowing for clinical management beyond conservative imaging surveillance [25].

3.2. Clinical Rationale for EUS-Guided Local Ablative Therapy of pNETs/Insulinomas

In general, pNETs exhibit heterogenous clinical behavior, spanning from incidental growths on imaging, to indolent and slow-growing masses, to aggressively metastatic lesions [26]. Recommendations for pNET management are provided by the National Comprehensive Cancer Network (NCCN) guidelines, which are largely based on tumor staging (including tumor size, nodal involvement, and presence of distal metastases) as well as histologic grading, which is generally defined by mitotic count and/or Ki-67 index on pathologic reporting [27]. Since tumor size remains an important correlate to malignant potential [28], all tumors greater than 2 cm are generally considered locally invasive and therefore warrant surgical resection along with regional lymphadenectomy [18].

However, given their unpredictable malignant potential, there remains great controversy surrounding the management of non-functional pNETs less than 2 cm in size, with some recommending a conservative "watch-and-wait" approach over invasive surgery [29]. Thus, there is a growing interest in EUS-guided ablation as a minimally invasive locoregional treatment modality that can balance the risks of overtreatment (i.e., surgical excision and its associated complications) and undertreatment (i.e., undetected malignancy in a patient undergoing conservative periodic surveillance) [30,31]. Additionally, since the prognosis of functional pNETs tends to be more favorable in comparison to non-functional tumors given their propensity to produce symptoms that contribute to earlier detection [32,33], EUS-guided ablation offers a therapeutic option for rapid symptom relief in those suffering from hormone over-production, especially when these patients may not be appropriate candidates for definitive cure with surgical intervention [34].

4. Mechanisms of Action for Select EUS-Guided Local Ablative Therapies

In 1992, the first case of EUS-guided FNA of a pancreatic head lesion was reported by Vilmann et al. [35], signifying a revolutionary step in the clinical diagnosis and staging of GI pathology. Through the decades, the techniques of EUS-guided FNA have been modified to serve an interventional role, resulting in the field of EUS-guided local ablative therapy. Although several ablative therapies have been described in the literature, this portion of this review article will largely focus on the mechanisms of the two most widely used techniques: chemical ablation (including EA and intratumoral drug delivery) and RFA.

4.1. Mechanisms of EUS-Guided EA

The use of ethanol as a chemical ablative substrate has a rich history in clinical medicine, spanning the spectrum from thyroid cyst therapy [36] to alcohol septal ablation for hypertrophic obstructive cardiomyopathy [37]. In the field of GI specifically, the efficacy of percutaneous ethanol lavage of cystic lesions in solid organs such as the liver [38] and spleen [39] has been reported for decades. Given the success of these therapies with evidence of significant reduction in cyst volume even after a single session [38], these techniques have evolved to address pancreatic pathology through endoscopic intervention.

In 2005, Gan et al. reported the first study in a human model that utilized EUS-guided ethanol ablation to treat pancreatic cystic lesions [5], demonstrating both the efficacy and clinical feasibility of this intervention. Ethanol's popularity as a chemical ablative agent has since persisted due to its low cost, abundant availability, and rapid-acting ablative capacity [15]. Ethanol is a short-chain alcohol that, at high concentrations, solubilizes the cell membrane and alters protein tertiary structure [40]. Thus, by injecting the toxic substrate into a cystic cavity or neoplastic lesion, ethanol promotes cellular death through a combination of membrane lysis, protein denaturation, and vascular occlusion [41]. Additionally, cytotoxicity of ethanol is enhanced through mitochondrial injury and disruption of intracellular signal transduction [42]. Together, these mechanisms generate tissue necrosis in target lesions, which can be localized to pathologic tissue under ultrasound guidance.

4.2. Mechanisms of EUS-Guided Intratumoral Drug Delivery

Intratumoral injection of chemotherapeutic or other biological antitumor agents has previously been described in the treatment of conditions such as endobronchial non-small cell lung tumors [43] and pediatric brain cancers [44]. Recently, EUS has made possible the local delivery of chemotherapeutic agents (namely, paclitaxel) to treat cystic tumors of the pancreas while mitigating systemic side effects [6,7]. Paclitaxel is a hydrophobic and viscous chemotherapeutic agent, thereby exerting a long-lasting antineoplastic effect on a closed, cystic cavity with low possibility of leakage into surrounding healthy tissue [6]. Oh et al. [7] initially reported the safety, feasibility, and efficacy of EUS-guided ethanol lavage with paclitaxel injection for PCNs through a prospective pilot study. They described a potential synergistic effect between the two chemical agents, with primary distortion of cystic epithelium by ethanol followed by secondary antitumor effect from microtubule inhibition with paclitaxel. Additionally, there is evidence that EUS-guided ethanol lavage with paclitaxel can alter mutant DNA (including KRAS mutations) present in pre-treated cystic fluid, potentially interrupting progression to malignancy [45].

4.3. Mechanisms of EUS-Guided RFA

RFA as an interventional technique has previously shown efficacy in the palliative treatment of solid, unresectable tumors throughout the body, including the lungs [46], bone [47], prostate [48], and kidneys [49]. The safety of EUS-guided RFA of the pancreatic head was first shown by Gaidhane et al. [50] in 2012 utilizing a porcine model, which demonstrated the targeted potential of RFA therapy to generate discrete areas of necrosis while minimizing focal acute pancreatitis in healthy tissue. Since this initial study, the use of EUS-guided RFA has expanded to include human subjects seeking therapy for a spectrum of pancreatic neoplasms, including PDAC [51].

RFA harnesses the antitumor effects of hyperthermia, inducing cellular protein denaturation and subsequent coagulative necrosis [52]. Since human cells cannot typically withstand temperatures above 50 °C, the use of high-frequency alternating current (usually 200–1200 kHz frequency) delivered via an ultrasound-guided electrode leads to local agitation and friction with subsequent heat generation to temperatures as high as 90 °C [51]. Since maximum heat is generated in the vicinity closest to the electrode, this leads to decreased tumor bulk while minimizing side effects on healthy adjacent parenchyma [53]. Additionally, RFA is believed to produce cellular debris that promotes antigen presentation to lymphocytes, thereby enhancing antitumor effect by stimulating tumor-specific T cells and activating systemic immunity [54].

5. Clinical Applications of EUS-Guided Ablative Therapies for Pancreatic Pathology: A Summary of Reviewed Studies

As the technical scope of EUS-guided ablation has expanded, so has the spectrum of pathology addressed by this minimally invasive intervention. The focus of this literature review will be the use of EUS-guided chemical ablation and RFA for the therapy of PCNs and pNETs, with a summary of outcomes and complications of select studies in the sections to follow.

5.1. EUS-Guided EA for the Treatment of PCNs

The efficacy and safety of EUS-guided EA for the treatment of PCNs has been reported in several observational trials [5,24,55–58] and a randomized trial [59] (Table 1). Gan et al. [5] published the first pilot study of EUS-guided EA of cystic lesions at Massachusetts General Hospital in 2005. In this prospective, single-center study, 25 asymptomatic patients with image-confirmed pancreatic cystic lesions (including MCNs, IPMNs, SCNs, and one pseudocyst) were selected to undergo EUS-guided cyst aspiration followed by ethanol lavage. The results were promising, revealing complete cyst resolution in 35% of participants at one year follow-up. When assessing outcomes according to pre-procedural diagnosis, 62.5% of MCNs were completely resolved at follow-up while 100% of IPMNs persisted despite therapy. Importantly, no documented adverse events were noted for 72 h post-procedure. Thus, in addition to proving the technical feasibility of this procedure, Gan et al. also showed that EUS-guided EA of PCNs is a safe intervention with a theoretically low risk of precipitating pancreatitis.

In 2009, DeWitt et al. [59] designed a prospective, multicenter, double-blind randomized controlled trial to compare the efficacy of EUS-guided ablation with ethanol to that of saline lavage in the treatment of a spectrum of pancreatic cysts (including MCNs, IPMNs, SCNs, and pseudocysts). The results revealed that lavage with 80% ethanol resulted in significant reduction in cyst size when compared to injection of saline solution alone, and that one or more sessions of EA led to complete cyst resolution in 33% of patients who completed follow-up. Evidence for the ablative potential of ethanol substrate was furthered by histopathologic examination: four patients in the study later underwent surgical resection of their mucinous cysts, revealing 0% cyst epithelial ablation in the participant treated with saline lavage alone versus 50–100% observed in those who received one or two sessions of EUS-guided EA. Although patients were randomized to receive either one or two sessions of EA, the study was underpowered to reveal any benefit in cyst reduction when comparing the two groups. In contrast to Gan et al., complications were observed in this study, with 12–16% of patients experiencing abdominal pain within one week of the procedure and two patients developing acute pancreatitis due to extravasation of ethanol from the cyst into adjacent parenchyma.

Table 1. Summary of Results for Selected Studies Utilizing EUS-Guided EA for PCN Therapy.

Author	Study Year	Ablative Strategy	Number of Treated Patients	Number of Treated Lesions			Efficacy on Follow-Up Imaging **, n (%)			Adverse Events, (n)
				MCN	IPMN	Other *	Incomplete Response	Partial Response	Complete Response	
Gan et al. [5]	2005	Ethanol (5–80%)	25	14	3	6	13 (56)	2 (9)	8 (35)	None
DeWitt et al. [59]	2009	Ethanol (80%)	25	10	10	5	13 (59)	0 (0)	9 (41)	Mild abdominal pain (7); Intra-cystic bleeding (1); Acute pancreatitis (1)
		Saline	17 ***	7	7	3	11 (79)	0 (0)	3 (21) ****	Mild abdominal pain (3)
DiMaio et al. [56]	2011	Ethanol (80%)	13	0	13	0	8 (62)	0 (0)	5 (38)	Mild abdominal pain (1)
Caillol et al. [24]	2012	Ethanol (99%)	13	14	0	0	2 (15)	0 (0)	11 (85)	None
Gómez et al. [57]	2016	Ethanol (80%)	23	4	15	4	11 (48)	10 (43)	2 (9)	Mild abdominal pain (1): Acute pancreatitis (1)
Park et al. [58]	2016	Ethanol (99%)	91	12	9	70	13 (14)	37 (41)	41 (45)	Mild abdominal pain (18); Fever without infection (8); Acute pancreatitis (3)

* The designation of "Other" includes patients treated in the above studies for cystic lesions that are non-neoplastic (i.e., pseudocysts), neoplastic without malignant potential (i.e., SCNs), or indeterminate based on pre-procedural analysis. Although the scope of this review focuses on the use of EUS-guided ablative procedures in the treatment of neoplastic cysts capable of malignant transformation (i.e., MCNs and IPMNs), this column is included in the table for the purpose of completeness. ** Complete response is defined as the radiographic absence of residual lesion on post-procedural imaging. Incomplete response is defined as either persistent or enlarged residual lesion on post-procedural imaging. If the study authors noted reduction in lesion size without resolution on post-procedural imaging, this is considered a partial response; if this was not recorded by the study authors, these lesions are categorized as incomplete response. *** Of the 17 patients initially treated with a session of saline lavage, 14 received a second follow-up session with ethanol lavage. **** All three patients with complete cyst resolution received initial saline lavage followed by a second session with ethanol lavage.

In 2010, the same group conducted a prospective cohort study that provided long-term follow-up of cysts that were successfully ablated with one or two sessions of EA in their original study [55]. Of the 12 patients in the initial study who experienced radiographically confirmed resolution of their PCNs after EUS-guided ablation, 9 participants underwent repeat CT scan at a median of 26 months after documentation of complete cyst ablation, demonstrating absence of recurrence in all patients. This study supported the long-term durability of cyst ablation using EUS-guided EA, revealing the potential for this intervention to "cure" individuals of their PCNs.

While these prior studies demonstrated the feasibility, safety, and durability of EUS-guided EA for PCNs, there remained a question regarding the potential therapeutic benefit of conducting multiple sessions of ethanol lavage in comparison to a single treatment course. Thus, in 2011, DiMaio et al. [56] conducted a retrospective review of 13 patients with asymptomatic, benign-appearing IPMNs who underwent two or more sessions of EA for cyst ablation given their status as poor surgical candidates. They observed a significantly greater decrease in cyst diameter and surface area after two sessions of EUS-guided EA in comparison to a single session. Although image-confirmed cyst resolution did not occur in any patient after a single EA session, it occurred in 5 patients (38% of participants) after their second course of EA. Additionally, the group noted only minor abdominal pain after the first and second EA sessions in a single patient, further supporting the safety of this intervention.

In 2012, Caillol et al. [24] sought to understand the efficacy of EUS-guided ablation of MCNs specifically, conducting a bi-center prospective cohort study of 13 patients who received EA for treatment of their mucinous cysts given their contraindications to surgery (including heart failure, hypertension, and recent cancer). At a follow-up of 26 months post-procedure, 85% of patients had complete cyst ablation on imaging, a high success rate that can likely be attributed to the low sample size and strict inclusion criteria (as ablated cysts were small in diameter and lacked septation). Later in 2016, Park et al. [58] completed a clinical study of 91 participants with unilocular or oligolocular pancreatic cysts (including an overwhelming majority of SCNs and indeterminate lesions) treated with a single session of EUS-guided EA. Although overall treatment response was high with 45% of participants experiencing complete resolution at 40-month follow-up, the success rate varied significantly according to pre-procedural cyst classification: while 50% of patients with MCNs achieved cyst resolution, only 11% of IPMNs were responsive to EA. The authors speculated that this was likely multi-factorial, including the presence of a complex papillary growth pattern in IPMNs as well as communication with the MPD (as the treated cysts were branch duct IPMNs) that may have collectively diminished the ablative effects of ethanol. In the absence of concrete evidence to support these speculations, the authors concluded that further investigations are required to determine how cystic fluid parameters can function as surrogate markers for predicting the success of EUS-guided EA for PCNs.

While these studies support the promising therapeutic efficacy of EUS-guided EA for PCNs, this is not the case for all trials. In 2015, Gómez et al. [57] conducted a single-center, prospective pilot study of 23 patients with cystic lesions (a majority of which were MCNs or IPMNs) treated with EUS-guided EA, reporting less than 80% cyst size reduction at 6-month follow-up in 10 patients and even a 73% increase in cyst volume in one treated patient. Additionally, surveillance imaging conducted at annual intervals post-procedure revealed an increase in cyst volume in 9 treated participants. Complete cyst resolution occurred only in two patients, one of whom was diagnosed with a presumed unilocular IPMN; otherwise, 93.3% of treated IPMNs persisted on follow-up imaging. When comparing participants who achieved 80% or greater initial reduction in cyst volume to those with less than 80% reduction, the authors reported no significant differences regarding patient demographics, cyst characteristics (including initial cyst volume, cyst CEA concentrations, or number of cystic locules), or ethanol concentration between the study groups. However, the authors did report that cysts presumed to be non-mucinous in composition experienced a greater reduction in size compared to those presumed to be mucinous, supporting the findings reported by Park et al. In terms of safety, only two participants experienced complications within 24 h of treatment, including one case of pancreatitis that resulted in hospitalization. Unfortunately, one patient with presumed IPMN was diagnosed with PDAC 41 months following EUS-guided EA, with the cancer likely arising from the treated cyst despite an initial observed reduction in cyst volume of 69% after endoscopic intervention. While median radiographic follow-up in this study was cited at 37.3 months, recent large studies of patients with branch-duct IPMNs have revealed a 5-year incidence rate of pancreatic malignancy of 3.3%, which increases to 15% at 15 years post-diagnosis [60]. Since the risk for malignant degeneration of IPMNs is elevated compared to the general population even after 5 years of surveillance [60], the follow-up period of this study (as well as the other studies reviewed in this section) was likely too brief to capture the cumulative risk of malignant conversion in the study population. This unfortunate outcome therefore highlights the need for sustained follow-up of PCNs with malignant potential treated with EA to effectively monitor for the clinical goal of preventing malignant conversion and progression.

5.2. EUS-Guided Intratumoral Drug Delivery for the Treatment of PCNs

The efficacy of EUS-guided intratumoral drug delivery for the treatment of PCNs has been reported in several observational trials [6,7,61–63] and a randomized trial [64] (Table 2). Oh et al. [7] first described the feasibility and safety of EUS-guided paclitaxel injection following EA of 14 PCNs at a single center in 2008. This procedure was safely performed in all but one patient, with only one reported case of mild acute pancreatitis that resolved with supportive care. Additionally, at mean follow-up of 9 months, complete resolution was observed in 11 patients, with the authors reporting better treatment response in smaller cysts less than 3 mL in volume. The same group subsequently performed a larger prospective study of 52 patients with PCNs in 2011 that observed the outcomes of a similar treatment algorithm of EA followed by paclitaxel injection [6]. At mean follow-up of 21.7 months, complete resolution was achieved in 29 patients, with univariate analysis describing smaller EUS-measured cyst diameter and volume as predictors of treatment success. Although this study did not reveal an association between the presence of cystic septa and the likelihood of post-treatment resolution, the same group performed a 2009 study of 10 patients with oligo-septated PCNs who underwent EUS-guided EA followed by paclitaxel injection [61]. While complete resolution was observed in 6 patients, post-operative evaluation of persistent cysts resected from two patients revealed remnant neoplastic epithelial lining in missed locules, suggesting that cyst morphology may play an important role in proper candidate selection for EUS-guided chemical ablation.

Table 2. Summary of Results for Selected Studies Utilizing EUS-Guided Intratumoral Drug Delivery for PCN Ablation.

Author	Study Year	Ablative Strategy	Number of Treated Patients	Number of Treated Lesions			Efficacy on Follow-Up Imaging **, n (%)			Adverse Events, (n)
				MCN	IPMN	Other *	Incomplete Response	Partial Response	Complete Response	
Oh et al. [7]	2008	Ethanol (88–99%) + Paclitaxel	14	2	0	12	1 (7)	2 (14)	11 (79)	Mild abdominal pain (1); Acute pancreatitis (1)
Oh et al. [61]	2009	Ethanol (99%) + Paclitaxel	10	3	0	7	2 (20)	2 (20)	6 (60)	Acute pancreatitis (1)
Oh et al. [6]	2011	Ethanol (99%) + Paclitaxel	52	9	0	43	12 (25)	6 (13)	29 (62)	Fever without infection (1); Mild abdominal pain (1); Acute pancreatitis (1); Splenic vein obliteration (1); Peri-cystic spillage (1)
Choi et al. [62]	2017	Ethanol (99%) + Paclitaxel	164	71	11	82	13 (8)	31 (20)	114 (72)	Fever without infection (1); Peri-cystic spillage (1); Intra-cystic bleeding (1); Acute pancreatitis (6); Pseudocyst formation (2); Abscess formation (2); Portal vein thrombosis (1); Splenic vein obliteration (1); MPD stricture (1)
Kim et al. [63]	2017	Ethanol (100%) or Ethanol (100%) + Paclitaxel	8 (Ethanol) 28 (Ethanol + Paclitaxel)	16	14	6	8 (24)	7 (20)	19 (56)	Mild abdominal pain (4); Acute pancreatitis (4); Intra-cystic bleeding (1)
Moyer et al. [64]	2017	Ethanol (80%) + Paclitaxel + Gemcitabine	18	9	27	3	3 (17)	4 (22)	11 (61)	Mild abdominal pain (4); Acute pancreatitis (1)
		Saline + Paclitaxel + Gemcitabine	21				4 (19)	3 (14)	14 (67)	None

* The designation of "Other" includes patients treated in the above studies for cystic lesions that are non-neoplastic (i.e., pseudocysts), neoplastic without malignant potential (i.e., SCNs), or indeterminate based on pre-procedural analysis. Although the scope of this review focuses on the use of EUS-guided ablative procedures in the treatment of neoplastic cysts capable of malignant transformation (i.e., MCNs and IPMNs), this column is included in the table for the purpose of completeness. ** Complete response is defined as the radiographic absence of residual lesion on post-procedural imaging. Incomplete response is defined as either persistent or enlarged residual lesion on post-procedural imaging. If the study authors noted reduction in lesion size without resolution on post-procedural imaging, this is considered a partial response; if this was not recorded by the study authors, these lesions are categorized as incomplete response.

In 2017, Choi et al. [62] investigated the long-term durability of EUS-guided chemical ablation of PCNs with ethanol and paclitaxel by conducting a single-center, prospective study of 164 patients with median follow-up of one- and 6-years duration. At one-year follow-up, the authors reported complete cyst resolution in 72.2% of participants, with subsequent multivariate analysis revealing cyst diameter less than 35 mm and absence of septation as significant predictors of complete response. Interestingly, cystic lesions presumed to be IPMNs based on pre-procedural fluid analysis displayed the lowest rate of complete resolution (only 50%, compared to 76.1% of MCNs), supporting the results previously reported by Park et al. [58] suggesting that therapy of an IPMN may not be the optimal indication for EUS-guided chemical ablation. Of the 114 patients with complete cyst resolution at one-year post-procedure, radiologic cyst recurrence was noted in only 2 patients at a median follow-up of 72 months with no reported cases of malignancy during this time. Given complete cyst resolution in 98.3% of participants at long-term follow-up, the authors concluded that EUS-guided chemical ablation of PCNs with ethanol and paclitaxel induces a durable treatment response; however, the presence of recurrence in a small number of patients indicates the need for surveillance imaging post-procedure.

In 2017, Kim et al. [63] sought to evaluate the sonographic and cytological changes associated with EUS-guided PCN ablation, designing a prospective, single-center study of 36 patients with benign-appearing cysts who received therapy with ethanol alone (8 patients) or with a combination of ethanol and paclitaxel (28 patients). Although not specifically designed to compare these two chemical ablative regimens, this study revealed that the combination of ethanol and paclitaxel increased the quantity but decreased the quality of cystic DNA after EUS-guided ablation. The authors owed this finding to likely increased epithelial cell turnover after ablation, as well as the potential influx of inflammatory cells into cystic fluid as a response to one or both ablative agents. These findings supported a previous observation that EUS-guided chemical ablation may eliminate mutant cystic DNA [45].

To determine whether alcohol is required for effective PCN ablation, Moyer et al. [64] conducted a single-center, double-blind, randomized controlled trial of 39 patients with mucinous-type pancreatic cysts who first received EUS-guided lavage with either ethanol or normal saline, followed by an infusion of paclitaxel and gemcitabine. Despite a previously postulated synergistic effect between the two substrates, there was no statistically significant difference in complete ablation rates at one-year follow-up between those who underwent alcohol-free chemical ablation versus those who first received ethanol lavage. Additionally, no serious adverse events were observed in the alcohol-free group, while one case of acute pancreatitis was reported in the ethanol arm. These results suggest that alcohol is not required for successful ablation if an effective antitumor chemical agent is used in its place, and that alcohol's addition to a chemotherapeutic substrate may incur a higher complication rate. Thus, the removal of ethanol from EUS-guided chemotherapeutic regimens may preserve clinical efficacy while mitigating side effects.

While these prior studies sought to measure the efficacy and durability of EUS-guided intratumoral drug delivery based on post-procedural radiographic cyst resolution, An et al. [65] recently reported the histopathologic characteristics of 12 surgically resected PCNs following EUS-guided local ablation with ethanol and/or paclitaxel. Based on pre-treatment imaging, a majority (84%) of these lesions were believed to be MCNs, with a mean cyst size that was similar pre- and post-procedure. Therefore, all 12 participants underwent surgical resection at a median of 18 months following initial ablation, with subsequent pathologic examination revealing 8 cases (67%) with either complete absence of or <5% residual lining epithelia. Based on these results, the authors concluded that, when compared to untreated MCNs, pancreatic cysts treated with EUS-guided local ablation may display wider areas of cystic walls free from covering lining epithelium. Although the clinical implications of the study cannot be extrapolated given the small sample size, these results suggest that EUS-guided chemical ablation with ethanol and/or paclitaxel likely induces histologic cystic changes on the tissue level that can be present even in the absence of a complete or partial radiographic response.

5.3. EUS-Guided RFA for the Treatment of PCNs

Although less studied than EA, the efficacy of EUS-guided RFA for the treatment of PCNs has been reported in several observational trials [11,66–68] (Table 3). In 2015,

Pai et al. [11] designed the first multicenter pilot study that investigated the safety and feasibility of using EUS-guided RFA to treat PCNs in the head of the pancreas of 6 patients. Follow-up imaging was obtained 3–6 months post-procedure, which revealed complete cyst resolution in 2 patients and partial response with 48.4% reduction in cyst size in 3 patients. In terms of safety, only 2 patients experienced mild abdominal pain that resolved within 3 days post-procedure, but there were no episodes of pancreatitis, perforation, or bleeding.

Table 3. Summary of Results for Selected Studies Utilizing EUS-Guided RFA for PCN Therapy.

Author	Study Year	Number of Treated Patients	Number of Treated Lesions			Efficacy on Follow-Up Imaging **, n (%)			Adverse Events, (n)
			MCN	IPMN	Other *	Incomplete Response	Partial Response	Complete Response	
Pai et al. [11]	2015	6	4	1	1	0 (0)	4 (67)	2 (33)	Mild abdominal pain (2)
Barthet et al. [66]	2019	17	1	16	0	5 (29)	1 (6)	11 (65)	Jejunal perforation (1)
Oh et al. [68]	2021	13	0	0	13	5 (38)	8 (62)	0 (0)	Mild abdominal pain (1)
Younis et al. [67]	2022	5	1	4	0	1 (20)	1 (20)	3 (60)	Mild abdominal pain (2); Acute pancreatitis (1)

* The designation of "Other" includes patients treated in the above studies for cystic lesions that are non-neoplastic (i.e., pseudocysts), neoplastic without malignant potential (i.e., SCNs), or indeterminate based on pre-procedural analysis. Although the scope of this review focuses on the use of EUS-guided ablative procedures in the treatment of neoplastic cysts capable of malignant transformation (i.e., MCNs and IPMNs), this column is included in the table for the purpose of completeness. ** Complete response is defined as the radiographic absence of residual lesion on post-procedural imaging. Incomplete response is defined as either persistent or enlarged residual lesion on post-procedural imaging. If the study authors noted reduction in lesion size without resolution on post-procedural imaging, this is considered a partial response; if this was not recorded by the study authors, these lesions are categorized as incomplete response.

In 2019, Barthet et al. [66] designed a multicenter, prospective study of 17 patients with either an IPMN or a MCN who were treated with EUS-guided RFA, a new procedure for two of the sites included in the investigation. The primary objective of this study was to assess for procedural safety, with a secondary outcome of observing antitumor effect. Due to post-procedural complications observed in the first two patients (one of whom was being treated for a pNET, not a PCN), the group introduced a procedural prophylaxis of rectal diclofenac and antibiotic coverage with amoxicillin-clavulanic acid for all subsequent patients. Overall, this resulted in improved outcomes, with no additional serious complications of pancreatitis, perforations, or infections in those receiving treatment for their PCNs. The procedure also proved to be efficacious, with a complete response observed in 8 patients at six-month follow-up that increased to 11 patients at one-year. Interestingly, the authors attributed this increased response at one-year to the immunostimulatory effects of residual tumoral antigen produced through RFA-induced necrosis and cell death.

In 2022, Younis et al. [67] conducted a prospective single-center study of 5 patients with either an IPMN or a MCN who were treated with EUS-guided RFA after prophylaxis with the same regimen described in Barthet et al. Results revealed complete response in 3 patients and only 3 cases of relatively minor complications. Taken together, these two studies support the safety and technical feasibility of EUS-guided RFA for the treatment of mucinous cysts, although their small sample sizes, short follow-up, and lack of a control arm limit their clinical impact.

Departing from these studies, Oh et al. [68] sought to evaluate the feasibility and safety of EUS-guided RFA for the treatment of SCNs in particular, designing a prospective study of 13 patients who underwent single or multiple sessions of RFA intervention with follow-up imaging approximately 9 months post-procedure. Although no participants had complete cyst resolution, partial response with cystic volume reduction by 66% was observed in 8 patients, along with an acceptable adverse event rate of one case of mild, self-resolving abdominal pain. The authors speculated that the seemingly lower efficacy observed in their study was due to the complex morphology of the treated cysts, as they all had a honeycomb appearance with multiple septations that may have prevented heat delivery into multiple locules.

5.4. EUS-Guided EA for the Treatment of pNETs

The feasibility, efficacy, and safety of EUS-guided local EA for the treatment of pNETs (especially insulinomas) has been reported in several observational trials [31,69–71] (Table 4). In 2012, Levy et al. [69] performed the first retrospective study of 5 patients with either sporadic or multiple endocrine neoplasia 1-associated insulinomas who underwent two or more sessions of EUS-guided chemical ablation with 95–99% ethanol. At median follow-up of 13 months following their last session, 3 patients reported complete resolution of their hypoglycemic symptoms (although one patient was still taking daily diazoxide), while the other 2 reported marked improvement in the frequency and severity of their symptoms. Additionally, there were no intraprocedural or postprocedural complications observed in these participants, thereby supporting the safety of this intervention. Nonetheless, the study was limited by its small sample size, its absence of standardized follow-up imaging to monitor for treatment-induced morphologic response, and its retrospective, uncontrolled design.

Table 4. Summary of Results for Selected Studies Utilizing EUS-Guided EA for pNET Therapy.

Author	Study Year	Ablative Strategy	Number of Treated Patients	Number of Treated Lesions		Efficacy on Follow-Up Imaging *, n (%)		Adverse Events, (n)
				Insulinoma	Non-Functional pNET	Incomplete Response	Complete Response	
Levy et al. [69]	2012	Ethanol (95–99%)	5	5	0	N/A **	N/A **	None
Park et al. [31]	2015	Ethanol (99%)	11	4	10	5 (38)	8 (62)	Mild abdominal pain (1); Acute pancreatitis (3); MPD stricture (1)
Choi et al. [70]	2018	Ethanol (99%) + Lipiodol	33	1	39	16 (40)	24 (60)	Acute pancreatitis (2)
Matsumoto et al. [71]	2020	Ethanol	5	0	5	1 (20)	4 (80)	None

* Complete response is defined as the radiographic absence of residual lesion on post-procedural imaging. Incomplete response is defined as either persistent or enlarged residual lesion on post-procedural imaging. ** No follow-up imaging was obtained to assess therapeutic efficacy, although 3 of 5 patients reported post-procedural resolution of hypoglycemic symptoms.

To assess the feasibility and safety of this intervention, Park et al. [31] performed a retrospective analysis of a prospectively collected database of 11 patients with 14 pNETs (4 insulinomas and 10 non-functional pNETs) who were treated with one or more sessions of EUS-guided EA. Of the patients who underwent a single treatment session, 3-month radiographic follow-up revealed complete resolution in 7 tumors; three tumors that had not resolved were subjected to re-ablation, after which the total number of tumors with complete response was increased to 8 (or, 61.5% of all tumors at follow-up). Additionally, both patients who received treatment for their insulinomas reported complete resolution of hypoglycemic symptoms at follow-up. Based on these results, the authors deemed EUS-guided EA a technically feasible intervention for the treatment of pNETs specifically in those who refuse surgery or who are deemed to be poor surgical candidates. In terms of safety, 3 patients experienced acute pancreatitis immediately post-procedure; one of these patients was subsequently found to have a MPD stricture requiring stent placement. Interestingly, all patients who developed pancreatitis received more than 2 mL of ethanol in a single session, suggesting a potential dose-dependent response to ethanol-related toxicity on local healthy parenchyma.

In an effort to mitigate these complications, Choi et al. [70] designed a prospective study of 33 patients with 40 pathologically confirmed pNETs who underwent one or more sessions of EUS-guided chemical ablation with a mixture of ethanol and lipiodol. When combined with ethanol, lipiodol (an iodized poppy seed oil) had previously shown promise as an ablative agent in the chemoembolization of unresectable hepatocellular carcinoma [72,73], working to occlude microvasculature while also serving as a contrast agent for detection of drug delivery. Compared to Park et al., Choi et al. reported a comparatively lower rate of adverse events (3.6%); the authors attributed this phenomenon to the presence of the fatty acid lipiodol, which enhanced chemical retention in the tumor without leakage into surrounding parenchyma. Furthermore, lipiodol retention within the tumor following EUS-guided EA served as a significant predictor of complete ablation (p = 0.004), thereby supporting the use of post-procedural lipiodol retention seen on CT or fluoroscopic imaging as an early predictor of interventional success.

More recently, Matsumoto et al. [71] sought to investigate the efficacy of early EUS-guided ethanol reinjection for patients with pNETs, designing a prospective pilot study of 5 patients with small pNETs who all underwent initial EA with subsequent contrast-enhanced CT imaging conducted 3 days post-procedure; for the 3 patients with residual enhancement, an additional session of EA was conducted while the patient was still hospitalized. Results revealed complete ablation without recurrence at one-year follow-up in 4 patients (80%), and there were no reported complications in those who received early reinjection. Although this study supported the safety and feasibility of this protocol, the absence of a large sample population, the lack of a comparative group, and the short follow-up duration limited its clinical impact.

5.5. EUS-Guided RFA for the Treatment of pNETs

There exists a robust and rapidly growing body of literature reporting the feasibility, safety, and efficacy of EUS-guided RFA for the treatment of pNETs, with a review of selected studies summarized below [11,66,74–77] (Table 5). Pai et al. [11] performed the first multicenter prospective pilot study assessing the feasibility of EUS-guided RFA for the treatment of 2 patients with non-functional NETs of the pancreatic head. On follow-up cross sectional imaging, a change in the tumor vascularity was noted in one patient, while two sessions of RFA in the second patient resulted in an area of central tumor necrosis. Importantly, no adverse events were noted in these patients, demonstrating the safety of the procedure. Several years later in 2019, Barthet et al. [66] conducted a larger prospective multicenter trial of 12 patients with 14 non-functional pNETs treated with EUS-guided RFA, reporting complete radiographic resolution at one-year follow-up in 85.7% of tumors. Two serious complications were noted in this study: one case of acute pancreatitis with an area of infected necrosis, which was observed in a patient who did not receive prophylaxis of amoxicillin-clavulanic acid and rectal diclofenac; the second was a case of MPD stenosis in a patient who did receive prophylaxis, requiring treatment with endoscopic stenting. Taken together, these studies supported the efficacy and favorable safety profile of using EUS-guided RFA to treat pre-malignant non-functional pNETs.

Oleinikov et al. [74] conducted an even larger retrospective multicenter study of 18 adult patients with 27 neuroendocrine lesions (including insulinomas and non-functional pNETs) treated with EUS-guided RFA. In terms of technical feasibility, 96% of tumors were successfully ablated based on EUS visualization immediately post-procedure, while one tumor experienced incomplete ablation due to its proximity to the MPD. Compared to prior studies, Oleinikov et al. included 7 patients with functional pNETs, thereby evaluating the efficacy of EUS-guided RFA in the treatment of symptoms related to hormone over-production. The authors reported that all study participants with insulinomas achieved immediate symptom relief and euglycemia within one hour of the procedure. Additionally, this treatment response was durable, as no symptom recurrence was noted by any of the patients at a mean follow-up of 9.7 months. Two cases of mild acute pancreatitis were noted and resolved with conservative treatment within an average of 3 days. Importantly, this study included 5 patients who were initially offered serial surveillance imaging of their incidentally diagnosed, small, and asymptomatic non-functional pNETs, but refused due to the emotional burden of a "wait and see" approach. Thus, while prior studies mainly included participants who were poor operative candidates, Oleinikov et al. demonstrated that EUS-guided RFA is a safe and feasible approach for those seeking a more definitive alternative to surveillance for the treatment of their incidental pNETs.

Table 5. Summary of Results for Selected Studies Utilizing EUS-Guided RFA for pNET Therapy.

Author	Study Year	Number of Treated Patients	Number of Treated Lesions		Efficacy on Follow-Up Imaging *, n (%)			Adverse Events, (n)
			Insulinoma	Non-Functional pNET	Incomplete Response	Partial Response	Complete Response	
Pai et al. [11]	2015	2	0	2	0 (0)	2 (100) **	0 (0)	None
Barthet et al. [66]	2019	12	0	14	2 (14)	0 (0)	12 (86)	Acute pancreatitis with necrosis and bacteremia (1); MPD stenosis (1)
Oleinikov et al. [74]	2019	18	9	18	1 (4)	0 (0)	26 (96)	Acute pancreatitis (2)
Marx et al. [75]	2022	7	7	0	0 (0)	0 (0)	6 (100)	Mild abdominal pain (1); Acute pancreatitis (2); Coagulation necrosis of the superior mesenteric vein (1); Retro-gastric collection resulting in death (1)
Marx et al. [76]	2022	27	0	27	0 (0)	2 (7)	25 (93)	Mild abdominal pain (3); Acute pancreatitis (4); Periprocedural bleeding (2); Pseudocyst formation (1); Pancreatic fistula formation (1); MPD stricture (1)
Figueiredo et al. [77]	2022	29 ***	13	10	2 (18)	3 (27)	6 (55)	Mild abdominal pain (4); Acute pancreatitis (3); MPD stenosis (1); Periprocedural bleeding (1); Gastric wall hematoma (1); Fever without infection (1)

* Complete response is defined as the radiographic absence of residual lesion on post-procedural imaging. Incomplete response is defined as either persistent or enlarged residual lesion on post-procedural imaging. If the study authors noted reduction in lesion size without resolution on post-procedural imaging, this is considered a partial response; if this was not recorded by the study authors, these lesions are categorized as incomplete response. ** Although complete lesion resolution was not observed, cross-sectional imaging revealed changes in tumor vascularity in one patient and central necrosis of the tumor in the other. *** This number of treated patients reflects the inclusion of one case of PDAC and 11 metastatic lesions in 6 patients who were subjected to EUS-guided RFA as part of the study population. These patients are not included in the columns displaying tumor efficacy but are included in the adverse events column.

Marx et al. [75] conducted a retrospective review of EUS-guided RFA specifically for the treatment of insulinomas at two tertiary referral centers, reporting the periprocedural safety and outcomes for 7 patients with radiographic follow-up via magnetic resonance imaging (MRI)/CT. Prior to the procedure, all participants endorsed episodic symptomatic hypoglycemia with significant impact on quality of life that necessitated frequent hospitalization. However, post-procedure, all patients reported immediate symptom relief accompanied by euglycemia that persisted throughout follow-up, with complete tumor resolution observed in 6 patients at 12–18 months post-procedure. However, safety was a concern in this study, with one patient developing acute pancreatitis despite preventive stent placement due to the tumor's proximity to the MPD, while another developed an area of coagulative necrosis because of the tumor's proximity to the superior mesenteric vein. Unfortunately, a frail elder patient was found to have a retro-gastric collection two weeks post-procedure, which ultimately resulted in her death prior to evaluation for treatment response.

The same group [76] conducted a much larger multicenter retrospective review of 27 patients with non-functional pNETs, reporting excellent efficacy with complete resolution of 93% of tumors after one or more sessions of EUS-guided RFA at a mean follow-up of 15.7 months. Relevant complications included three cases of acute pancreatitis, one of which resulted in pseudocyst formation and two of which required cystogastrostomy for drainage of retro-gastric/retro-splenic collections. The authors could not identify a single unequivocal risk factor for the development of pancreatitis, although they suggested the possibility of exploring a step-up approach for larger lesions to reduce adverse events generated by single sessions aimed at complete ablation.

Most recently, Figueiredo et al. [77] conducted a large, prospective multicenter study that evaluated the safety and clinical efficacy of EUS-guided RFA of 29 patients with a spectrum of 35 pancreatic and peripancreatic tumors, including 10 non-functional pNETs, 13 insulinomas, 1 PDAC, and 11 intra-pancreatic and extra-pancreatic metastatic lesions (largely arising from metastatic lung and renal carcinoma). Of the 15 pNETs with 6-month follow-up, 73.3% showed a significant response to intervention with either complete necrosis or greater than 50% size reduction on imaging. In terms of clinical response for those receiving therapy of their functional pNETs, 100% of cases resulted in immediate resolution of hypoglycemia post-procedure, with no symptom recurrence during median follow-up of 9.5 months. Thus, Figueiredo et al. concluded that functional pNETs were seemingly the best indication for EUS-guided RFA therapy, reporting high efficacy in symptom reduction along with an acceptable safety profile.

6. Complications of EUS-Guided Local Ablative Therapies

As detailed in the above studies, EUS-guided local ablative therapies are associated with a spectrum of mild to severe adverse events. Complications may arise from the endoscopic technique, including perforation, infection, and hemorrhage [66]. Additionally, treatment of cystic structures with chemical substrate can lead to peri-cystic spillage and intra-cystic hemorrhage [62,63]. While ultrasound-guidance allows for targeted delivery of ablative substrates to pathologic tissue, complications can also arise when normal parenchyma is damaged. Acute pancreatitis is a commonly described complication that is largely responsive to supportive treatment; however, progression to pancreatic necrosis [66] or MPD stenosis requiring stent placement [31,62,66] has been described. In particular, EUS-guided EA of branch duct IPMNs raises concern for extravasation given the presence of a widely patent communication with the adjacent ductal system, thereby increasing the risk of complications such as MPD stenosis [5]; as a result, some consensus guidelines have considered the presence of communicating IPMNs as a contraindication to EUS-guided EA [20]. Pancreatic pseudocyst formation has been described as a complication of EUS-guided RFA [76], which can increase the risk of future infection, hemorrhage, rupture, or ductal disruption. Finally, given the proximity of the pancreas to the portal venous system, EUS-guided treatment of cysts close to venous structures can lead to chemical extravasation and subsequent portal vein thrombosis [62] or splenic vein obstruction [6,62].

7. Limitations in EUS-Guided Local Ablative Therapies for Pancreatic Pathology

Despite the promising results of EUS-guided local ablative therapies as detailed in the above studies, there are important considerations that limit the quality of evidence in the current literature. Several of the aforementioned studies suffer from a limited, unrandomized sample population, thereby reducing the generalizability and clinical impact of their reported results. Additionally, many studies lack the long-term follow-up that is necessary to adequately monitor for PCN or pNET resolution post-procedure. As in Gómez et al. [57], there exists the possibility of malignant progression despite initial EUS-guided therapy, which may not be observed within the limited follow-up reported in the current literature. In fact, for PCNs of malignant potential in particular, some guidelines recommend surveillance cross-sectional imaging at 6-month intervals for the first year post-procedure, followed by annual imaging until patient co-morbidities and age limit the survival benefit of surveillance [25]; unfortunately, the vast majority of the above studies do not provide this duration of follow-up, and therefore the results may overstate the efficacy of ablation in the short term. Nearly all studies are observational in nature and are thereby limited by the absence of a control arm, which would be useful for comparing outcomes among those who opt for surgical management or conservative surveillance over EUS-guided local therapy. Finally, treatment response in the literature is typically monitored via interval change in tumor dimensions on cross-sectional imaging. Since this method does not necessarily confirm complete histopathologic ablation on the tissue level, it may be inadequate to assess the true efficacy of EUS-guided intervention in generating complete tumor necrosis and regression.

As a technique, EUS-guided ablation is limited in its therapeutic scope by important technical and safety considerations. Firstly, although procedural side effects are typically manageable, there remains a risk for serious complications, including MPD stenosis, pancreatic necrosis, bowel perforation, and even death. More data are necessary to assess how clinician expertise and institutional volume affect the frequency of these observed complications. Secondly, EUS-guided local ablation is limited in its ability to definitively address advanced local and metastatic disease, as extensive lymph node dissection is not yet technically feasible with endoscopy. Finally, in comparison to surgical intervention, the absence of resected specimen that can be assessed for tumor margins limits the extent to which EUS-guided ablative therapy can be considered as a form of definitive management for neoplastic pathology.

While many of the above studies sought to investigate the safety, technical feasibility, and efficacy of EUS-guided local ablative therapies, their results raised important inquiries for future clinical research. There remains a question of the efficacy of EUS-guided alcohol ablation specifically for the indication of pancreatic IPMNs, with evidence suggesting a decreased propensity for cyst reduction following intervention when compared to outcomes for MCN ablation [58,62]. Perhaps more importantly, the malignant progression of a treated IPMN observed in Gómez et al. [57] highlights the notion that size reduction does not necessarily correlate with decreased risk of future malignancy [25]; therefore, post-procedural surveillance remains an important consideration for future investigation to determine the long-term outcomes and clinical utility of EUS-guided ablation for IPMNs. Together, these results have led some international consensus guidelines to avoid recommending EUS-guided EA for the treatment of IPMNs outside of the context of a controlled research protocol until future data is available [20]. Additionally, data is limited concerning the proper course of action for therapeutic intervention of cysts in close proximity to the MPD, with some studies reporting prophylactic placement of an endoscopic stent to prevent acute pancreatitis post-treatment [75]. Finally, while some studies reported the apparent effects of cyst morphology (especially the presence of septations [61,68]) on treatment efficacy, comparative trials are necessary to understand the specific clinical features that predict treatment success to optimize candidate selection.

8. New Horizons: Future Applications of EUS-Guided Local Ablation

While this study has largely focused on the literature of EUS-guided chemical ablation and RFA for the treatment of PCNs and pNETs, there are exciting new horizons for the technical and therapeutic scope of this minimally invasive intervention.

8.1. New Ablative Techniques to Address Pancreatic Pathology

Apart from RFA and chemical ablation with ethanol and/or paclitaxel/gemcitabine, new ablative techniques are currently being investigated and are in various stages of clinical application. In addition to the intratumoral injection of chemotherapeutic agents, chemical ablation with the sclerosant agent lauromacrogol has recently shown efficacy in the local therapy of PCNs [78]. By inducing severe local inflammation and intramural fibrosis of vascular structures, lauromacrogol has previously been utilized in the mechanical obliteration of gastric varices in patients with liver cirrhosis [79]. It has also been applied to the clinical treatment of hepatic cysts [80] and the experimental therapy of endometrial cysts in an animal model [81]. In 2017, Linghu et al. [78] was the first group to assess the safety and efficacy of EUS-guided PCN ablation with lauromacrogol in 29 patients with imaging follow-up at a mean of 9 months post-procedure. The authors reported complete resolution in 37.9% of participants, with mild procedural complications occurring in 3 patients. Given the absence of severe adverse events, the authors concluded that EUS-guided local ablation with lauromacrogol is a safe intervention, with the potential added benefit of providing intra- and post-operative pain relief due to its mild anesthetic effect. The same group [82] conducted a study of the long-term outcomes of EUS-guided lauromacrogol ablation in 55 patients with median follow-up of 15 months, reporting a similar rate of complete cyst resolution of 47.3%. Despite its promising safety profile, the resolution rate noted in the aforementioned studies appears to be similar to the lower rates of effective ablation seen with ethanol [25,83], and therefore chemical ablation with ethanol or chemotherapeutic substrate largely remains the preferred technique. Additionally, both studies specifically excluded patients with IPMNs, thereby limiting the therapeutic scope of this modality.

The feasibility of EUS-guided laser ablation (LA) of pancreatic tissue with the neodymium-doped yttrium aluminum garnet laser was initially demonstrated in a pig model in 2010, where it was shown to induce localized tissue necrosis with the advantage of great precision [84]. By utilizing a finer needle, EUS-guided LA has become an attractive option for the treatment of lesions in high-risk areas or locations that are more technically difficult to access [85]. In 2018, Di Matteo et al. [86] proved the feasibility of this intervention in 9 patients with unresectable PDAC, demonstrating technical success in all patients without adverse events. Since its introduction to clinical application, EUS-guided LA has undergone changes in technical design, including the development of cylindrical interstitial laser ablation (CILA). This technique uses a diffusing application to help ablate tissue in a circular shape, thereby minimizing thermal damage to healthy parenchyma [87]. Although not in clinical use, EUS-guided CILA was demonstrated to be technically feasible in a porcine model of locally advanced PDAC, generating large areas of uniform ablation without significant complications [88].

Microwave ablation (MWA) is based on the production of frictional heat through the oscillation of dipole molecules, thereby inducing consistent and homogenous energy delivery to a discrete area of tissue [89]. Despite several studies demonstrating the safety and feasibility of percutaneous MWA on locally advanced pancreatic head cancer [90,91], EUS-guided MWA remains largely in the experimental phase of investigation, with one case report reporting technical success of the intervention in a poor surgical candidate with an unresectable neuroendocrine tumor of the pancreas [89].

Finally, EUS-guided cryoablation, often used in combination with RFA, was initially shown to be technically feasible in a porcine pancreas in 2008 [92], with subsequent studies demonstrating its safety and efficacy in patients with local advanced pancreatic cancer [93].

8.2. Growing Pathologic Scope of EUS-Guided Ablative Application

EUS-guided local ablation has been shown to be a technically feasible therapeutic option for patients with unresectable PDAC [94,95]. PDAC generally has a poor prognosis, with a 5-year overall survival of approximately 9% [96]. In large part, this is because most patients present with locally advanced or metastatic disease at the time of diagnosis, which limits therapeutic options including surgery, chemotherapy, or chemoradiation. EUS-guided local ablative therapies (namely, RFA) have emerged as promising treatment alternatives for PDAC, especially for those who are poor surgical candidates or with surgically unresectable tumors. When used in combination with other conventional antitumor interventions such as chemotherapy, EUS-guided RFA has been shown to potentially improve survival outcomes in patients with PDAC [97]. By shrinking tumor size, EUS-guided therapy has the added benefit of controlling local complications of malignancy bulk including pain and biliary obstruction, improving patient quality of life and providing a form of palliation for those who do not desire aggressive therapy [98].

9. Conclusions

EUS-guided local ablative therapies have shown promising technical feasibility, safety, and efficacy in the treatment of neuroendocrine and cystic neoplasms of the pancreas. In harnessing the antitumor effects of chemical toxicity and hyperthermia, EUS-guided chemical ablation and RFA balance targeted tissue necrosis with potential side effects on adjacent healthy parenchyma. These complications are mitigated by the benefits of real-time image guidance, close clinical follow-up, and careful selection of appropriate procedural candidates. To date, observational studies have demonstrated high clinical success of EUS-guided RFA and chemical ablation in the treatment of lesions with malignant potential, and emerging evidence highlights the growing technical and therapeutic scope of this minimally invasive intervention. Additional research is needed to determine the optimal procedural, demographic, and pathologic features that predict positive clinical outcomes.

Author Contributions: Conceptualization, A.M.P. and T.A.G.; methodology, A.M.P. and T.A.G.; investigation, A.M.P.; resources, T.A.G.; writing—original draft preparation, A.M.P.; writing—review and editing, A.M.P. and T.A.G.; visualization, A.M.P.; supervision, T.A.G.; project administration, T.A.G. All authors have read and agreed to the published version of the manuscript.

Funding: This research received no external funding.

Institutional Review Board Statement: Not applicable.

Informed Consent Statement: Not applicable.

Data Availability Statement: Not applicable.

Conflicts of Interest: The authors declare no conflict of interest.

References

1. Kahl, S.; Glasbrenner, B.; Zimmermann, S.; Malfertheiner, P. Endoscopic ultrasound in pancreatic diseases. *Dig. Dis.* **2002**, *20*, 120–126. [CrossRef] [PubMed]
2. Mekky, M.A.; Abbas, W.A. Endoscopic ultrasound in gastroenterology: From diagnosis to therapeutic implications. *World J. Gastroenterol.* **2014**, *20*, 7801–7807. [CrossRef] [PubMed]
3. Saraireh, H.A.; Bilal, M.; Singh, S. Role of endoscopic ultrasound in liver disease: Where do we stand in 2017? *World J. Hepatol.* **2017**, *9*, 1013–1021. [CrossRef] [PubMed]
4. Gonzalo-Marin, J.; Vila, J.J.; Perez-Miranda, M. Role of endoscopic ultrasound in the diagnosis of pancreatic cancer. *World J. Gastrointest. Oncol.* **2014**, *6*, 360–368. [CrossRef] [PubMed]
5. Gan, S.I.; Thompson, C.C.; Lauwers, G.Y.; Bounds, B.C.; Brugge, W.R. Ethanol lavage of pancreatic cystic lesions: Initial pilot study. *Gastrointest. Endosc.* **2005**, *61*, 746–752. [CrossRef]
6. Oh, H.-C.; Seo, D.W.; Song, T.J.; Moon, S.; Park, D.H.; Lee, S.S.; Lee, S.K.; Kim, M.; Kim, J. Endoscopic ultrasonography-guided ethanol lavage with paclitaxel injection treats patients with pancreatic cysts. *Gastroenterology* **2011**, *140*, 172–179. [CrossRef]
7. Oh, H.-C.; Seo, D.W.; Lee, T.Y.; Kim, J.Y.; Lee, S.S.; Lee, S.K.; Kim, M.-H. New treatment for cystic tumors of the pancreas: EUS-guided ethanol lavage with paclitaxel injection. *Gastrointest. Endosc.* **2008**, *67*, 636–642. [CrossRef]
8. Lakhtakia, S.; Seo, D.W. Endoscopic ultrasonography-guided tumor ablation. *Dig. Endosc.* **2017**, *29*, 486–494. [CrossRef]
9. Cho, M.K.; Choi, J.H.; Seo, D.W. Endoscopic ultrasound-guided ablation therapy for pancreatic cysts. *Endosc. Ultrasound* **2015**, *4*, 293–298. [CrossRef]
10. Adamska, A.; Domenichini, A.; Falasca, M. Pancreatic Ductal Adenocarcinoma: Current and Evolving Therapies. *Int. J. Mol. Sci.* **2017**, *18*, 1338. [CrossRef]
11. Pai, M.; Habib, N.; Senturk, H.; Lakhtakia, S.; Reddy, N.; Cicinnati, V.R.; Kaba, I.; Beckebaum, S.; Drymousis, P.; Kahaleh, M.; et al. Endoscopic ultrasound guided radiofrequency ablation, for pancreatic cystic neoplasms and neuroendocrine tumors. *World J. Gastrointest. Surg.* **2015**, *7*, 52–59. [CrossRef]
12. Birkmeyer, J.D.; Sun, Y.; Wong, S.L.; Stukel, T.A. Hospital volume and late survival after cancer surgery. *Ann. Surg.* **2007**, *245*, 777–783. [CrossRef]
13. Jürgensen, C.; Schuppan, D.; Neser, F.; Ernstberger, J.; Junghans, U.; Stölzel, U. EUS-guided alcohol ablation of an insulinoma. *Gastrointest. Endosc.* **2006**, *63*, 1059–1062. [CrossRef]
14. Zanini, N.; Giordano, M.; Smerieri, E.; D'Abruzzo, G.C.; Guidi, M.; Pazzaglini, G.; De Luca, F.; Chiaruzzi, G.; Vitullo, G.; Piva, P.; et al. Estimation of the prevalence of asymptomatic pancreatic cysts in the population of San Marino. *Pancreatology* **2015**, *15*, 417–422. [CrossRef]
15. Zhang, W.Y.; Li, Z.S.; Jin, Z.D. Endoscopic ultrasound-guided ethanol ablation therapy for tumors. *World J. Gastroenterol.* **2013**, *19*, 3397–3403. [CrossRef]
16. Levink, I.; Bruno, M.J.; Cahen, D.L. Management of Intraductal Papillary Mucinous Neoplasms: Controversies in Guidelines and Future Perspectives. *Curr. Treat. Options Gastroenterol.* **2018**, *16*, 316–332. [CrossRef]
17. Yao, J.C.; Eisner, M.P.; Leary, C.; Dagohoy, C.; Phan, A.; Rashid, A.; Hassan, M.; Evans, D.B. Population-based study of islet cell carcinoma. *Ann. Surg. Oncol.* **2007**, *14*, 3492–3500. [CrossRef]
18. Ma, Z.-Y.; Gong, Y.-F.; Zhuang, H.-K.; Zhou, Z.-X.; Huang, S.-Z.; Zou, Y.-P.; Huang, B.; Sun, Z.-H.; Zhang, C.-Z.; Tang, Y.-Q.; et al. Pancreatic neuroendocrine tumors: A review of serum biomarkers, staging, and management. *World J. Gastroenterol.* **2020**, *26*, 2305–2322. [CrossRef]

19. Fernández-del Castillo, C.; Targarona, J.; Thayer, S.P.; Rattner, D.W.; Brugge, W.R.; Warshaw, A.L. Incidental pancreatic cysts: Clinicopathologic characteristics and comparison with symptomatic patients. *Arch. Surg.* **2003**, *138*, 427–434. [CrossRef]
20. Tanaka, M.; Fernández-del Castillo, C.; Kamisawa, T.; Jang, J.Y.; Levy, P.; Ohtsuka, T.; Salvia, R.; Shimizu, Y.; Tada, M.; Wolfgang, C.L. Revisions of international consensus Fukuoka guidelines for the management of IPMN of the pancreas. *Pancreatology* **2017**, *17*, 738–753. [CrossRef]
21. Cho, C.S.; Russ, A.J.; Loeffler, A.G.; Rettammel, R.J.; Oudheusden, G.; Winslow, E.R.; Weber, S.M. Preoperative classification of pancreatic cystic neoplasms: The clinical significance of diagnostic inaccuracy. *Ann. Surg. Oncol.* **2013**, *20*, 3112–3119. [CrossRef] [PubMed]
22. Buerlein, R.C.D.; Shami, V.M. Management of pancreatic cysts and guidelines: What the gastroenterologist needs to know. *Ther. Adv. Gastrointest. Endosc.* **2021**, *14*, 26317745211045769. [CrossRef] [PubMed]
23. Scheiman, J.M.; Hwang, J.H.; Moayyedi, P. American gastroenterological association technical review on the diagnosis and management of asymptomatic neoplastic pancreatic cysts. *Gastroenterology* **2015**, *148*, 824–848.e22. [CrossRef]
24. Caillol, F.; Poincloux, L.; Bories, E.; Cruzille, E.; Pesenti, C.; Darcha, C.; Poizat, F.; Monges, G.; Raoul, J.L.; Bommelaer, G.; et al. Ethanol lavage of 14 mucinous cysts of the pancreas: A retrospective study in two tertiary centers. *Endosc. Ultrasound* **2012**, *1*, 48–52. [CrossRef] [PubMed]
25. Teoh, A.Y.-B.; Seo, D.W.; Brugge, W.; Dewitt, J.; Kongkam, P.; Linghu, E.; Moyer, M.T.; Ryu, J.K.; Ho, K.Y. Position statement on EUS-guided ablation of pancreatic cystic neoplasms from an international expert panel. *Endosc. Int. Open* **2019**, *7*, E1064–E1077. [CrossRef] [PubMed]
26. Perri, G.; Prakash, L.R.; Katz, M.H.G. Pancreatic neuroendocrine tumors. *Curr. Opin. Gastroenterol.* **2019**, *35*, 468–477. [CrossRef] [PubMed]
27. Shah, M.H.; Goldner, W.S.; Benson, A.B.; Bergsland, E.; Blaszkowsky, L.S.; Brock, P.; Chan, J.; Das, S.; Dickson, P.V.; Fanta, P.; et al. Neuroendocrine and Adrenal Tumors, Version 2.2021, NCCN Clinical Practice Guidelines in Oncology. *J. Natl. Compr. Cancer Netw.* **2021**, *19*, 839–868. [CrossRef]
28. Sallinen, V.; Le Large, T.Y.; Galeev, S.; Kovalenko, Z.; Tieftrunk, E.; Araujo, R.; Ceyhan, G.O.; Gaujoux, S. Surveillance strategy for small asymptomatic non-functional pancreatic neuroendocrine tumors—A systematic review and meta-analysis. *HPB* **2017**, *19*, 310–320. [CrossRef]
29. Falconi, M.; Bartsch, D.K.; Eriksson, B.; Klöppel, G.; Lopes, J.M.; O'Connor, J.M.; Salazar, R.; Taal, B.G.; Vullierme, M.P.; O'Toole, D. ENETS Consensus Guidelines for the management of patients with digestive neuroendocrine neoplasms of the digestive system: Well-differentiated pancreatic non-functioning tumors. *Neuroendocrinology* **2012**, *95*, 120–134. [CrossRef]
30. Larghi, A.; Rizzatti, G.; Rimbaş, M.; Crino, S.F.; Gasbarrini, A.; Costamagna, G. EUS-guided radiofrequency ablation as an alternative to surgery for pancreatic neuroendocrine neoplasms: Who should we treat? *Endosc. Ultrasound* **2019**, *8*, 220–226. [CrossRef]
31. Park, D.H.; Choi, J.-H.; Oh, D.; Lee, S.S.; Seo, D.-W.; Lee, S.K.; Kim, M.-H. Endoscopic ultrasonography-guided ethanol ablation for small pancreatic neuroendocrine tumors: Results of a pilot study. *Clin. Endosc.* **2015**, *48*, 158–164. [CrossRef] [PubMed]
32. Howe, J.R.; Merchant, N.B.; Conrad, C.; Keutgen, X.M.; Hallet, J.; Drebin, J.A.; Minter, R.M.; Lairmore, T.C.; Tseng, J.F.; Zeh, H.J.; et al. The North American Neuroendocrine Tumor Society Consensus Paper on the Surgical Management of Pancreatic Neuroendocrine Tumors. *Pancreas* **2020**, *49*, 1–33. [CrossRef] [PubMed]
33. Halfdanarson, T.R.; Rabe, K.G.; Rubin, J.; Petersen, G.M. Pancreatic neuroendocrine tumors (PNETs): Incidence, prognosis and recent trend toward improved survival. *Ann. Oncol.* **2008**, *19*, 1727–1733. [CrossRef] [PubMed]
34. El Sayed, G.; Frim, L.; Franklin, J.; McCrudden, R.; Gordon, C.; Al-Shamma, S.; Kiss, S.; Hegyi, P.; Erőss, B. Endoscopic ultrasound-guided ethanol and radiofrequency ablation of pancreatic insulinomas: A systematic literature review. *Therap. Adv. Gastroenterol.* **2021**, *14*, 17562848211042171. [CrossRef] [PubMed]
35. Vilmann, P.; Jacobsen, G.K.; Henriksen, F.W.; Hancke, S. Endoscopic ultrasonography with guided fine needle aspiration biopsy in pancreatic disease. *Gastrointest. Endosc.* **1992**, *38*, 172–173. [CrossRef]
36. Bennedbaek, F.N.; Hegedüs, L. Treatment of recurrent thyroid cysts with ethanol: A randomized double-blind controlled trial. *J. Clin. Endocrinol. Metab.* **2003**, *88*, 5773–5777. [CrossRef]
37. El Masry, H.; Breall, J.A. Alcohol septal ablation for hypertrophic obstructive cardiomyopathy. *Curr. Cardiol. Rev.* **2008**, *4*, 193–197. [CrossRef]
38. Larssen, T.B.; Jensen, D.K.; Viste, A.; Horn, A. Single-session alcohol sclerotherapy in symptomatic benign hepatic cysts. Long-term results. *Acta Radiol.* **1999**, *40*, 636–638. [CrossRef]
39. Völk, M.; Rogler, G.; Strotzer, M.; Lock, G.; Manke, C.; Feuerbach, S. Post-traumatic pseudocyst of the spleen: Sclerotherapy with ethanol. *Cardiovasc. Interv. Radiol.* **1999**, *22*, 246–248. [CrossRef]
40. Schurmann, P.; Peñalver, J.; Valderrábano, M. Ethanol for the treatment of cardiac arrhythmias. *Curr. Opin. Cardiol.* **2015**, *30*, 333–343. [CrossRef]
41. Gelczer, R.K.; Charboneau, J.W.; Hussain, S.; Brown, D.L. Complications of percutaneous ethanol ablation. *J. Ultrasound Med.* **1998**, *17*, 531–533. [CrossRef]
42. Baker, R.C.; Kramer, R.E. Cytotoxicity of short-chain alcohols. *Annu. Rev. Pharmacol. Toxicol.* **1999**, *39*, 127–150. [CrossRef]

43. Celikoglu, S.I.; Celikoglu, F.; Goldberg, E.P. Endobronchial intratumoral chemotherapy (EITC) followed by surgery in early non-small cell lung cancer with polypoid growth causing erroneous impression of advanced disease. *Lung Cancer* 2006, *54*, 339–346. [CrossRef]
44. Hader, W.J.; Steinbok, P.; Hukin, J.; Fryer, C. Intratumoral therapy with bleomycin for cystic craniopharyngiomas in children. *Pediatr. Neurosurg.* 2000, *33*, 211–218. [CrossRef]
45. DeWitt, J.M.; Al-Haddad, M.; Sherman, S.; LeBlanc, J.; Schmidt, C.M.; Sandrasegaran, K.; Finkelstein, S.D. Alterations in cyst fluid genetics following endoscopic ultrasound-guided pancreatic cyst ablation with ethanol and paclitaxel. *Endoscopy* 2014, *46*, 457–464. [CrossRef]
46. Akhan, O.; Güler, E.; Akıncı, D.; Çiftçi, T.; Köse, I.Ç. Radiofrequency ablation for lung tumors: Outcomes, effects on survival, and prognostic factors. *Diagn. Interv. Radiol.* 2016, *22*, 65–71. [CrossRef]
47. Koo, J.S.; Chung, S.H. The Efficacy of Radiofrequency Ablation for Bone Tumors Unsuitable for Radical Excision. *Clin. Orthop. Surg.* 2021, *13*, 278–285. [CrossRef]
48. Jindal, G.; Friedman, M.; Locklin, J.; Wood, B.J. Palliative radiofrequency ablation for recurrent prostate cancer. *Cardiovasc. Interv. Radiol.* 2006, *29*, 482–485. [CrossRef]
49. Wah, T.M.; Irving, H.C.; Gregory, W.; Cartledge, J.; Joyce, A.D.; Selby, P.J. Radiofrequency ablation (RFA) of renal cell carcinoma (RCC): Experience in 200 tumours. *BJU Int.* 2014, *113*, 416–428. [CrossRef]
50. Gaidhane, M.; Smith, I.; Ellen, K.; Gatesman, J.; Habib, N.; Foley, P.; Moskaluk, C.; Kahaleh, M. Endoscopic Ultrasound-Guided Radiofrequency Ablation (EUS-RFA) of the Pancreas in a Porcine Model. *Gastroenterol. Res. Pract.* 2012, *2012*, 431451. [CrossRef]
51. Yousaf, M.N.; Ehsan, H.; Muneeb, A.; Wahab, A.; Sana, M.K.; Neupane, K.; Chaudhary, F.S. Role of Radiofrequency Ablation in the Management of Unresectable Pancreatic Cancer. *Front. Med.* 2021, *7*, 624997. [CrossRef] [PubMed]
52. Matsui, Y.; Nakagawa, A.; Kamiyama, Y.; Yamamoto, K.; Kubo, N.; Nakase, Y. Selective thermocoagulation of unresectable pancreatic cancers by using radiofrequency capacitive heating. *Pancreas* 2000, *20*, 14–20. [CrossRef] [PubMed]
53. Girelli, R.; Frigerio, I.; Giardino, A.; Regi, P.; Gobbo, S.; Malleo, G.; Salvia, R.; Bassi, C. Results of 100 pancreatic radiofrequency ablations in the context of a multimodal strategy for stage III ductal adenocarcinoma. *Langenbecks Arch. Surg.* 2013, *398*, 63–69. [CrossRef] [PubMed]
54. Dromi, S.A.; Walsh, M.P.; Herby, S.; Traughber, B.; Xie, J.; Sharma, K.V.; Sekhar, K.P.; Luk, A.; Liewehr, D.J.; Dreher, M.R.; et al. Radiofrequency ablation induces antigen-presenting cell infiltration and amplification of weak tumor-induced immunity. *Radiology* 2009, *251*, 58–66. [CrossRef] [PubMed]
55. DeWitt, J.; DiMaio, C.J.; Brugge, W.R. Long-term follow-up of pancreatic cysts that resolve radiologically after EUS-guided ethanol ablation. *Gastrointest. Endosc.* 2010, *72*, 862–866. [CrossRef]
56. DiMaio, C.J.; DeWitt, J.M.; Brugge, W.R. Ablation of pancreatic cystic lesions: The use of multiple endoscopic ultrasound-guided ethanol lavage sessions. *Pancreas* 2011, *40*, 664–668. [CrossRef]
57. Gómez, V.; Takahashi, N.; Levy, M.J.; McGee, K.P.; Jones, A.; Huang, Y.; Chari, S.T.; Clain, J.E.; Gleeson, F.C.; Pearson, R.K.; et al. EUS-guided ethanol lavage does not reliably ablate pancreatic cystic neoplasms (with video). *Gastrointest. Endosc.* 2016, *83*, 914–920. [CrossRef]
58. Park, J.K.; Song, B.J.; Ryu, J.K.; Paik, W.H.; Park, J.M.; Kim, J.; Lee, S.H.; Kim, Y.-T. Clinical Outcomes of Endoscopic Ultrasonography-Guided Pancreatic Cyst Ablation. *Pancreas* 2016, *45*, 889–894. [CrossRef]
59. DeWitt, J.; McGreevy, K.; Schmidt, C.M.; Brugge, W.R. EUS-guided ethanol versus saline solution lavage for pancreatic cysts: A randomized, double-blind study. *Gastrointest. Endosc.* 2009, *70*, 710–723. [CrossRef]
60. Oyama, H.; Tada, M.; Takagi, K.; Tateishi, K.; Hamada, T.; Nakai, Y.; Hakuta, R.; Ijichi, H.; Ishigaki, K.; Kanai, S.; et al. Long-term Risk of Malignancy in Branch-Duct Intraductal Papillary Mucinous Neoplasms. *Gastroenterology* 2020, *158*, 226–237.e5. [CrossRef]
61. Oh, H.-C.; Seo, D.W.; Kim, S.C.; Yu, E.; Kim, K.; Moon, S.-H.; Park, D.H.; Lee, S.S.; Lee, S.K.; Kim, M.-H. Septated cystic tumors of the pancreas: Is it possible to treat them by endoscopic ultrasonography-guided intervention? *Scand. J. Gastroenterol.* 2009, *44*, 242–247. [CrossRef]
62. Choi, J.-H.; Seo, D.W.; Song, T.J.; Park, D.H.; Lee, S.S.; Lee, S.K.; Kim, M.-H. Long-term outcomes after endoscopic ultrasound-guided ablation of pancreatic cysts. *Endoscopy* 2017, *49*, 866–873. [CrossRef]
63. Kim, K.H.; McGreevy, K.; La Fortune, K.; Cramer, H.; DeWitt, J. Sonographic and cyst fluid cytologic changes after EUS-guided pancreatic cyst ablation. *Gastrointest. Endosc.* 2017, *85*, 1233–1242. [CrossRef]
64. Moyer, M.T.; Sharzehi, S.; Mathew, A.; Levenick, J.M.; Headlee, B.D.; Blandford, J.T.; Heisey, H.D.; Birkholz, J.H.; Ancrile, B.B.; Maranki, J.L.; et al. The Safety and Efficacy of an Alcohol-Free Pancreatic Cyst Ablation Protocol. *Gastroenterology* 2017, *153*, 1295–1303. [CrossRef]
65. An, S.; Sung, Y.N.; Kim, S.J.; Seo, D.W.; Jun, S.Y.; Hong, S.M. Pancreatic Cysts after Endoscopic Ultrasonography-Guided Ethanol and/or Paclitaxel Ablation Therapy: Another Mimic of Pancreatic Pseudocysts. *Pathobiology* 2022, *89*, 49–55. [CrossRef]
66. Barthet, M.; Giovannini, M.; Lesavre, N.; Boustiere, C.; Napoleon, B.; Koch, S.; Gasmi, M.; Vanbiervliet, G.; Gonzalez, J.-M. Endoscopic ultrasound-guided radiofrequency ablation for pancreatic neuroendocrine tumors and pancreatic cystic neoplasms: A prospective multicenter study. *Endoscopy* 2019, *51*, 836–842. [CrossRef]
67. Younis, F.; Shor, D.B.-A.; Lubezky, N.; Geva, R.; Osher, E.; Shibolet, O.; Phillips, A.; Scapa, E. Endoscopic ultrasound-guided radiofrequency ablation of premalignant pancreatic-cystic neoplasms and neuroendocrine tumors: Prospective study. *Eur. J. Gastroenterol. Hepatol.* 2022, *34*, 1111–1115. [CrossRef]

68. Oh, D.; Ko, S.W.; Seo, D.-W.; Hong, S.-M.; Kim, J.H.; Song, T.J.; Park, D.H.; Lee, S.K.; Kim, M.-H. Endoscopic ultrasound-guided radiofrequency ablation of pancreatic microcystic serous cystic neoplasms: A retrospective study. *Endoscopy* **2021**, *53*, 739–743. [CrossRef]
69. Levy, M.J.; Thompson, G.B.; Topazian, M.D.; Callstrom, M.R.; Grant, C.S.; Vella, A. US-guided ethanol ablation of insulinomas: A new treatment option. *Gastrointest. Endosc.* **2012**, *75*, 200–206. [CrossRef]
70. Choi, J.; Park, D.H.; Kim, M.; Hwang, H.S.; Hong, S.; Song, T.J.; Lee, S.S.; Seo, D.; Lee, S.K. Outcomes after endoscopic ultrasound-guided ethanol-lipiodol ablation of small pancreatic neuroendocrine tumors. *Dig. Endosc.* **2018**, *30*, 652–658. [CrossRef]
71. Matsumoto, K.; Kato, H.; Kawano, S.; Fujiwara, H.; Nishida, K.; Harada, R.; Fujii, M.; Yoshida, R.; Umeda, Y.; Hinotsu, S.; et al. Efficacy and safety of scheduled early endoscopic ultrasonography-guided ethanol reinjection for patients with pancreatic neuroendocrine tumors: Prospective pilot study. *Dig. Endosc.* **2020**, *32*, 425–430. [CrossRef] [PubMed]
72. Yu, S.C.; Hui, J.W.; Hui, E.P.; Mo, F.; Lee, P.S.; Wong, J.; Lee, K.F.; Lai, P.B.; Yeo, W. Embolization efficacy and treatment effectiveness of transarterial therapy for unresectable hepatocellular carcinoma: A case-controlled comparison of transarterial ethanol ablation with lipiodol-ethanol mixture versus transcatheter arterial chemoembolization. *J. Vasc. Interv. Radiol.* **2009**, *20*, 352–359. [CrossRef] [PubMed]
73. Yu, S.C.; Hui, E.P.; Wong, J.; Wong, H.; Mo, F.; Ho, S.S.; Wong, Y.Y.; Yeo, W.; Lai, P.B.; Chan, A.T.; et al. Transarterial ethanol ablation of hepatocellular carcinoma with lipiodol ethanol mixture: Phase II study. *J. Vasc. Interv. Radiol.* **2008**, *19*, 95–103. [CrossRef] [PubMed]
74. Oleinikov, K.; Dancour, A.; Epshtein, J.; Benson, A.; Mazeh, H.; Tal, I.; Matalon, S.; A Benbassat, C.; Livovsky, D.M.; Goldin, E.; et al. Endoscopic Ultrasound-Guided Radiofrequency Ablation: A New Therapeutic Approach for Pancreatic Neuroendocrine Tumors. *J. Clin. Endocrinol. Metab.* **2019**, *104*, 2637–2647. [CrossRef]
75. Marx, M.; Trosic-Ivanisevic, T.; Caillol, F.; Demartines, N.; Schoepfer, A.; Pesenti, C.; Ratone, J.-P.; Robert, M.; Giovannini, M.; Godat, S. EUS-guided radiofrequency ablation for pancreatic insulinoma: Experience in 2 tertiary centers. *Gastrointest. Endosc.* **2022**, *95*, 1256–1263. [CrossRef]
76. Marx, M.; Godat, S.; Caillol, F.; Poizat, F.; Ratone, J.; Pesenti, C.; Schoepfer, A.; Hoibian, S.; Dahel, Y.; Giovannini, M. Management of non-functional pancreatic neuroendocrine tumors by endoscopic ultrasound-guided radiofrequency ablation: Retrospective study in two tertiary centers. *Dig. Endosc.* **2022**, *34*, 1207–1213. [CrossRef]
77. Ferreira, M.F.; Garces-Duran, R.; Eisendrath, P.; Devière, J.; Deprez, P.; Monino, L.; Van Laethem, J.-L.; Borbath, I. EUS-guided radiofrequency ablation of pancreatic/peripancreatic tumors and oligometastatic disease: An observational prospective multicenter study. *Endosc. Int. Open* **2022**, *10*, E1380–E1385. [CrossRef]
78. Linghu, E.; Du, C.; Chai, N.; Li, H.; Wang, Z.; Sun, Y.; Xu, W.; Guo, X.; Ning, B.; Sun, L.; et al. A prospective study on the safety and effectiveness of using lauromacrogol for ablation of pancreatic cystic neoplasms with the aid of EUS. *Gastrointest. Endosc.* **2017**, *86*, 872–880. [CrossRef]
79. Luo, X.; Ma, H.; Yu, J.; Zhao, Y.; Wang, X.; Yang, L. Efficacy and safety of balloon-occluded retrograde transvenous obliteration of gastric varices with lauromacrogol foam sclerotherapy: Initial experience. *Abdom. Radiol.* **2018**, *43*, 1820–1824. [CrossRef]
80. Xue, J.; Geng, X. Curative effect of lauromacrogol and absolute ethyl alcohol injection guided by ultrasound on simplex hepatic cyst. *Pak. J. Pharm. Sci.* **2015**, *28*, 697–700.
81. Liu, W.; Wang, L.; Guo, C.X. The effects of lauromacrogol injection into rat endometrial cysts: A preliminary experimental study. *Arch. Gynecol. Obstet.* **2016**, *294*, 555–559. [CrossRef]
82. Du, C.; Chai, N.; Linghu, E.; Li, H.; Feng, X.; Ning, B.; Wang, X.; Tang, P. Long-term outcomes of EUS-guided lauromacrogol ablation for the treatment of pancreatic cystic neoplasms: 5 years of experience. *Endosc. Ultrasound* **2022**, *11*, 44–52. [CrossRef]
83. Gaballa, D.; Moyer, M. Thoughts of the safety and efficacy of EUS-guided cyst ablation with the use of lauromacrogol. *Gastrointest. Endosc.* **2018**, *87*, 1367. [CrossRef]
84. Di Matteo, F.; Martino, M.; Rea, R.; Pandolfi, M.; Rabitti, C.; Masselli, G.M.P.; Silvestri, S.; Pacella, C.M.; Papini, E.; Panzera, F.; et al. EUS-guided Nd:YAG laser ablation of normal pancreatic tissue: A pilot study in a pig model. *Gastrointest. Endosc.* **2010**, *72*, 358–363. [CrossRef]
85. Francica, G.; Petrolati, A.; Di Stasio, E.; Pacella, S.; Stasi, R.; Pacella, C.M. Effectiveness, safety, and local progression after percutaneous laser ablation for hepatocellular carcinoma nodules up to 4 cm are not affected by tumor location. *AJR Am. J. Roentgenol.* **2012**, *199*, 1393–1401. [CrossRef]
86. Di Matteo, F.M.; Saccomandi, P.; Martino, M.; Pandolfi, M.; Pizzicannella, M.; Balassone, V.; Schena, E.; Pacella, C.M.; Silvestri, S.; Costamagna, G. Feasibility of EUS-guided Nd:YAG laser ablation of unresectable pancreatic adenocarcinoma. *Gastrointest. Endosc.* **2018**, *88*, 168–174.e1. [CrossRef]
87. Truong, V.G.; Jeong, S.; Park, J.-S.; Tran, V.N.; Kim, S.M.; Lee, D.H.; Kang, H.W. Endoscopic ultrasound (EUS)-guided cylindrical interstitial laser ablation (CILA) on *in vivo* porcine pancreas. *Biomed. Opt. Express* **2021**, *12*, 4423–4437. [CrossRef]
88. Lim, S.; Truong, V.G.; Choi, J.; Jeong, H.J.; Oh, S.-J.; Park, J.-S.; Kang, H.W. Endoscopic Ultrasound-Guided Laser Ablation Using a Diffusing Applicator for Locally Advanced Pancreatic Cancer Treatment. *Cancers* **2022**, *14*, 2274. [CrossRef]
89. Robles-Medranda, C.; Arevalo-Mora, M.; Oleas, R.; Alcivar-Vasquez, J.; Del Valle, R. Novel EUS-guided microwave ablation of an unresectable pancreatic neuroendocrine tumor. *VideoGIE* **2022**, *7*, 74–76. [CrossRef]
90. Carrafiello, G.; Ierardi, A.M.; Fontana, F.; Petrillo, M.; Floridi, C.; Lucchina, N.; Cuffari, S.; Dionigi, G.; Rotondo, A.; Fugazzola, C. Microwave ablation of pancreatic head cancer: Safety and efficacy. *J. Vasc. Interv. Radiol.* **2013**, *24*, 1513–1520. [CrossRef]

91. Vogl, T.J.; Panahi, B.; Albrecht, M.H.; Naguib, N.N.N.; Nour-Eldin, N.-E.A.; Gruber-Rouh, T.; Thompson, Z.M.; Basten, L.M. Microwave ablation of pancreatic tumors. *Minim. Invasive Ther. Allied Technol.* **2018**, *27*, 33–40. [CrossRef] [PubMed]
92. Carrara, S.; Arcidiacono, P.G.; Albarello, L.; Addis, A.; Enderle, M.D.; Boemo, C.; Campagnol, M.; Ambrosi, A.; Doglioni, C.; Testoni, P.A. Endoscopic ultrasound-guided application of a new hybrid cryotherm probe in porcine pancreas: A preliminary study. *Endoscopy* **2008**, *40*, 321–326. [CrossRef] [PubMed]
93. Arcidiacono, P.G.; Carrara, S.; Reni, M.; Petrone, M.C.; Cappio, S.; Balzano, G.; Boemo, C.; Cereda, S.; Nicoletti, R.; Enderle, M.D.; et al. Feasibility and safety of EUS-guided cryothermal ablation in patients with locally advanced pancreatic cancer. *Gastrointest. Endosc.* **2012**, *76*, 1142–1151. [CrossRef] [PubMed]
94. Song, T.J.; Seo, D.W.; Lakhtakia, S.; Reddy, N.; Oh, D.W.; Park, D.H.; Lee, S.S.; Lee, S.K.; Kim, M.-H. Initial experience of EUS-guided radiofrequency ablation of unresectable pancreatic cancer. *Gastrointest. Endosc.* **2016**, *83*, 440–443. [CrossRef]
95. Scopelliti, F.; Pea, A.; Conigliaro, R.; Butturini, G.; Frigerio, I.; Regi, P.; Giardino, A.; Bertani, H.; Paini, M.; Pederzoli, P.; et al. Technique, safety, and feasibility of EUS-guided radiofrequency ablation in unresectable pancreatic cancer. *Surg. Endosc.* **2018**, *32*, 4022–4028. [CrossRef]
96. Siegel, R.L.; Miller, K.D.; Jemal, A. Cancer statistics, 2020. *CA Cancer J. Clin.* **2020**, *70*, 7–30. [CrossRef]
97. Oh, D.; Seo, D.W.; Song, T.J.; Park, D.H.; Lee, S.K.; Kim, M.H. Clinical outcomes of EUS-guided radiofrequency ablation for unresectable pancreatic cancer: A prospective observational study. *Endosc. Ultrasound* **2022**, *11*, 68–74. [CrossRef]
98. Hwang, J.S.; Joo, H.D.; Song, T.J. Endoscopic Ultrasound-Guided Local Therapy for Pancreatic Neoplasms. *Clin. Endosc.* **2020**, *53*, 535–540. [CrossRef]

Disclaimer/Publisher's Note: The statements, opinions and data contained in all publications are solely those of the individual author(s) and contributor(s) and not of MDPI and/or the editor(s). MDPI and/or the editor(s) disclaim responsibility for any injury to people or property resulting from any ideas, methods, instructions or products referred to in the content.

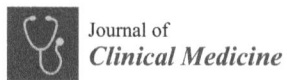

Review

The Latest Advancements in Diagnostic Role of Endosonography of Pancreatic Lesions

Jagoda Oliwia Rogowska *, Łukasz Durko and Ewa Malecka-Wojciesko

Department of Digestive Tract Diseases, Medical University of Lodz, 90-647 Lodz, Poland; lukasz.durko@umed.lodz.pl (Ł.D.); ewa.malecka-panas@umed.lodz.pl (E.M.-W.)
* Correspondence: jagoda.rogowska@stud.umed.lodz.pl

Abstract: Endosonography, a minimally invasive imaging technique, has revolutionized the diagnosis and management of pancreatic diseases. This comprehensive review highlights the latest advancements in endosonography of the pancreas, focusing on key technological developments, procedural techniques, clinical applications and additional techniques, which include real-time elastography endoscopic ultrasound, contrast-enhanced-EUS, EUS-guided fine-needle aspiration or EUS-guided fine-needle biopsy. EUS is well established for T-staging and N-staging of pancreaticobiliary malignancies, for pancreatic cyst discovery, for identifying subepithelial lesions (SEL), for differentiation of benign pancreaticobiliary disorders or for acquisition of tissue by EUS-guided fine-needle aspiration or EUS-guided fine-needle biopsy. This review briefly describes principles and application of EUS and its related techniques.

Keywords: endoscopic ultrasound; endoscopic ultrasound guided biopsy; pancreas; review

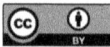

Citation: Rogowska, J.O.; Durko, Ł.; Malecka-Wojciesko, E. The Latest Advancements in Diagnostic Role of Endosonography of Pancreatic Lesions. *J. Clin. Med.* **2023**, *12*, 4630. https://doi.org/10.3390/jcm12144630

Academic Editor: Antonio M Caballero-Mateos

Received: 18 May 2023
Revised: 29 June 2023
Accepted: 5 July 2023
Published: 12 July 2023

Copyright: © 2023 by the authors. Licensee MDPI, Basel, Switzerland. This article is an open access article distributed under the terms and conditions of the Creative Commons Attribution (CC BY) license (https://creativecommons.org/licenses/by/4.0/).

1. Introduction

The origin of endoscopic ultrasound (EUS) dates to 1980, when images were obtained in dogs according to DiMagno et al. [1]. Since then, there has been significant progression in the diagnostic role of EUS, not only in its wide range of usage in pancreatic pathology but also in its safety [1]. Due to its innovative mechanism, which combines fibre-optic endoscopic and ultrasonic capabilities, EUS has become an enormously indispensable diagnostic tool for differentiation of subepithelial lesions [2]. What is more, a review of 66 studies showed that EUS was the most sensitive and specific investigation technique in identifying subepithelial lesions (SEL) < 2 cm compared to other imaging modalities such as computed tomography (CT) or magnetic resonance imaging (MRI), the sensitivities of EUS, CT and MRI were 93%, 53% and 67%, respectively [3,4].

Numerous studies have shown high sensitivity (92–100%), specificity (89–100%) and accuracy (86–99%) of EUS in the detection of pancreatic malignancies, which is higher than that of CT scan, particularly with small diameter lesions (Table 1) [5].

The increasing incidence of incidental pancreatic lesions has prompted a focus on their accurate diagnosis. These lesions, referred to as focal pancreatic lesions, can manifest as solid, cystic or mixed tumours. Solid lesions encompass a spectrum from benign (serous pancreatic cystadenoma, papillary cysts, lymphoepithelial cysts) to precancerous (intraductal papillary mucinous neoplasm (IPMN) with low-grade dysplasia, mucinous cystic neoplasm (MCN) with low-grade dysplasia, benign neuroendocrine tumours) and malignant (ductal adenocarcinoma, acinar cell carcinoma, IPMN with invasive carcinoma, cystadenocarcinoma, neuroendocrine tumours) [6,7]. Comparative diagnostic studies have evaluated various imaging techniques for characterizing focal pancreatic lesions, as presented in Table 2 of the multi-centre study by Best LM et al. [8].

Furthermore, there is an urgent need for advanced tools that not only aid in diagnosis but also facilitate tissue acquisition, forming the basis for therapeutic procedures [2]. EUS has introduced related techniques such as contrast-enhanced EUS, EUS elastography and

EUS-guided fine-needle aspiration biopsy (EUS-FNA) for tissue sampling [9]. Contrast-enhanced EUS employs contrast agents to enhance visualization of blood flow within pancreatic lesions, assisting in the differentiation of malignant and benign lesions. EUS elastography provides information about tissue stiffness, aiding in the characterization of solid and cystic lesions [10]. EUS-FNA enables real-time ultrasound-guided sampling of tissue for histological and cytological analysis, enabling a definitive diagnosis [11].

Once a diagnosis is established, the treatment approach for focal pancreatic lesions varies depending on the nature of the lesion. Benign and precancerous lesions may be managed conservatively with regular monitoring, while malignant lesions often require intervention. Treatment options encompass surgical resection, endoscopic resection, ablation techniques and systemic therapies tailored to the specific diagnosis and disease stage.

To sum up, the diagnosis of focal pancreatic lesions is crucial, and various imaging techniques have been compared for their diagnostic capabilities. EUS-related techniques, such as contrast-enhanced EUS, EUS elastography and EUS-FNA, offer valuable tools for both diagnosis and tissue acquisition. The treatment strategy depends on the nature of the lesion, ranging from conservative management to invasive interventions, ensuring personalized care for patients with focal pancreatic lesions.

Table 1. Studies on diagnostic performance of EUS versus CT for detection of pancreatic malignancy.

Study, Year	Cases	Sensitivity, EUS vs. CT (%)	Specificity, EUS vs. CT (%)
Due et al., 2017 [12]	68	98 vs. 73	NA
Kamata et al., 2014 [13]	35	100 vs. 56	100 vs. 100
Kitana et al., 2012 [14]	277	91 vs. 71	94 vs. 92

CT—computed tomography, EUS—endoscopic ultrasound, NA—not applicable.

Table 2. Different imaging techniques in characterizing pancreatic focal lesions according to Best et al. [8].

Diagnostic Technique	Cases	Sensitivity	Specificity	Post-Test Probability of Positive Test	Post-Test Probability of Negative Test
PET	99	92%	65%	86%	22%
EUS	133	95%	53%	82%	18%
EUS-FNA (cytology)	147	79%	100%	99%	32%
CT	123	98%	76%	90%	6%
MRI	29	80%	89%	94%	34%

PET—positron emission tomography, EUS—endoscopic ultrasound, FNA—fine-needle aspiration, CT—computed tomography, MRI—magnetic resonance imaging.

2. Principles of EUS-Related Techniques

2.1. Real-Time Elastography EUS (RTE-EUS)

Elastography is an imaging technique based on the evaluation of tissue stiffness, which leads to a better classification of lesions [15,16]. The principle of this method is explained by using the spring model. Under compression, hard springs are remotely deformed while soft springs compress significantly [16]. Malignant tumours are harder than benign ones [17]. There are two semi-quantitative elastography methods: SH (mean strain histograms) and strain ratio (SR) [18]. The mean strain histogram value corelates with the hardness of the lesion depicted by the colour on the scale from hardest (0) to softest (255). The system is set up to use a colour map (red-green-blue), where hard tissue areas appear as dark blue, medium hard tissue areas as cyan, intermediate tissue areas as green, medium soft tissue areas as yellow and soft tissue areas as red [15]. Elastography imaging of the normal pancreas is characterized by a homogenous green colour distribution (representing intermediate stiffness) [15]. Neuroendocrine tumours tend to be stiffer when compared to the pancreatic parenchyma, especially if they are malignant. When it comes to acute pancreatitis, the necrotic zones appear softer as compared to the stiffer surroundings [19].

In initial stages of chronic pancreatitis, a honeycomb pattern dominated by hard strands is reflected in elastography images [20].

Shear-wave elastography (SWE) is a newly introduced imaging technique that allows quantification of mechanical and elastic tissue properties. SWE uses an acoustic radiation force pulse sequence to generate shear waves, which propagate perpendicular to the ultrasound beam, causing transient displacements. What is more, shear waves propagate faster through stiffer contracted tissue [21]. SWE is able to assess the biomechanical properties of tissue; generally, malignant lesions are stiffer than the healthy parenchyma. Principal applications are determination of fibrosis and autoimmune pancreatic diseases, characterization of pancreatic lesions, guiding biopsy in the stiff part of a focal area or characterization of pancreatic gland stiffness in suspected chronic pancreatitis [22].

Giovannini et al., in a multi-centre study including 121 patients, demonstrated that the sensitivity and specificity of EUS elastography for malignancy in pancreas were 92.3% and 80%, respectively.

2.2. Contrast-Enhanced-EUS

CE-EUS is a remotely new established diagnostic examination that contains both high-resolution ultrasound and the administration of ultrasound contrast agents [23]. The technique was invented by using two different methods: contrast-enhanced endoscopic Doppler ultrasound with a high-mechanical index (CEHMI-EUS) (this one does not require special software) or the second one, which runs on the specific mode, contrast-enhanced low-MI EUS (CELMI-EUS) [23]. The introduction of contrast enhancers could provide additional information about the vascularization of the organ, which resulted in increased value of the method, especially for diagnosing necrotic pancreatic areas [23]. There are three contrast agents that are currently available: sulphur hexafluoride (SF6) gas with a lipid stabilizer shell, octafluoropropane (C3F8) with a lipid stabilizer shell or perfluorobutane (C4F10) with a lipid stabilizer shell; the last one is not available in Europe, apart from Norway and Denmark [24,25]. When the agents are administered through a peripheral vein, the microbubbles in the contrast agent receive transmitted US waves and are disrupted or stimulated to resonate, thereby producing the signal detected in the US image, which has low interferences [4]. The main elements and advantages of CE-EUS include real-time imaging of microvascularity and microperfusion, real-time intervention guidance, on-site performance ability and impressively good detail resolution [23].

Clinical applications include differential diagnosis of focal pancreatic masses and evaluation of acute and chronic pancreatitis, particularly complications associated with pancreatitis, assessment of cystic lesions, characterization of intraductal biliary/pancreatic structures gallbladder lesions, SEL, lymph node assessment and others [26,27]. Kamata et al. [13] reported that CE-EUS identified mural nodules more accurately than conventional EUS, providing sensitivity and specificity values of 97% and 75% for CE-EUS and 97% and 40% for conventional EUS. This differentiation between mural nodules and mucous clots is crucial to distinguish MCNs from IPMN [4].

CE-EUS is believed to be beneficial in differentiating pancreatic adenocarcinoma and neuroendocrine tumours [22]. According to Ishikawa T et al. [28] CE-EUS has been reported to have a high sensitivity in identifying PNETs compared to CT with values of 95% and 81%, respectively. What is more, CE-EUS detects a heterogeneous tumour texture, which is a significant sign of malignancy [29]. Due to the study conducted by Leem G et al. [30], CEH-EUS of the pancreatic solid masses showed higher sensitivity and specificity in differentiating pancreatic adenocarcinoma and neuroendocrine tumours (82.0% and 87.9% for pancreatic adenocarcinoma and 81.1% and 90.9% for neuroendocrine tumours, respectively) [13].

Less than 5% of pancreatic masses represent metastases and their differentiation from primary tumours using conventional EUS is difficult [31]. CH-EUS, due to its ability to provide information about the vascularization of the organ, can detect pancreatic metastatic lesions, which according to Teodorescu C et al. [31] are mostly hypervascular. These metastases can have a hyperenhanced aspect (renal cell carcinoma or melanoma) or a hypovascular aspect (colon cancer, breast carcinoma).

What is more CE-EUS has been reported to have better accuracy than contrast-enhanced multidetector CT (MDCT) for early diagnosis of small pancreatic cancer. In the Japanese study from 2020, the sensitivity of CE-EUS and MDCT was 91.2% and 70.6%, respectively [27,32]. CE-EUS was also significantly more accurate than the standard EUS in diagnosing malignant cysts with accuracy (84% vs. 64%).

2.3. EUS-Guided Fine-Needle Aspiration (EUS-FNA)

This technique has been used as a gastroenterological standard for sampling pancreatic solid masses, SEL and lymph nodes since 1992 [33,34]. When the aspirate is sufficient for cytology, it's accuracy ranges from 77% to 95% for pancreatic masses [35,36]. In general, 19 G–25 G calibre needles are inserted under EUS guidance for the pathological diagnosis of pancreatic cancer and lymph nodes [4]. EUS-FNA is often performed in the evaluation of pancreatic cystic lesions (PCL) for a better preoperative characterization [37]. One of the most crucial limitations of EUS-FNA is the fact that it does not provide core tissue specimens with preserved architecture, therefore immunohistochemical staining and histologic diagnosis cannot be assessed [38]. Rapid on-site evaluation (ROSE) refers to the immediate cytologic assessment after FNA by a cytopathologist, and is useful for increasing the accuracy and sample acquisition and reducing the number of needle passes in EUS-FNA [39]. Observational studies demonstrated that ROSE improved the diagnostic accuracy and tissue adequacy of EUS-FNA, particularly in solid pancreatic lesions. However, four meta-analyses suggested a modest improvement in sensitivity with ROSE, but the difference was not statistically significant, while other meta-analyses did not support the advantages of ROSE in terms of specimen adequacy and diagnostic yield [40]. Therefore, The European Society of Gastrointestinal Endoscopy panel recommends EUS-FNA with or without ROSE equally, given the conflicting evidence [41].

2.4. EUS-Guided Fine-Needle Biopsy (EUS-FNB)

In order to overcome the limitations of EUS-FNA, in the early 2000s, EUS-FNB was introduced to obtain a tissue specimen and a molecular analysis [33]. The pooled data showed EUS-guided pancreas biopsy could be a safe approach for the diagnosis of pancreatic tumours [4]. EUS-guided fine-needle biopsy uses a Franseen needle to sample considerable material with a small number of punctures [34].

Table 3 presents superiority of EUS-FNB over EUS-FNA in the diagnosis of pancreatic cancer, however, they are equivalent when it comes to detecting SEL [34].

Table 3. Comparison of EUS-FNA and EUS-FNB of diagnostic accuracy in pancreatic cancer and SEL.

Study	Cases	Ethology	Sensitivity	Specificity	Accuracy	PPV	NPV	Comments
Kuroka N et al. [34]	94	Pancreatic cancer	78.1%	100%	81.6%	-	-	EUS-FNA
Kuroka N et al. [34]	36	Pancreatic cancer	85%	100%	85.7%	-	-	EUS-FNB
Kuroka N et al. [34]	94	SEL	100%	N/A	100%	-	-	EUS-FNA
Kuroka N et al. [34]	36	SEL	100%	N/A	100%	-	-	EUS-FNB
Oppong KW et al. [42]	108	SEL	71%	-	64%	-	-	EUS-FNA
Oppong KW et al. [42]	108	SEL	82%	-	79%	-	-	EUS-FNB
De Moura DTH et al. [43]	229	SEL	51.92%	98.39%	77.19%	96.43%	70.93%	EUS-FNA
De Moura DTH et al. [43]	229	SEL	79.41%	100%	88.03%	100%	77.78%	EUS-FNB

SEL—subepithelial lesions, N/A—not assessed, PPV—positive predictive value, NPV—negative predictive value, EUS-FNA—endoscopic ultrasound guided fine-needle aspiration, EUS-FNB—endoscopic ultrasound guided fine-needle biopsy.

Although EUS-guided tissue acquisition is a standard modality for establishing a conclusive diagnosis and individualized therapeutic plan for pancreatic solid tumours, the diagnostic performance has been reported to have a wide range according to the needle type [44,45].

Based on the systematic review and network meta-analysis [46] conducted on the comparative diagnostic performance of end-cutting fine-needle biopsy (FNB) needles for tissue sampling of pancreatic masses, several key findings emerged. Franseen needles and Fork-tip needles exhibited superior diagnostic accuracy and sample adequacy compared to reverse-bevel needles and FNA needles. Among the different needle sizes, 25-gauge Franseen and Fork-tip needles did not show superiority over 22-gauge reverse-bevel needles. Importantly, when rapid onsite cytologic evaluation was available, none of the tested FNB needles demonstrated significant superiority over other FNB devices or FNA needles. Overall, Franseen and Fork-tip needles, particularly in 22-gauge size, showed the highest performance for tissue sampling of pancreatic masses. However, it is essential to note that the confidence in these estimates was low, underscoring the need for further research and validation in this field [47].

2.5. EUS-Guided Rendezvous Technique (EUS-RV)

The endoscopic ultrasound-guided rendezvous technique (EUS-RV) is a promising procedure used in gastrointestinal endoscopy when conventional methods like endoscopic retrograde cholangiopancreatography (ERCP) are not successful. EUS-RV combines EUS imaging with therapeutic intervention to achieve access to the biliary system [48].

By creating a connection between the biliary and gastrointestinal tracts, EUS-RV enables successful biliary access for diagnostic and therapeutic purposes. Using a specialized linear array echoendoscope, this technique provides high-resolution ultrasound imaging and targeted interventions. EUS-RV overcomes anatomical challenges and offers a less invasive option for patients who may not be suitable candidates for ERCP [49].

The procedure involves inserting the echoendoscope, visualizing the biliary tree and puncturing the gastrointestinal wall under ultrasound guidance. A guidewire is then placed into the bile duct, creating a pathway for subsequent interventions. EUS-RV has shown success in cases of difficult biliary cannulation, altered anatomy and previous surgeries [49].

EUS-RV is a valuable technique used in the management of pancreatic ascites resulting from pancreatic duct (PD) leaks. While PD disruption and resultant ascites are more commonly associated with chronic pancreatitis, it is rare in cases of acute necrotizing pancreatitis. Medical therapy, surgical management or endotherapy are the available options for managing pancreatic ascites [50,51].

Factors that contribute to a successful EUS-RV procedure have been identified, with a dilated PD being essential for optimal outcomes. However, the literature lacks reports on EUS-guided rendezvous in a nondilated PD. The procedure offers a potential solution for cases where ERCP fails to achieve selective cannulation, allowing for successful access to the PD and subsequent endotherapy [50,51].

EUS-RV has shown promise as an effective technique for managing pancreatic ascites associated with PD leaks. By utilizing the capabilities of EUS, this procedure provides a minimally invasive approach to accessing the PD and facilitating appropriate intervention. Further research and clinical experience are necessary to refine the technique and identify the optimal patient selection criteria for successful EUS-RV in both dilated and nondilated PDs [50].

3. EUS in Pancreatic Pathologies

3.1. Pancreatic Cancer

Pancreatic cancer is currently the seventh leading cause of cancer death worldwide [52]. The five-year survival rate is exceptionally low—less than 10% [53]. Unfortunately, due to the huge progress in surgery, most of the cases are diagnosed at an advanced stage, so as a result only few patients can be qualified for surgery. What is more, this kind of treatment is still associated with high post-operative morbidity [52]. The commonly used term "pancreatic cancer" usually refers to ductal adenocarcinoma (PDAC), which represents 85% of all pancreatic tumours. Despite the ongoing developments, surgery is still associated with high post-operative morbidity [54].

EUS is considered to be the most sensitive technique to detect early neoplasia in the pancreas, which is presented as a hypoechoic mass with irregular borders. Typically, the dilatation of the proximal PD occurs. Unfortunately, when it comes to evaluation of distant metastasis, CT is superior to EUS [54]. The most widely used technique for the initial evaluation is the CT scan, with a sensitivity between 76% and 92%. Nonetheless, the sensitivity of EUS in detecting pancreatic lesions is around 98%, therefore it is the most sensitive technique for the detection of small pancreatic tumours [55]. Maguchi et al. [56] compared different imaging techniques for pancreatic cancer with a diameter < 2 cm and found that transabdominal ultrasound, CT and EUS had a sensitivity of 52.4%, 42.8% and 95.2%, respectively. What is more, EUS is superior to conventional imaging techniques due to such advantages as the lack of dosing ionizing radiation to the patient and the absence of contraindications such as metal implants or claustrophobia [57].

Since the EUS was invented, it has been also used to visualize a pancreas mass directly, secure a definitive cytologic or histologic diagnosis, define the degree of tumour-vascular involvement and more [58].

Conventional EUS functions may be enhanced by the newer related technique—EUS elastography. For instance, to obtain a histologic diagnosis and to provide material for molecular testing, EUS elastography can be merged with EUS-FNB in order to guide the biopsy. What is more, one of the recent prospective single-centre studies showed that EUS-FNA had a sensitivity, specificity and accuracy of 77.8%, 100% and 84% for pancreatic cancer diagnosis, respectively [59]. However, there is a possibility to achieve a higher diagnostic rate by combining real-time tissue elastography (RTE) with EUS-FNA, which was reported to have diagnostic accuracy, sensitivity and specificity of 94.4%, 93.4% and 100%, respectively [60].

According to recent clinical research, EUS-elastography, based on mean strain histogram and mass elasticity, is able to distinguish benign from malignant pancreatic tumours with a high sensitivity (Table 4) [15,61]. During EUS elastography, one trapezoidal region of interest (ROI) containing at least 50% of the lesion is manually selected. To calculate SH, a smaller round ROI is selected at the level of the focal lesion without the need to include a reference area [18]. The mean SH value represents the overall hardness of a lesion, with lower values (<80) being predictive of malignancy and higher values (>80) predictive of benign lesions. Combined CE-EUS (where the lesion is hypovascular) and SH with a cut-off value of 80 have shown to be the most specific and sensitive diagnostic method (98.6% and 81.4%, respectively) for detecting pancreatic carcinoma, according to Costache MI et al. [18] the average sensitivity of mean SH values ranges from 85% to 96%, while specificity ranges from 64% to 76% in detecting pancreatic tumours [18].

Table 4. Meta-analysis in EUS-elastography to distinguish benign from malignant solid pancreatic masses.

Study	Cases	Sensitivity	Specificity	Diagnostic Odds Ratio	Comments
Zhang B et al. [62]	1044	95%	67%	42.28%	EUS elastography
Lu Y et al. [63]	1544 lesions	97%	67%	-	Qualitative methods
Lu Y et al. [63]	1544 lesions	97%	67%	-	Strain histograms
Lu Y et al. [63]	1544 lesions	98%	62%	-	Strain ratio

EUS—endoscopic ultrasound.

Figure 1 presents pancreatic adenocarcinoma adjacent tdetected using EUS-elastography.

The results of a recent meta-analysis showed pooled estimates of sensitivity and specificity of CEH EUS for pancreatic cancer diagnosis at 93% and 80%, respectively [57].

Moreover, to discriminate tumour lesions from inflammatory pancreatic masses, contrast-enhanced EUS may be used. When it generates an acoustic signal, as mentioned above, it helps in the assessment of vascularity of pancreatic masses in addition to providing information about the echogenicity of the lesions [5]. Iso-enhancement or hypo-enhancement, arterial irregularity and absent venous vasculature within a mass are typical for pancreatic PDAC, whereas hyper-enhanced lesions with the preserved architecture point to chronic pancreatitis [64–66]. CE-EUS can differentiate pancreatitis from pancreatic cancer with sensitivity, specificity, positive predictive value and negative predictive values of 91%, 93%, 100% and 88%, respectively [5].

The differences in diagnostic abilities of RTE-EUS and CE-EUS are shown in Table 5.

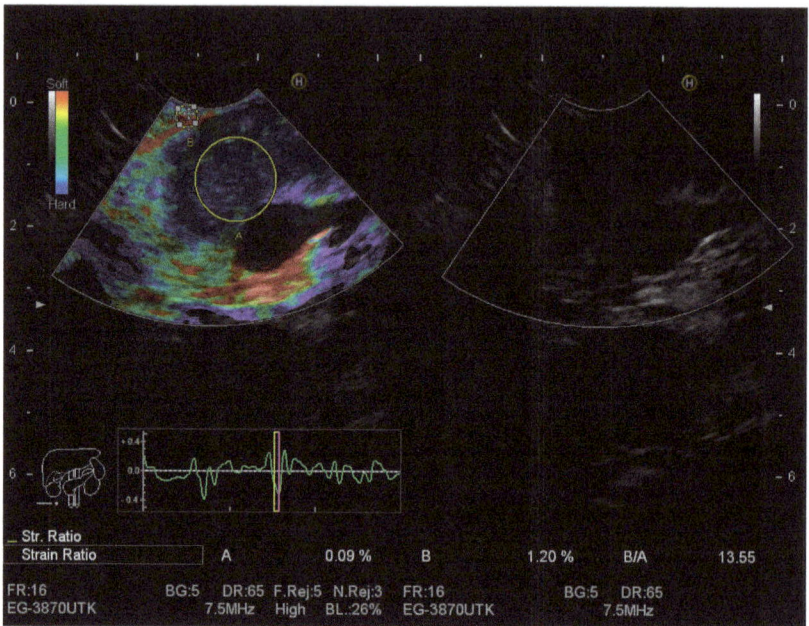

Figure 1. EUS–elastography; A. pancreatic adenocarcinoma adjacent to the splenic vein (yellow circle) with strain ratio on; B. without strain ratio.

Table 5. Studies in CE-EUS and real-time elastography for pancreatic cancer.

Study	Cases	Ethology	Sensitivity	Specificity	Accuracy	PPV	NPV	Comments
Costache MI et al. [18]	97	Pancreatic cancer	100%	29.63%	80.41%	78.65%	100%	Real-time EUS elastography
Costache MI et al. [18]	97	Pancreatic cancer	98.57%	77.78%	92.78%	92%	95.45%	CE-EUS
Costache MI et al. [18]	97	Pancreatic cancer	98.57%	98.57%	93.81%	-	-	Combining CE-EUS and EUS elastography

EUS-endoscopic ultrasound, N/A-not assessed, PPV-positive predictive value, NPV-negative predictive value, CE-EUS-contrast enhanced endoscopic ultrasound.

3.2. Pancreatic Neuroendocrine Tumours

Pancreatic neuroendocrine tumours (PNETS) are 7–10% of all pancreatic solid lesions. A majority of them (50–60%) are not secreting NETS [14]. Neuroendocrine tumours are malignant lesions that arise from neuroendocrine cells. They mostly occur in the gastrointestinal tract (48%), lung (25%) and pancreas (9%) [67]. Among the secreting endocrine tumours affecting the pancreas, insulinomas and gastrinomas tend to be the most common [68].

The use of EUS in the diagnosis and localization of PNETs has become increasingly a routine procedure [69]. With EUS, PNETs can be found at a low grade, what translates to a prompt surgery and a higher survival rate. According to the study conducted by Fujimori N et al. [70], EUS showed significantly higher sensitivity (96.7%) for identifying PNETs than CT (85.2%), MRI (70.2%) and ultrasonography (75.5%). What is more, the sensitivity of EUS-FNA for the diagnosis of PNET was 89.2%. The smaller size of the tumour was (<2 cm) the higher the concordance between EUS-FNA and surgical specimens, which is 87.5% [70]. EUS findings can differentiate between G1 and G2/G3 PNETs, with G2/G3 tumours more likely to be larger in size (>20 mm), heterogeneous and associated with main pancreatic duct (MPD) obstruction. Large tumour diameter and MPD obstruction are significantly associated with G2/G3 tumours, indicating a more advanced grade. EUS and EUS-FNA are considered highly sensitive and accurate diagnostic methods for PNETs. Characteristic EUS findings, such as large tumour size and MPD obstruction, can help in the grading of PNETs, particularly identifying G2/G3 tumours. To conclude, EUS and EUS-FNA are valuable tools for the diagnosis and grading of PNETs, providing important clinical information for treatment planning and management decisions [70].

Hypervascularization is another feature typical for PNETs, which used in imaging studies. According to the recent research by Battistella A et al. [71], hypervascularization is a common characteristic of PNETs and aids in their identification during imaging studies. However, the density of microvessels within PNETs can vary depending on their biological behaviour, and lower microvessel density is associated with more aggressive disease. The study found that a low microvessel density is indicative of aggressive behaviour in patients with nonfunctioning PNETs. Additionally, contrast-enhanced CT and contrast-enhanced EUS were identified as reliable and readily accessible methods for preoperatively assessing microvessel density in these tumours [71].

According to Deguelte S et al. [72], EUS is the most sensitive examination for PNET diagnosis with a detection rate of 86%. It can detect PNETs smaller than 2 cm with a great specificity. Therefore, EUS became part of the surveillance protocol for patients with hereditary syndromes (such as MEN-1 syndrome—multiple endocrine neoplasia-1) [72]. What is substantial to mention is the fact that the main risk factor for metastases in MEN-1 is the pancreatic tumour size [73]. According to the study conducted by the Endocrine tumour group, EUS detected nearly 85% of PNETs larger than 1 cm, whereas MRI visualized only 67% of them [73]. In addition, in pancreatic solid tumours, EUS can be combined with trans-gastric or trans-duodenal FNB [72]. Due to their rich vascularization, PNETs typically enhance with contrast for all modalities of imaging with early arterial enhancement like CE-EUS [72].

EUS should play a part in preoperative assessment, especially when there is an indication to perform a pancreatic parenchyma-sparing surgery, because it can define the anatomic relationship of the PNET to the PD and vascular structures [5]. Assessment of the distance between the PNET and the MPD is important before considering enucleation (where a distance of 2–3 mm between the lesion and the duct is usually recommended to limit the risk of ductal deformation and postoperative pancreatic fistula) [72].

Figure 2 presents images obtained from EUS-elastography detecting neuroendocrine tumour with high hardness strain ratio; while Figure 3 NET of the pancreas, enhancing after contrast administration was detected.

3.3. Pancreatic Cysts

Nowadays, PCL has become commonly recognized with an increasing frequency, so that the detection rate is rising with the advances in imaging technology, and there is an increased incidence of detection of unsuspected small PCLs [37,74]. Cystic lesions of the pancreas are classified into simple retention cysts, pseudocysts and cystic tumours [75]. The most common pancreatic cystic tumours include the IPMN, MCN and serous cystic adenoma. Numerous international guidelines recommend the qualification for surgical treatment of patients with a pancreatic cyst with a diameter of more than 30 mm, with the presence of adjacent tissue masses and concomitant dilatation of the Wirsung duct. The presence of such changes is associated with an increased risk of malignant transformation [76].

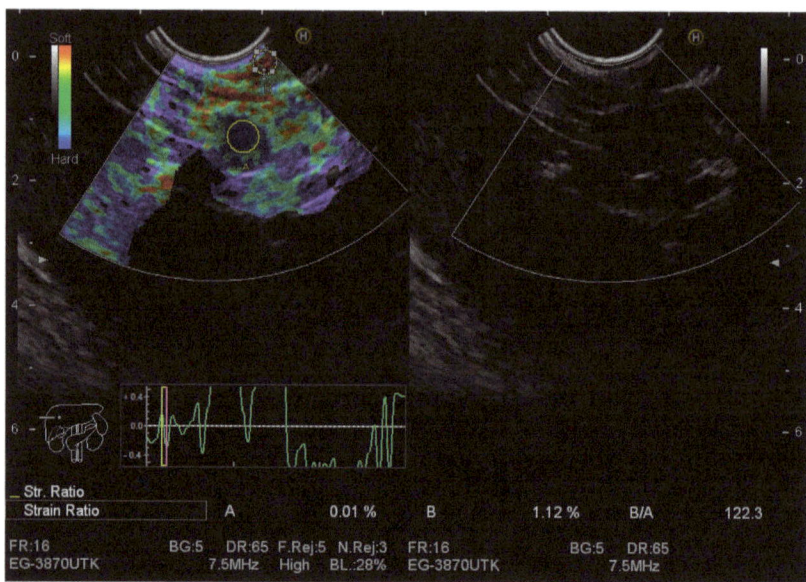

Figure 2. EUS elastography A. neuroendocrine tumour with high hardness strain ratio–SR = 122 is in the yellow circle); B. without strain ratio.

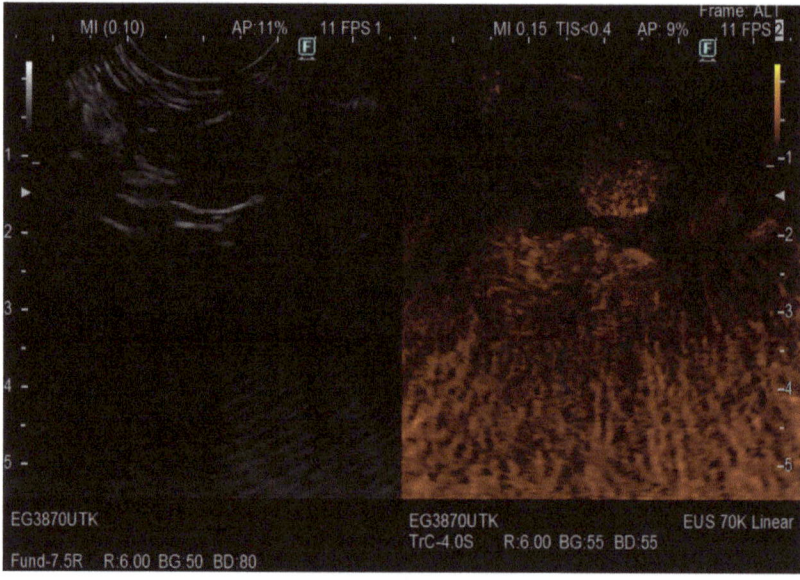

Figure 3. CE–EUS, NET of the pancreas, enhancing after contrast administration.

3.3.1. Intraductal Papillary Mucinous Neoplasm

The European Study Group on Cystic Tumours of the Pancreas recommends EUS and MRI as a method to diagnose the type of PCL [66]. Additionally, CH-EUS might detect hyperenhancement of a mural nodule, solid mass or septations, which point to malignancy. EUS-fine-needle aspiration (FNA) helps to determine the type of PCL [66]. The aspirated cystic fluid can be assessed for carcinoembryonic antigen (CEA), amylase levels and cytology. These parameters have the highest accuracy for differential diagnosis of mucinous from non-mucinous PCNs [77].

Mutations in the GNAS gene play a significant role in the diagnosis of IPMN of the pancreas. The study conducted by Kadayifci A et al. [78] demonstrates that GNAS testing, in combination with KRAS and CEA testing, enhances the accuracy of diagnosing IPMN. The presence of a GNAS mutation is highly specific to IPMN, with 47.2% of IPMN patients showing a positive GNAS result. When GNAS testing is added to CEA and KRAS testing, the overall diagnostic accuracy significantly increases to 86.2%. However, while the addition of GNAS to CEA improves accuracy, it does not surpass the diagnostic superiority of KRAS testing alone. In conclusion, the GNAS mutation serves as a valuable molecular marker in distinguishing IPMN and its inclusion in testing panels enhances the accuracy of IPMN diagnosis [78].

Numerous guidelines have been published to provide clear diagnostic and therapeutic recommendations for IPMNs. One of them is the Fukuoka Guidelines, which have been the current diagnostic and treatment standard for these tumours since 2017 [79]. This classification distinguishes three different types of IPMNs:

1. Fukuoka-positive IPMNs—that have high-risk stigmata for malignancy (localized in pancreatic head leading to obstructive icterus, with mural nodules 5 mm in size and with dilation of the MPD to 10 mm).
2. IPMNs with Fukuoka "worrisome features" (clinical signs of pancreatitis, dilation of the MPD to 5–9 mm, increased serum CA 19-9 values, clinical signs of pancreatitis).
3. Fukuoka-negative IPMNs—without high-risk stigmata and without the "worrisome features" described above.

The treatment recommendations were also included. In resectable tumours, Fukuoka-positive IPMNs should be treated surgically. "Worrisome features", EUS signs of mural nodules 5 mm, evidence of ductal changes or cytology suspicious for malignancy or even malignancy should also be indication for surgery. If neither of these is true, CT/MRI or EUS studies should be performed at intervals depending on the size of the IPMN [79].

The American Gastroenterological Association (AGA) presented the official recommendations on the management of pancreatic cysts in 2015 [80]. The most crucial recommendation is that patients with pancreatic cysts measuring less than 3 cm, without a solid component or a dilated PD, should undergo MRI surveillance after one year and then every two years for a total of five years, as long as there are no changes in size or characteristics.

For pancreatic cysts with at least two high-risk features, such as a size of 3 cm or larger, a dilated MPD or the presence of an associated solid component, the recommendation is to perform an examination using EUS-FNA.

Patients who receive non-concerning results from EUS-FNA should continue with MRI surveillance after one year and then undergo subsequent MRIs every two years to ensure that there are no changes in the risk of malignancy.

In cases where patients have both a solid component and a dilated PD, along with concerning features on EUS and FNA, surgery is recommended to reduce the risk of mortality from carcinoma [74].

These guidelines provided by the AGA offer valuable guidance on the surveillance and management of pancreatic cysts, taking into account specific criteria and risk factors. It is important for clinicians to follow these recommendations in order to make well-informed decisions regarding the appropriate management strategy for patients with pancreatic cysts.

3.3.2. EUS-FNA

The gold standard in differentiating PCLs is EUS-FNA, which enables the use of aspirated samples for cytopathology examination and biochemical analyses, which provide an opportunity to further enhance diagnosis and medical decision making [81]. However, some sonographic findings of PCLs are indicative of malignancy, including a thick wall, septations and the presence of mural nodules, unfortunately, sonographic appearance or cytopathological examination has still a low predictive value for its diagnosis [82].

Nevertheless, the meta-analysis study conducted by Wang QX et al. [83] found that the pooled sensitivity and specificity for malignant cytology were 51% and 94%, respectively.

The aim of the biopsy is to distinguish premalignant lesions from malignant and it is usually performed for better preoperative characterization of the lesion [37].

To sum up, EUS-FNA is a useful tool for the differential diagnosis of benign (mucinous) and probably malignant cysts (non-mutinous), which is clearly presented in Table 6.

Table 6. Studies using EUS-FNA in diagnosis of mucinous and non-mucinous pancreatic cysts.

Study	Cases	Sensitivity	Specificity	Year of the Study
Park et al. [84]	124	60%	93%	2011
Nagashio et al. [85]	68	89.2%	77.8%	2014
Okasha et al. [86]	77	73%	60%	2015

One of the main conclusions of the study conducted by Rogart et al. [87] was the fact that cyst wall puncture and aspiration during routine EUS-FNA may be a safe and easily applied. In the study, among patients with CEA < 192 ng/mL, 31% showed positive cytology for mucinous epithelium when CWP was employed. Additionally, when CEA analysis was not feasible due to insufficient fluid, CWP identified positive cytology for mucinous epithelium in 47% of the cysts. This cumulative approach using CWP resulted in an additional diagnostic yield of 37% for mucinous cysts. These findings demonstrate that incorporating CWP into the diagnostic process enhances the detection and characterization of mucinous cysts. Moreover, EUS-FNA enables clinicians to perform molecular analysis of cyst fluid, like KRAS mutation analysis. The latter increased the diagnostic accuracy of IPMNs to 81% [87,88].

However, EUS-FNA plays a significant role in the assessment of pancreatic cyst histotype, it also carries a notable risk of adverse events (AEs). To better understand the predictors for TTNB-related AEs and develop a prognostic model, a multi-centre retrospective analysis was conducted on 506 patients with PCLs who underwent TTNB. The study found that age, the number of TTNB passes, complete aspiration of the cyst and a diagnosis of IPMN were independent predictors of AEs. These findings were validated through logistic regression and random forest analyses. A hierarchical risk classification system was generated, identifying highrisk (IPMN with multiple microforcep passes), low-risk (patients < 64 years with non-IPMN diagnosis, ≤2 microforcep passes and complete cyst aspiration) and middle-risk groups. The study concludes that TTNB should be used selectively in patients with IPMN, and the developed model can assist in optimizing the benefit–risk balance of TTNB by aiding in patient selection [89].

The new disposable Moray micro forceps biopsy (MFB) device allows tissue sampling from the pancreatic cyst wall/septum and aims to improve diagnosis [90]. Recent meta-analyses have demonstrated that this instrument can significantly enhance the diagnostic accuracy of tissue sampling in patients with PCLs. Due to its effectiveness, MFB has been suggested as a valuable tool for diagnosing, characterizing and stratifying PCL. This disposable micro forceps can be inserted through a 19-gauge needle to obtain tissue samples from the cyst wall and/or septations. It enables histological examination of the architectural features and subepithelial stroma [91].

In the current study conducted by Zhang ML et al. [90], the diagnostic performance of PCF analysis and MFB was found to be similar in terms of diagnostic yield, mucinous cyst diagnosis and detection of high-risk cysts, with both methods achieving a diagnostic yield of over 70%. However, MFB outperformed PCF analysis in diagnosing specific types of cysts. Notably, MFB allowed for the diagnosis of 2.7 times more specific cysts compared to PCF analysis, across all cysts and specifically among those measuring less than 3 cm in size. In summary, the MFB allow for pancreatic cystic sampling with a higher level of precision.

EUS-FNB has revolutionized sampling techniques for pancreatic and nonpancreatic lesions, enabling histological evaluation and immunohistochemical staining. Two popular techniques, slow-pull and wet-suction, have been compared to the standard suction method. Slow-pull involves gradual withdrawal of the stylet to create negative pressure, while wet-suction flushes the needle with saline and applies suction using a pre-vacuum syringe. Previous studies have focused on comparing the standard suction and slow-pull techniques, showing similar adequacy and accuracy, with lower blood contamination in slow-pull. However, the wet-suction technique, introduced more recently, has demonstrated promising results in terms of specimen cellularity, adequacy and accuracy for both pancreatic and nonpancreatic lesions [92].

The findings from the study conducted by Crinò SF et al. [92] indicate that wet-suction showed a higher rate of tissue core acquisition, particularly in nonpancreatic lesions, suggesting that suction during the biopsy procedure may improve tissue quantity. Although the slow-pull technique did not significantly differ in tissue core acquisition, it demonstrated lower blood contamination, which may impact histological evaluation. Other strategies, such as the use of macroscopic on-site evaluation (MOSE), were not evaluated in this study. The choice between wet-suction and slow-pull should consider lesion characteristics, pathologist preference and operator experience. Further research and evidence are needed to comprehensively assess and compare the efficacy, safety and diagnostic yield of different sampling strategies.

The study conducted by Mangiavillano B et al. [93] compared the use of MOSE during EUS-guided fine-needle biopsy (EUS-FNB) with conventional EUS-FNB with three needle passes for pancreatic masses. The results showed that MOSE was noninferior to conventional EUS-FNB in terms of diagnostic accuracy, sample adequacy and safety. MOSE reliably assessed sample adequacy and reduced the number of needle passes required for diagnosis using a 22G Franseen needle. Incorporating MOSE into tissue sampling strategies for pancreatic masses can potentially optimize the procedure by improving efficiency without compromising diagnostic accuracy. Further research is needed to validate the role and benefits of MOSE in pancreatic tissue sampling.

3.3.3. Carcinoembryonic Antigen

CEA is currently considered the most accurate marker for differentiating mucinous, from non-mucinous cysts. Initially, the accuracy of cystic fluid CEA has been superior to EUS, cytology or other tumour markers. The optimal cut-off for differentiating mucinous from non-mucinous cysts was identified to be 192 ng/mL, which was associated with 75% sensitivity, and 84% specificity. Nevertheless, the recent meta-analysis of 18 studies with 1438 patients proved that CEA has 63% sensitivity and 88% specificity for identifying mucinous cysts. Another issue with this marker involves obtaining sufficient cyst fluid to assess CEA levels, which is often not possible, particularly in exceedingly small cysts [94].

3.3.4. Amylase

Its cyst fluid level can be useful in excluding a pseudocyst from other types of pancreatic cysts. A large meta-analysis [95] found that a level of < 250 IU/L had a remarkably high specificity of 98% for excluding a pseudocyst. According to Thornton GD et al. [96] cyst fluid amylase level is similar in IPMNs and MCNs, therefore, its elevated level cannot be used to differentiate these two types of cysts.

3.3.5. Cytology

Cyst fluid for cytology usually has a low diagnostic yield and less than 50% sensitivity for mucosal lesions, but is useful if positive for a specific diagnosis. Similarly, cytology is highly specific for malignancy, with at best a 60% sensitivity for malignancy [97].

3.3.6. Glucose

Cyst fluid glucose levels have shown promise as a valuable diagnostic marker for mucinous cysts and may be more accurate than CEA for mucinous cysts. Cyst fluid glucose levels tend to be significantly lower in mucinous cysts compared to non-mucinous cysts. A cut-off value of <50 mg/dL has been proposed to optimize diagnostic accuracy. According to a recent meta-analysis, glucose has a sensitivity of 91% and a specificity of 75%, while CEA has a sensitivity of 67% and a specificity of 80% [98].

3.3.7. CH-EUS

The quantum leap in diagnosing PCLs' malignancy is said to be CH-EUS. It has a better ability to detect mural nodules, which can be a sign of a malignant cyst. Its improved ability can be assigned to the injected second-generation ultrasound contrast agents, which can detect microcirculation with better resolution and fewer artefacts than Doppler EUS images [6]. According to a prospective Zhong L et al. [99] study on CE-EUS for differential diagnosis of PCL, CE-EUS demonstrated greater accuracy in identifying PCNs than did CT, MRI or EUS-FB (fundamental B-mode)—CE-EUS vs. CT: 92.3% vs. 76.9%; CE-EUS vs. MRI: 93.0% vs. 78.9%; CE-EUS vs. FB-EUS: 92.7% vs. 84.2%. In the study conducted by Ohno E et al. [100], MPD involvement was diagnosed using CH-EUS in 90 patients with a sensitivity, specificity and accuracy of 83.5%, 87.0% and 84.9%, respectively. These results favoured it enough to be recommended by The European Study Group on Cystic Tumours of the Pancreas for being considered for further evaluation of mural nodules and assessing vascularity within the cyst and septations [66].

3.3.8. EUS-nCLE

Confocal laser endomicroscopy (CLE) is a newly developed endoscopic technique that enables both the endoscopist and the pathologist, real-time imaging of tissue and vascular microstructures [101,102]. In this examination, a 19 G EUS needle is used, in which the stylet is replaced by the confocal mini-probe [102]. According to research conducted by Napoleon B et al. [101], there are three ample pieces of clinical evidence for an added benefit of the application of nCLE to EUS-FNA in the management of PCLs:

1. EUS-nCLE provides better differentiation of mucinous and non-mucinous PCLs compared to the current standard of care.
2. EUS-nCLE can improve the accuracy of diagnosis of PCLs, therefore reducing the rate of unnecessary follow-up investigations or inappropriate resections.
3. The interobserver agreement for EUS-nCLE to differentiate mucinous from non-mucinous PCLs is high.

According to Giovannini M [102], the presence of epithelial villous structures based on nCLE was associated with pancreatic cystic neoplasm (IPMN) and provided a sensitivity of 59%, specificity of 100%, positive predictive value of 100%, and negative predictive value of 50%. Although, these data suggested that nCLE has a high specificity in the detection of IPMN, it may be limited by a low sensitivity.

3.4. Autoimmune Pancreatitis

Autoimmune pancreatitis (AIP) is an inflammatory process of the pancreas with a presumed autoimmune ethology, which is regarded as a separate type of chronic pancreatitis [103]. Two distinct types of AIP have been identified: AIP type 1 (AIP-1), considered the pancreatic manifestation of an IgG, related multiorgan disease, and AIP type 2 and is characterized by lymphoplasmacytic sclerosing pancreatitis (LPSP), pancreatic swelling, PD narrowing, obliterative phlebitis and IgG4-positive plasma cell infiltration [104–106]. However, AIP-2 is considered as a pancreatic-specific disease unrelated to IgG and is characterized by idiopathic duct-centric chronic pancreatitis, which is histopathologically represented by granulocytic epithelial lesions [104,106]. Clinical presentation of AIP, such as obstructive jaundice, abdominal pain and weight loss, mimics misleadingly pancreatic cancer (PC). What is more, AIP can also cause peripancreatic lymphadenopathy and vascular invasion, which makes differentiating AIP from PC challenging [103].

Diagnostic criteria are based on imaging findings of the pancreatic parenchyma, serological findings and response to steroid therapy [75]. Although diagnostic criteria are very similar, however, the method for analysing each finding varies depending on the country. For instance, in Japan endoscopic retrograde pancreatography (ERCP) is performed, while, in contrast, in the United States pancreatic core biopsy is routine for diagnosing AIP [75]. However, there is a common consensus that histology is a key criterion for the diagnosis of AIP. According to Matsubayashi H et al. [75], IgG4 ($\geq$135 mg/dL) is the most specific serum marker for type 1 AIP with 86% sensitivity and 96% specificity to AIP against PC. Nevertheless, IgG4 is not actually specific for AIP.

According to Ishikawa T et al. [107], EUS can reveal pancreatic parenchymal and ductal features in much more detail than any other existing imaging modality. However, differentiating AIP and PC based on hypoechoic masses using conventional EUS is difficult, there may be some finding representative of AIP. It has been reported that diffuse hypoechoic areas, diffuse enlargement, bile duct wall thickening and peripancreatic hypoechoic margins on conventional EUS are characteristic features of AIP, and the frequencies of these findings are significantly higher in AIP than in PC [107].

3.4.1. Conventional EUS

Hoki N et al. [108] reported that few conventional EUS features of chronic pancreatitis (CP) were seen in patients with AIP. What is more, the frequencies of diffuse hypoechoic areas, diffuse enlargement, bile duct wall thickening and peripancreatic hypoechoic margins were significantly higher in AIP than in PC.

3.4.2. CH-EUS

Hocke M et al. [109] reported that contrast-enhanced endosonography showed a unique vascularization pattern for AIP, which makes it easy to discriminate from lesions caused by PC. According to the mentioned research, lesions caused by AIP and the surrounding pancreas typically showed hypervascularization, whereas lesions caused by PC were hypovascularized [109]. Moreover, the study conducted by Ishikawa T et al. [107] CH-EUS revealed focal or diffuse iso-enhancement in most AIP cases and hypo-enhancement in most PC cases. Features of CH-EUS have been also proved to be useful in distinguishing AIP from PC in the Korean study conducted by Cho MK et al. [110]. Accordingly, it was demonstrated that, in differentiating AIP from PC, in the arterial phase of contrast agent distribution, the sensitivity and specificity of hyper- to iso-enhancement were 89% and 87%, respectively [110].

3.4.3. Elastography

Dietrich CF et al. [111] in their study found that elastography of the pancreas shows a typical and unique finding with homogenous stiffness of the whole organ, and this distinguishes AIP from the circumscribed mass lesion in PDAC.

3.4.4. EUS-FNA

Despite excellent results in terms of sensitivity for PC, the data are disappointing regarding the diagnosis of AIP. Previous EUS-FNA studies have reported poor to modest diagnostic performance. A prospective, a multi-centre study evaluating 50 patients with suspected AIP using a 22-gauge FNA needle reported a sensitivity of 7.9% [112]. Therefore, considering that the histological diagnosis is difficult, there is a conclusion that FNA may be used to rule out malignancy in patients with AIP. According to Matsubayashi H et al. [75], the diagnosis of pancreatic mass lesions by EUS-FNA provides a sensitivity for detecting PC tissue that exceeds 90%, making EUS-FNA the most effective tool for excluding pancreatic malignancies.

3.4.5. EUS-FNB

According to the study conducted by Mizuno N et al. [113], histological diagnosis of AIP was achieved only in 37% with FNA and in all (100%) with FNB. New FNB needles, such as Franseen and Fork-tip needles [113], enabled achievement of better results in a histological diagnosis of AIP than FNA [114]. What is more, in Noguchi K et al.'s [105] study EUS-FNB was associated with a higher adverse event rate than EUS-FNA, statistically by 20%.

3.4.6. Duodenal Papilla Biopsy

In 2010, Kim MH et al. [115] conducted a prospective research study to confirm the clinical validity of endoscopically accessible ampullary tissue, by evaluating IgG4 immunostaining to diagnose AIP and to distinguish it from other pancreatobiliary diseases. It confirmed the 100% specificity of positive IgG4 immunostaining of the major duodenal papilla in distinguishing AIP from pancreatobiliary malignancies.

3.5. Chronic Pancreatitis

CP is characterized by irreversible morphological changes, fibrosis, calcification and exocrine and endocrine insufficiency [116]. There are four modalities typically used to assess CP. The first one includes MRI. Ultrasonography (USG) is a widely and most commonly used modality for the initial diagnosis of CP. USG provides a non-invasive and cost-effective approach to evaluate the pancreas and detect structural abnormalities associated with chronic inflammation. CT is also a common imaging tool used for the initial diagnosis; however, its findings mostly appear in the advanced stages of CP, making it difficult to detect early CP. Even though, MRI allows detection of the morphological presentations of pancreatic fibrotic change, it is EUS that is believed to be the most sensitive modality for diagnosing early CP [117,118].

It is well known that advanced CP is an irreversible condition, nevertheless, Ito T. et al. [119] state that early diagnosis and intervention are crucial in managing CP and preventing further damage. By following the Clinical Practice Guidelines, healthcare professionals can implement strategies to alleviate symptoms, optimize treatment approaches and minimize complications, ultimately aiming to improve patient outcomes and potentially prevent disease progression [120]. Therefore, it is clinically crucial to diagnose CP in its early stages in order to prevent pancreatic fibrosis, progression and other complications [118]. EUS has emerged as an important imaging modality for the detection of early morphologic changes in CP/ [118]. The group of EUS experts introduced the Rosemont classification (RC) [121]. Major criteria for CP are hyperechoic foci with shadowing and MPD calculi and lobularity with honeycombing, whereas minor criteria are cysts, dilated ducts ≥3.5 mm, irregular PD contour, dilated side branches ≥1 mm, hyperechoic duct wall, strands, non-shadowing hyperechoic foci and lobularity with non-contiguous lobules [121].

EUS elastography enhances the diagnosis of CP due to its ability of measuring tissue hardness, therefore evaluation of tissue stiffness can be used to assess fibrosis of the pancreas in CP [118]. The EUS strain elastography was reported as another diagnostic method for CP, and it was shown to be correlated with the CP stages of RC [122]. However, due to its several limitations (unable to measure absolute value of hardness or is affected by the size and/or position of ROI), EUS shear-wave measurement (EUS-SWM) is a more precise tool for diagnosing CP, since it provides absolute value of pancreatic hardness [122]. A recent study conducted by Domínguez-Muñoz JE et al. [123] demonstrated that EUS-SWM was significantly positively correlated with RC stages and the number of EUS features in the RC, therefore, values obtained with EUS-SWM may reflect pancreatic fibrosis without performing histologic examinations. They came up also with data that showed the diagnostic ability of EUS-SWM for CP, the sensitivity and specificity were 100% and 94%, respectively. In 2013 Iglesias-Garcia J et al. [124] reported the sensitivity and specificity of conventional strain EUS elastography to be 91.2%, 91%, respectively. Comparing these two, EUS-SWM seems superior to conventional strain EUS elastography.

Since CP is one of the major risks for pancreatic PDAC development, it is enormously crucial to differentiate these two. Unfortunately, the diagnosis is a real challenge due to the low specificity of symptoms, imaging signs and biological markers [125]. According to Le Cosquer G et al. [125], EUS-FNAB is believed to be the technique that should provide the best information, however, its accuracy may be limited by the presence of calcifications and fibrosis of pancreatic parenchyma. To clear this limitation, artificial intelligence systems were suggested to enhance the detection of PDAC [126]. In a retrospective multi-centre study, the ability of EUS-FNAB to distinguish CP from cancer was evaluated with the sensitivity ranging from 75 to 85% and the good negative predictive value ranging from 85 to 95% [44,126–128]. Nonetheless, imaging of CP and PC is difficult, EUS-FNAB tends to be a helpful modality to assess the suspicious areas.

A subset of patients presents a unique diagnostic challenge as they exhibit symptoms suggestive of CP but do not show definitive abnormalities in the structure of the pancreas. These patients are commonly referred to as having early or minimal-change chronic pancreatitis (MCCP). Symptoms almost always include pain, and later exocrine pancreatic insufficiency [129]. Identifying this condition provides a distinct opportunity for early diagnosis and intervention prior to the extensive destruction of acinar cells becoming apparent on cross-sectional imaging [130]. A growing body of literature has examined alternative test to diagnose CP and MCCP—the secretin endoscopic pancreatic function test (ePFT). It detects mild exocrine dysfunction which has been considered a surrogate marker of early fibrosis [131]. In the study conducted by Albashir S et al. [132], where the patients were undergoing surgery for CP, a combined EUS with ePFT offered 100% sensitivity for detecting CP. In the recent retrospective cohort study, the ability of EUS and ePFT to predict disease progression in patients with suspected MCCP was determined [131]. The baseline ePFT result was recorded as the peak bicarbonate concentration (peak bicarbonate < 80 mmol is abnormal). Prior to collection, an intravenous dose of synthetic secretin (0.2 mcg/kg) was administered. Duodenal samples were collected at 15, 30 and 45 min after secretin stimulation and analysed for bicarbonate concentration on a hospital auto-analyser. The study found that a hazard ratio for peak bicarbonate was 4.7 for predicting future radiographic changes of CP, indicating its helpful predictive ability. To summarize EUS combined with ePFT may be helpful tests to diagnose suspected MCCP, given that they are predictive of eventual "obvious" structural changes of CP.

The sum up of the main features of different pancreatic pathologies coud be found in the Table 7.

Table 7. Presents the main features of different pancreatic pathologies mentioned above.

Pathology	Examination	Features
Pancreatic cancer	EUS	Hypoechoic mass with irregular borders, dilatation of the proximal PD
	EUS elastography	The mean SH value (the overall hardness of a lesion) is lower than 80
	CE-EUS	Iso-enhancement or hypo-enhancement, arterial irregularity and absent venous vasculature within a mass
Chronic pancreatitis	EUS-elastography	Hyperechoic foci with shadowing and MPD calculi and lobularity with honeycombing
	CE-EUS	Hyper-enhanced lesions with preserved architecture
PNETs	CE-EUS	Hypervascularization, a low microvessel architecture
Autoimmune pancreatitis	EUS	Diffuse hypoechoic areas, diffuse enlargement, bile duct wall thickening and peripancreatic hypoechoic margins
	CE-EUS	Hypervascularization, focal or diffuse iso-enhancement
	EUS-elastography	Homogeneous stiffness of the whole organ

EUS—endoscopic ultrasound, CE-EUS—contrast-enhanced endoscopic ultrasound, PNETs—pancreatic neuroendocrine tumours.

3.6. Artificial Intelligence (AI)

AI is a growing field with a wide range of applications to augment the currently available modalities. AI refers to computer systems designed to imitate the human brain. Machine learning (ML) is a subset of AI that leverages vast amounts of data to identify patterns. In medical diagnostics, supervised learning methods, such as artificial neural networks (ANNs) or neural networks (NN), and support vector machines (SVM), have been investigated. Deep learning (DL), an advanced concept derived from ANN, utilizes complex layers inspired by human neurons, with convolutional neural networks (CNNs) being an example. SVM, a type of supervised ML, categorizes data based on predefined boundaries. While SVM is simpler and more generalizable than ANN, it requires significant data and development time [133].

The use of AI in EUS has the potential to enhance its diagnostic capabilities and improve the recognition of pancreatic malignancies, even in the presence of CP. In a systematic review, SVM demonstrated high sensitivity, specificity and diagnostic accuracy in distinguishing PC from CP and normal pancreas, while CNN showed slightly lower specificity. In differentiating benign and malignant IPMNs, CNN performed better than conventional EUS alone. However, the performance of AI-assisted EUS in real time and its generalizability across endoscopists of varying experience levels require further investigation. The limitations of the review include small sample sizes, retrospective designs and heterogeneity in AI methodologies.

Despite these limitations, AI outperformed conventional EUS in differentiating PC from CP and non-cancerous conditions. SVM, with its simplicity and high performance, shows promise in recognizing cancer in the presence of chronic pancreatic inflammation and in screening high-risk individuals. Prospective and real-time studies are needed to establish the role of AI in routine EUS procedures for endoscopists at all levels of training. If AI development continues to progress, it may eventually enable accurate differentiation of PC from CP and other non-cancerous conditions using EUS imaging alone, potentially revolutionizing PC screening in high-risk patients without a consensus on effective screening methods [133].

What is more AI-assisted EUS models can serve as a valuable tool for endosonographers, improving diagnostic accuracy and aiding in composite imaging for vascular staging of PCs. Additionally, AI can facilitate EUS-guided fine-needle injection for the treatment of deep pancreatic lesions. While most studies on AI are retrospective in nature, large-scale prospective clinical trials are necessary to evaluate the diagnostic accuracy of AI algorithms in real-world clinical settings. If successful, AI-assisted EUS models have the potential to become an indispensable tool in the management of patients with PC [134].

4. Conclusions

In summary, EUS is an indispensable tool in the diagnostic approach to gastrointestinal diseases, particularly for pancreatic conditions. Its ability to detect small lesions, differentiate various pancreatic diseases and facilitate guided interventions has revolutionized the field of gastroenterology. As technology and research progress, the future of EUS looks promising, with the potential for even greater precision and efficacy in diagnosing and managing pancreatic pathologies.

Author Contributions: Conceptualization, J.O.R., Ł.D. and E.M.-W.; writing—original draft preparation, J.O.R., Ł.D. and E.M.-W.; writing—review and editing, J.O.R., Ł.D. and E.M.-W.; supervision, Ł.D., E.M.-W.; funding acquisition, E.M.-W. All authors have read and agreed to the published version of the manuscript.

Funding: The study was supported by grant No. 503/1-002-01/503-11-001-19-00 from the Medical University of Lodz, Poland.

Institutional Review Board Statement: Not applicable.

Informed Consent Statement: Not applicable.

Data Availability Statement: Not applicable.

Conflicts of Interest: The authors declare no conflict of interest.

References

1. DiMagno, E.P.; DiMagno, M.J. Endoscopic Ultrasonography: From the Origins to Routine EUS. *Dig. Dis. Sci.* **2016**, *61*, 342–353. [CrossRef] [PubMed]
2. Ang, T.L.; Kwek, A.B.E.; Wang, L.M. Diagnostic Endoscopic Ultrasound: Technique, Current Status and Future Directions. *Gut Liver* **2018**, *12*, 483–496. [CrossRef] [PubMed]

3. Chong, C.C.N.; Tang, R.S.Y.; Wong, J.C.T.; Chan, A.W.H.; Teoh, A.Y.B. Endoscopic ultrasound of pancreatic lesions. *J. Vis. Surg.* **2016**, *2*, 119. [CrossRef]
4. Kitano, M.; Yoshida, T.; Itonaga, M.; Tamura, T.; Hatamaru, K.; Yamashita, Y. Impact of endoscopic ultrasonography on diagnosis of pancreatic cancer. *J. Gastroenterol.* **2019**, *54*, 19–32. [CrossRef] [PubMed]
5. Yousaf, M.N.; Chaudhary, F.S.; Ehsan, A.; Suarez, A.L.; Muniraj, T.; Jamidar, P.; Aslanian, H.R.; Farrell, J.J. Endoscopic ultrasound (EUS) and the management of pancreatic cancer. *BMJ Open Gastroenterol.* **2020**, *7*, e000408. [CrossRef] [PubMed]
6. Jin, Z.; Sun, L.; Huang, H. Application of EUS-based techniques in the evaluation of pancreatic cystic neoplasms. *Endosc. Ultrasound* **2021**, *10*, 230–240. [CrossRef] [PubMed]
7. Dite, P.; Novotny, I.; Dvorackova, J.; Kianicka, B.; Blaho, M.; Svoboda, P.; Uvirova, M.; Rohan, T.; Maskova, H.; Kunovsky, L. Pancreatic Solid Focal Lesions: Differential Diagnosis between Autoimmune Pancreatitis and Pancreatic Cancer. *Dig. Dis.* **2019**, *37*, 416–421. [CrossRef] [PubMed]
8. Best, L.M.; Rawji, V.; Pereira, S.P.; Davidson, B.R.; Gurusamy, K.S. Imaging modalities for characterising focal pancreatic lesions. *Cochrane Database Syst. Rev.* **2017**, *2017*, CD010213. [CrossRef]
9. Gollapudi, L.A.; Tyberg, A. EUS-RFA of the pancreas: Where are we and future directions. *Transl. Gastroenterol. Hepatol.* **2022**, *7*, 18. [CrossRef] [PubMed]
10. Kamata, K.; Kitano, M. Endoscopic diagnosis of cystic lesions of the pancreas. *Dig. Endosc.* **2018**, *31*, 5–15. [CrossRef]
11. Dhar, J.; Samanta, J. The expanding role of endoscopic ultrasound elastography. *Clin. J. Gastroenterol.* **2022**, *15*, 841–858. [CrossRef]
12. Du, C.; Chai, N.-L.; Linghu, E.-Q.; Li, H.-K.; Sun, L.-H.; Jiang, L.; Wang, X.-D.; Tang, P.; Yang, J. Comparison of endoscopic ultrasound, computed tomography and magnetic resonance imaging in assessment of detailed structures of pancreatic cystic neoplasms. *World J. Gastroenterol.* **2017**, *23*, 3184–3192. [CrossRef]
13. Kamata, K.; Kitano, M.; Kudo, M.; Sakamoto, H.; Kadosaka, K.; Miyata, T.; Imai, H.; Maekawa, K.; Chikugo, T.; Kumano, M.; et al. Value of EUS in early detection of pancreatic ductal adenocarcinomas in patients with intraductal papillary mucinous neoplasms. *Endoscopy* **2014**, *46*, 22–29. [CrossRef]
14. Kitano, M.; Kudo, M.; Yamao, K.; Takagi, T.; Sakamoto, H.; Komaki, T.; Kamata, K.; Imai, H.; Chiba, Y.; Okada, M.; et al. Characterization of Small Solid Tumors in the Pancreas: The Value of Contrast-Enhanced Harmonic Endoscopic Ultrasonography. *Am. J. Gastroenterol.* **2012**, *107*, 303–310. [CrossRef] [PubMed]
15. Lee, T.H.; Cha, S.-W.; Cho, Y.D. EUS Elastography: Advances in Diagnostic EUS of the Pancreas. *Korean J. Radiol.* **2012**, *13*, S12–S16. [CrossRef] [PubMed]
16. Dietrich, C.; Săftoiu, A.; Jenssen, C. Real time elastography endoscopic ultrasound (RTE-EUS), a comprehensive review. *Eur. J. Radiol.* **2014**, *83*, 405–414. [CrossRef] [PubMed]
17. Ophir, J.; Céspedes, I.; Ponnekanti, H.; Yazdi, Y.; Li, X. Elastography: A quantitative method for imaging the elasticity of biological tissues. *Ultrason. Imaging* **1991**, *13*, 111–134. [CrossRef] [PubMed]
18. Saftoiu, A.; Costache, M.I.; Cazacu, I.M.; Dietrich, C.F.; Petrone, M.C.; Arcidiacono, P.G.; Giovannini, M.; Bories, E.; Garcia, J.I.; Siyu, S.; et al. Clinical impact of strain histogram EUS elastography and contrast-enhanced EUS for the differential diagnosis of focal pancreatic masses: A prospective multicentric study. *Endosc. Ultrasound* **2020**, *9*, 116–121. [CrossRef]
19. Dietrich, C.F.; Bibby, E.; Jenssen, C.; Saftoiu, A.; Iglesias-Garcia, J.; Havre, R.F. EUS elastography: How to do it? *Endosc. Ultrasound* **2018**, *7*, 20–28. [CrossRef]
20. Janssen, J.; Schlörer, E.; Greiner, L. EUS elastography of the pancreas: Feasibility and pattern description of the normal pancreas, chronic pancreatitis, and focal pancreatic lesions. *Gastrointest. Endosc.* **2007**, *65*, 971–978. [CrossRef]
21. Taljanovic, M.S.; Gimber, L.H.; Becker, G.W.; Latt, L.D.; Klauser, A.S.; Melville, D.M.; Gao, L.; Witte, R.S. Shear-Wave Elastography: Basic Physics and Musculoskeletal Applications. *RadioGraphics* **2017**, *37*, 855–870. [CrossRef]
22. Ferraioli, G.; Barr, R.G.; Farrokh, A.; Radzina, M.; Cui, X.W.; Dong, Y.; Rocher, L.; Cantisani, V.; Polito, E.; D'onofrio, M.; et al. How to perform shear wave elastography. Part II. *Med. Ultrason.* **2022**, *24*, 196–210. [CrossRef]
23. Dietrich, C.F.; Sharma, M.; Hocke, M. Contrast-Enhanced Endoscopic Ultrasound. *Endosc. Ultrasound* **2012**, *1*, 130–136. [CrossRef] [PubMed]
24. Sidhu, P.S.; Cantisani, V.; Dietrich, C.F.; Gilja, O.H.; Saftoiu, A.; Bartels, E.; Bertolotto, M.; Calliada, F.; Clevert, D.-A.; Cosgrove, D.; et al. The EFSUMB Guidelines and Recommendations for the Clinical Practice of Contrast-Enhanced Ultrasound (CEUS) in Non-Hepatic Applications: Update 2017 (Long Version). *Ultraschall Med.* **2018**, *39*, e2–e44. [CrossRef]
25. Reddy, N.K.; Ioncică, A.M.; Săftoiu, A.; Vilmann, P.; Bhutani, M.S. Contrast-enhanced endoscopic ultrasonography. *World J. Gastroenterol.* **2011**, *17*, 42–48. [CrossRef]
26. Giovannini, M.; Thomas, B.; Erwan, B.; Christian, P.; Fabrice, C.; Benjamin, E.; Geneviève, M.; Paolo, A.; Pierre, D.; Robert, Y.; et al. Endoscopic ultrasound elastography for evaluation of lymph nodes and pancreatic masses: A multicenter study. *World J. Gastroenterol.* **2009**, *15*, 1587–1593. [CrossRef]
27. Saftoiu, A.; Napoleon, B.; Arcidiacono, P.G.; Braden, B.; Burmeister, S.; Carrara, S.; Cui, X.W.; Fusaroli, P.; Gottschalk, U.; Hocke, M.; et al. Do we need contrast agents for EUS? *Endosc. Ultrasound* **2020**, *9*, 361–368. [PubMed]
28. Ishikawa, T.; Itoh, A.; Kawashima, H.; Ohno, E.; Matsubara, H.; Itoh, Y.; Nakamura, Y.; Nakamura, M.; Miyahara, R.; Hayashi, K.; et al. Usefulness of EUS combined with contrast-enhancement in the differential diagnosis of malignant versus benign and preoperative localization of pancreatic endocrine tumors. *Gastrointest. Endosc.* **2010**, *71*, 951–959. [CrossRef]

29. Lee, L.; Ito, T.; Jensen, R.T. Imaging of pancreatic neuroendocrine tumors: Recent advances, current status, and controversies. *Expert Rev. Anticancer Ther.* **2018**, *18*, 837–860. [CrossRef]
30. Leem, G.; Chung, M.J.; Park, J.Y.; Bang, S.; Song, S.Y.; Chung, J.B.; Park, S.W. Clinical Value of Contrast-Enhanced Harmonic Endoscopic Ultrasonography in the Differential Diagnosis of Pancreatic and Gallbladder Masses. *Clin. Endosc.* **2018**, *51*, 80–88. [CrossRef] [PubMed]
31. Teodorescu, C.; Bolboaca, S.D.; Rusu, I.; Pojoga, C.; Seicean, R.; Mosteanu, O.; Sparchez, Z.; Seicean, A. Contrast enhanced endoscopic ultrasound in the diagnosis of pancreatic metastases. *Med. Ultrason.* **2022**, *24*, 277–283. [CrossRef] [PubMed]
32. Yamashita, Y.; Tanioka, K.; Kawaji, Y.; Tamura, T.; Nuta, J.; Hatamaru, K.; Itonaga, M.; Yoshida, T.; Ida, Y.; Maekita, T.; et al. Utility of Contrast-Enhanced Harmonic Endoscopic Ultrasonography for Early Diagnosis of Small Pancreatic Cancer. *Diagnostics* **2020**, *10*, 23. [CrossRef] [PubMed]
33. Levine, I.; Trindade, A.J. Endoscopic ultrasound fine needle aspiration vs. fine needle biopsy for pancreatic masses, subepithelial lesions, and lymph nodes. *World J. Gastroenterol.* **2021**, *27*, 4194–4207. [CrossRef]
34. Kuraoka, N.; Hashimoto, S.; Matsui, S.; Terai, S. Effectiveness of EUS-Guided Fine-Needle Biopsy versus EUS-Guided Fine-Needle Aspiration: A Retrospective Analysis. *Diagnostics* **2021**, *11*, 965. [CrossRef]
35. Bang, J.Y.; Hebert-Magee, S.; Trevino, J.; Ramesh, J.; Varadarajulu, S. Randomized trial comparing the 22-gauge aspiration and 22-gauge biopsy needles for EUS-guided sampling of solid pancreatic mass lesions. *Gastrointest. Endosc.* **2012**, *76*, 321–327. [CrossRef]
36. Dumonceau, J.-M.; Deprez, P.H.; Jenssen, C.; Iglesias-Garcia, J.; Larghi, A.; Vanbiervliet, G.; Aithal, G.P.; Arcidiacono, P.G.; Bastos, P.; Carrara, S.; et al. Indications, results, and clinical impact of endoscopic ultrasound (EUS)-guided sampling in gastroenterology: European Society of Gastrointestinal Endoscopy (ESGE) Clinical Guideline—Updated January 2017. *Endoscopy* **2017**, *49*, 695–714. [CrossRef] [PubMed]
37. Iglesias-Garcia, J.; Lariño-Noia, J.; de la Iglesia-Garcia, D.; Dominguez-Muñoz, J. EUS-FNA in cystic pancreatic lesions: Where are we now and where are we headed in the future? *Endosc. Ultrasound* **2018**, *7*, 102–109. [CrossRef]
38. Khan, M.A.; Grimm, I.S.; Ali, B.; Nollan, R.; Tombazzi, C.; Ismail, M.K.; Baron, T.H. A meta-analysis of endoscopic ultrasound–fine-needle aspiration compared to endoscopic ultrasound–fine-needle biopsy: Diagnostic yield and the value of onsite cytopathological assessment. *Endosc. Int. Open* **2017**, *5*, E363–E375. [CrossRef] [PubMed]
39. Seo, D.-W.; So, H.; Hwang, J.; Ko, S.; Oh, D.; Song, T.; Park, D.; Lee, S.; Kim, M.-H. Macroscopic on-site evaluation after EUS-guided fine needle biopsy may replace rapid on-site evaluation. *Endosc. Ultrasound* **2021**, *10*, 111–115. [CrossRef] [PubMed]
40. Sun, S.; Yang, F.; Liu, E. Rapid on-site evaluation (ROSE) with EUS-FNA: The ROSE Slooks beautiful. *Endosc. Ultrasound* **2019**, *8*, 283–287. [CrossRef]
41. Polkowski, M.; Jenssen, C.C.; Kaye, P.V.; Carrara, S.; Deprez, P.; Ginès, A.; Fernández-Esparrach, G.G.; Eisendrath, P.; Aithal, G.P.; Arcidiacono, P.P.; et al. Technical aspects of endoscopic ultrasound (EUS)-guided sampling in gastroenterology: European Society of Gastrointestinal Endoscopy (ESGE) Technical Guideline—March 2017. *Endoscopy* **2017**, *49*, 989–1006. [CrossRef] [PubMed]
42. Oppong, K.W.; Bekkali, N.L.H.; Leeds, J.S.; Johnson, S.J.; Nayar, M.K.; Darné, A.; Egan, M.; Bassett, P.; Haugk, B. Fork-tip needle biopsy versus fine-needle aspiration in endoscopic ultrasound-guided sampling of solid pancreatic masses: A randomized crossover study. *Endoscopy* **2020**, *52*, 454–461. [CrossRef]
43. De Moura, D.T.; McCarty, T.R.; Jirapinyo, P.; Ribeiro, I.B.; Flumignan, V.K.; Najdawai, F.; Ryou, M.; Lee, L.S.; Thompson, C.C. EUS-guided fine-needle biopsy sampling versus FNA in the diagnosis of subepithelial lesions: A large multicenter study. *Gastrointest. Endosc.* **2020**, *92*, 108–119.e3. [CrossRef]
44. Grassia, R.; Imperatore, N.; Capone, P.; Cereatti, F.; Forti, E.; Antonini, F.; Tanzi, G.P.; Martinotti, M.; Buffoli, F.; Mutignani, M.; et al. EUS-guided tissue acquisition in chronic pancreatitis: Differential diagnosis between pancreatic cancer and pseudotumoral masses using EUS-FNA or core biopsy. *Endosc. Ultrasound* **2020**, *9*, 122–129. [CrossRef]
45. Yang, M.J.; Kim, J.; Park, S.W.; Cho, J.H.; Kim, E.J.; Lee, Y.N.; Lee, D.W.; Park, C.H.; Lee, S.S. Comparison between three types of needles for endoscopic ultrasound-guided tissue acquisition of pancreatic solid masses: A multicenter observational study. *Sci. Rep.* **2023**, *13*, 3677. [CrossRef] [PubMed]
46. Gkolfakis, P.; Crinò, S.F.; Tziatzios, G.; Ramai, D.; Papaefthymiou, A.; Papanikolaou, I.S.; Triantafyllou, K.; Arvanitakis, M.; Lisotti, A.; Fusaroli, P.; et al. Comparative diagnostic performance of end-cutting fine-needle biopsy needles for EUS tissue sampling of solid pancreatic masses: A network meta-analysis. *Gastrointest. Endosc.* **2022**, *95*, 1067–1077.e15. [CrossRef] [PubMed]
47. Tian, G.; Ye, Z.; Zhao, Q.; Jiang, T. Complication incidence of EUS-guided pancreas biopsy: A systematic review and meta-analysis of 11 thousand population from 78 cohort studies. *Asian J. Surg.* **2020**, *43*, 1049–1055. [CrossRef]
48. Will, U.; Meyer, F.; Manger, T.; Wanzar, I. Endoscopic Ultrasound-Assisted Rendezvous Maneuver to Achieve Pancreatic Duct Drainage in Obstructive Chronic Pancreatitis. *Endoscopy* **2005**, *37*, 171–173. [CrossRef]
49. Mallery, S.; Matlock, J.; Freeman, M.L. EUS-guided rendezvous drainage of obstructed biliary and pancreatic ducts: Report of 6 cases. *Gastrointest. Endosc.* **2004**, *59*, 100–107. [CrossRef] [PubMed]
50. Khalsa, B.S.; Imagawa, D.K.; Chen, J.I.; Dermirjian, A.N.; Yim, D.B.; Findeiss, L.K. Evolution in the Treatment of Delayed Postpancreatectomy Hemorrhage: Surgery to interventional radiology. *Pancreas* **2015**, *44*, 953–958. [CrossRef] [PubMed]
51. Okuno, N.; Hara, K.; Mizuno, N.; Hijioka, S.; Tajika, M.; Tanaka, T.; Ishihara, M.; Hirayama, Y.; Onishi, S.; Niwa, Y.; et al. Endoscopic Ultrasound-guided Rendezvous Technique after Failed Endoscopic Retrograde Cholangiopancreatography: Which Approach Route Is the Best? *Intern. Med.* **2017**, *56*, 3135–3143. [CrossRef] [PubMed]

52. Tonini, V.; Zanni, M. Pancreatic cancer in 2021: What you need to know to win. *World J. Gastroenterol.* **2021**, *27*, 5851–5889. [CrossRef] [PubMed]
53. Oldfield, L.E.; Connor, A.A.; Gallinger, S. Molecular Events in the Natural History of Pancreatic Cancer. *Trends Cancer* **2017**, *3*, 336–346. [CrossRef]
54. Ilic, M.; Ilic, I. Epidemiology of pancreatic cancer. *World J. Gastroenterol.* **2016**, *22*, 9694–9705. [CrossRef]
55. Iglesias-Garcia, J.; de la Iglesia-Garcia, D.; Olmos-Martinez, J.M.; Lariño-Noia, J.; Dominguez-Muñoz, J.E. Differential diagnosis of solid pancreatic masses. *Minerva Gastroenterol. Dietol.* **2020**, *66*, 70–81. [CrossRef]
56. Maguchi, H.; Takahashi, K.; Osanai, M.; Katanuma, A. Small pancreatic lesions: Is there need for EUS-FNA preoperatively? What to do with the incidental lesions? *Endoscopy* **2006**, *38*, S53–S56. [CrossRef] [PubMed]
57. Yamashita, Y.; Shimokawa, T.; Napoléon, B.; Fusaroli, P.; Gincul, R.; Kudo, M.; Kitano, M. Value of contrast-enhanced harmonic endoscopic ultrasonography with enhancement pattern for diagnosis of pancreatic cancer: A meta-analysis. *Dig. Endosc.* **2019**, *31*, 125–133. [CrossRef]
58. Park, W.; Chawla, A.; O'Reilly, E.M. Pancreatic Cancer. A Review. *JAMA* **2021**, *326*, 851–862, Erratum in *JAMA* **2021**, *326*, 2081. [CrossRef]
59. Wu, L.; Guo, W.; Li, Y.; Cheng, T.; Yao, Y.; Zhang, Y.; Liu, B.; Zhong, M.; Li, S.; Deng, X.; et al. Value of endoscopic ultrasound-guided fine needle aspiration in pretest prediction and diagnosis of pancreatic ductal adenocarcinoma. *Nan Fang Yi Ke Da Xue Xue Bao* **2018**, *38*, 1171–1178. [CrossRef]
60. Facciorusso, A.; Martina, M.; Buccino, R.V.; Nacchiero, M.C.; Muscatiello, N. Diagnostic accuracy of fine-needle aspiration of solid pancreatic lesions guided by endoscopic ultrasound elastography. *Ann. Gastroenterol.* **2018**, *31*, 513–518. [CrossRef]
61. Conti, C.B.; Mulinacci, G.; Salerno, R.; Dinelli, M.E.; Grassia, R. Applications of endoscopic ultrasound elastography in pancreatic diseases: From literature to real life. *World J. Gastroenterol.* **2022**, *28*, 909–917. [CrossRef]
62. Zhang, B.; Zhu, F.; Li, P.; Yu, S.; Zhao, Y.; Li, M. Endoscopic ultrasound elastography in the diagnosis of pancreatic masses: A meta-analysis. *Pancreatology* **2018**, *18*, 833–840. [CrossRef]
63. Lu, Y.; Chen, L.; Li, C.; Chen, H.; Chen, J. Diagnostic utility of endoscopic ultrasonography-elastography in the evaluation of solid pancreatic masses: A meta-analysis and systematic review. *Med. Ultrason.* **2017**, *19*, 150–158. [CrossRef]
64. Kanda, M.; Knight, S.; Topazian, M.; Syngal, S.; Farrell, J.; Lee, J.; Kamel, I.; Lennon, A.M.; Borges, M.; Young, A.; et al. Mutant Gnas detected in duodenal collections of secretin-stimulated pancreatic juice indicates the presence or emergence of pancreatic cysts. *Gut* **2013**, *62*, 1024–1033. [CrossRef] [PubMed]
65. Tanaka, M.; Heckler, M.; Liu, B.; Heger, U.; Hackert, T.; Michalski, C.W. Cytologic Analysis of Pancreatic Juice Increases Specificity of Detection of Malignant IPMN–A Systematic Review. *Clin. Gastroenterol. Hepatol.* **2019**, *17*, 2199–2211.e21. [CrossRef] [PubMed]
66. European Study Group on Cystic Tumours of the Pancreas. European evidence-based guidelines on pancreatic cystic neoplasms. *Gut* **2018**, *67*, 789–804. [CrossRef]
67. Raphael, M.J.; Chan, D.L.; Law, C.; Singh, S. Principles of diagnosis and management of neuroendocrine tumours. *Can. Med. Assoc. J.* **2017**, *189*, E398–E404. [CrossRef]
68. Rösch, T.; Lightdale, C.J.; Botet, J.F.; Boyce, G.A.; Sivak, M.V.; Yasuda, K.; Heyder, N.; Palazzo, L.; Dancygier, H.; Schusdziarra, V.; et al. Localization of Pancreatic Endocrine Tumors by Endoscopic Ultrasonography. *N. Engl. J. Med.* **1992**, *326*, 1721–1726. [CrossRef]
69. Anderson, M.A.; Carpenter, S.; Thompson, N.W.; Nostrant, T.T.; Elta, G.H.; Scheiman, J.M. Endoscopic ultrasound is highly accurate and directs management in patients with neuroendocrine tumors of the pancreas. *Am. J. Gastroenterol.* **2000**, *95*, 2271–2277. [CrossRef] [PubMed]
70. Fujimori, N.; Osoegawa, T.; Lee, L.; Tachibana, Y.; Aso, A.; Kubo, H.; Kawabe, K.; Igarashi, H.; Nakamura, K.; Oda, Y.; et al. Efficacy of endoscopic ultrasonography and endoscopic ultrasonography-guided fine-needle aspiration for the diagnosis and grading of pancreatic neuroendocrine tumors. *Scand. J. Gastroenterol.* **2016**, *51*, 245–252. [CrossRef]
71. Battistella, A.; Partelli, S.; Andreasi, V.; Marinoni, I.; Palumbo, D.; Tacelli, M.; Lena, M.S.; Muffatti, F.; Mushtaq, J.; Capurso, G.; et al. Preoperative assessment of microvessel density in nonfunctioning pancreatic neuroendocrine tumors (NF-PanNETs). *Surgery* **2022**, *172*, 1236–1244. [CrossRef]
72. Deguelte, S.; de Mestier, L.; Hentic, O.; Cros, J.; Lebtahi, R.; Hammel, P.; Kianmanesh, R. Preoperative imaging and pathologic classification for pancreatic neuroendocrine tumors. *J. Visc. Surg.* **2018**, *155*, 117–125. [CrossRef]
73. Barbe, C.; Murat, A.; Dupas, B.; Ruszniewski, P.; Tabarin, A.; Vullierme, M.-P.; Penfornis, A.; Rohmer, V.; Baudin, E.; Le Rhun, M.; et al. Magnetic resonance imaging versus endoscopic ultrasonography for the detection of pancreatic tumours in multiple endocrine neoplasia type 1. *Dig. Liver Dis.* **2012**, *44*, 228–234. [CrossRef]
74. Okasha, H.H.; Awad, A.; El-Meligui, A.; Ezzat, R.; Aboubakr, A.; AbouElenin, S.; El-Husseiny, R.; Alzamzamy, A. Cystic pancreatic lesions, the endless dilemma. *World J. Gastroenterol.* **2021**, *27*, 2664–2680. [CrossRef]
75. Matsubayashi, H.; Kakushima, N.; Takizawa, K.; Tanaka, M.; Imai, K.; Hotta, K.; Ono, H. Diagnosis of autoimmune pancreatitis. *World J. Gastroenterol.* **2014**, *20*, 16559–16569. [CrossRef]
76. Falqueto, A.; Pelandré, G.L.; Da Costa, M.Z.G.; Nacif, M.S.; Marchiori, E. Prevalence of pancreatic cystic neoplasms on imaging exams: Association with signs of malignancy risk. *Radiol. Bras.* **2018**, *51*, 218–224. [CrossRef]
77. Jabłońska, B.; Szmigiel, P.; Mrowiec, S. Pancreatic intraductal papillary mucinous neoplasms: Current diagnosis and management. *World J. Gastrointest. Oncol.* **2021**, *13*, 1880–1895. [CrossRef]

78. Kadayifci, A.; Atar, M.; Wang, J.L.; Forcione, D.G.; Casey, B.W.; Pitman, M.B.; Brugge, W.R. Value of adding *GNAS* testing to pancreatic cyst fluid *KRAS* and carcinoembryonic antigen analysis for the diagnosis of intraductal papillary mucinous neoplasms. *Dig. Endosc.* **2017**, *29*, 111–117. [CrossRef]
79. Tanaka, M.; Fernández-del Castillo, C.; Kamisawa, T.; Jang, J.Y.; Levy, P.; Ohtsuka, T.; Salvia, R.; Shimizu, Y.; Tada, M.; Wolfgang, C.L. Revisions of international consensus Fukuoka guidelines for the management of IPMN of the pancreas. *Pancreatology* **2017**, *17*, 738–753. [CrossRef]
80. Vege, S.S.; Ziring, B.; Jain, R.; Moayyedi, P.; Clinical Guidelines Committee; American Gastroenterology Association. American Gastroenterological Association Institute Guideline on the Diagnosis and Management of Asymptomatic Neoplastic Pancreatic Cysts. *Gastroenterology* **2015**, *148*, 819–822. [CrossRef]
81. Kovacevic, B.; Vilmann, P. EUS tissue acquisition: From A to B. *Endosc. Ultrasound* **2020**, *9*, 225–231. [CrossRef]
82. Abdelkader, A.; Hunt, B.; Hartley, C.P.; Panarelli, N.C.; Giorgadze, T. Cystic Lesions of the Pancreas: Differential Diagnosis and Cytologic-Histologic Correlation. *Arch. Pathol. Lab. Med.* **2020**, *144*, 47–61. [CrossRef]
83. Wang, Q.-X.; Xiao, J.; Orange, M.; Zhang, H.; Zhu, Y.-Q. EUS-Guided FNA for Diagnosis of Pancreatic Cystic Lesions: A Meta-Analysis. *Cell. Physiol. Biochem.* **2015**, *36*, 1197–1209. [CrossRef]
84. Park, W.G.-U.; Mascarenhas, R.M.; Palaez-Luna, M.; Smyrk, T.C.; O'Kane, D.; Clain, J.E.; Levy, M.J.; Pearson, R.K.; Petersen, B.T.; Topazian, M.D.; et al. Diagnostic Performance of Cyst Fluid Carcinoembryonic Antigen and Amylase in Histologically Confirmed Pancreatic Cysts. *Pancreas* **2011**, *40*, 42–45. [CrossRef]
85. Nagashio, Y.; Hijioka, S.; Mizuno, N.; Hara, K.; Imaoka, H.; Bhatia, V.; Niwa, Y.; Tajika, M.; Tanaka, T.; Ishihara, M.; et al. Combination of cyst fluid CEA and CA 125 is an accurate diagnostic tool for differentiating mucinous cystic neoplasms from intraductal papillary mucinous neoplasms. *Pancreatology* **2014**, *14*, 503–509. [CrossRef]
86. Okasha, H.H.; Ashry, M.; Imam, H.M.K.; Ezzat, R.; Naguib, M.; Farag, A.H.; Gemeie, E.H.; Khattab, H.M. Role of endoscopic ultrasound-guided fine needle aspiration and ultrasound-guided fine-needle aspiration in diagnosis of cystic pancreatic lesions. *Endosc. Ultrasound* **2015**, *4*, 132–136. [CrossRef] [PubMed]
87. Rogart, J.N.; Loren, D.E.; Singu, B.S.; Kowalski, T.E. Cyst Wall Puncture and Aspiration During EUS-guided Fine Needle Aspiration May Increase the Diagnostic Yield of Mucinous Cysts of the Pancreas. *J. Clin. Gastroenterol.* **2011**, *45*, 164–169. [CrossRef]
88. Bournet, B.; Vignolle-Vidoni, A.; Grand, D.; Roques, C.; Breibach, F.; Cros, J.; Muscari, F.; Carrère, N.; Selves, J.; Cordelier, P.; et al. Endoscopic ultrasound-guided fine-needle aspiration plus KRAS and GNAS mutation in malignant intraductal papillary mucinous neoplasm of the pancreas. *Endosc. Int. Open* **2016**, *4*, E1228–E1235. [CrossRef] [PubMed]
89. Facciorusso, A.; Kovacevic, B.; Yang, D.; Vilas-Boas, F.; Martínez-Moreno, B.; Stigliano, S.; Rizzatti, G.; Sacco, M.; Arevalo-Mora, M.; Villarreal-Sanchez, L.; et al. Predictors of adverse events after endoscopic ultrasound-guided through-the-needle biopsy of pancreatic cysts: A recursive partitioning analysis. *Endoscopy* **2022**, *54*, 1158–1168. [CrossRef] [PubMed]
90. Zhang, M.L.; Arpin, R.N.; Brugge, W.R.; Forcione, D.G.; Basar, O.; Pitman, M.B. Moray micro forceps biopsy improves the diagnosis of specific pancreatic cysts. *Cancer Cytopathol.* **2018**, *126*, 414–420. [CrossRef]
91. Tacelli, M.; Celsa, C.; Magro, B.; Barchiesi, M.; Barresi, L.; Capurso, G.; Arcidiacono, P.G.; Cammà, C.; Crinò, S.F. Diagnostic performance of endoscopic ultrasound through-the-needle microforceps biopsy of pancreatic cystic lesions: Systematic review with meta-analysis. *Dig. Endosc.* **2020**, *32*, 1018–1030. [CrossRef]
92. Crinò, S.F.; Bellocchi, M.C.C.; Di Mitri, R.; Inzani, F.; Rimbaş, M.; Lisotti, A.; Manfredi, G.; Teoh, A.Y.B.; Mangiavillano, B.; Sendino, O.; et al. Wet-suction versus slow-pull technique for endoscopic ultrasound-guided fine-needle biopsy: A multicenter, randomized, crossover trial. *Endoscopy* **2022**, *55*, 225–234. [CrossRef]
93. Mangiavillano, B.; Crinò, S.F.; Facciorusso, A.; Di Matteo, F.; Barbera, C.; Larghi, A.; Rizzatti, G.; Carrara, S.; Spadaccini, M.; Auriemma, F.; et al. Endoscopic ultrasound-guided fine-needle biopsy with or without macroscopic on-site evaluation: A randomized controlled noninferiority trial. *Endoscopy* **2022**, *55*, 129–137. [CrossRef]
94. Ngamruengphong, S.; Lennon, A.M. Analysis of Pancreatic Cyst Fluid. *Surg. Pathol. Clin.* **2016**, *9*, 677–684. [CrossRef]
95. Van der Waaij, L.A.; van Dullemen, H.M.; Porte, R.J. Cyst fluid analysis in the differential diagnosis of pancreatic cystic lesions: A pooled analysis. *Gastrointest. Endosc.* **2005**, *62*, 383–389. [CrossRef]
96. Thornton, G.D.; McPhail, M.J.; Nayagam, S.; Hewitt, M.J.; Vlavianos, P.; Monahan, K.J. Endoscopic ultrasound guided fine needle aspiration for the diagnosis of pancreatic cystic neoplasms: A meta-analysis. *Pancreatology* **2012**, *13*, 48–57. [CrossRef]
97. Lee, L.S. Updates in diagnosis and management of pancreatic cysts. *World J. Gastroenterol.* **2021**, *27*, 5700–5714. [CrossRef]
98. Faias, S.; Cravo, M.M.; Chaves, P.; Pereira, L. A comparative analysis of glucose and carcinoembryonic antigen in diagnosis of pancreatic mucinous cysts: A systematic review and meta-analysis. *Gastrointest Endosc.* **2021**, *94*, 235–247. [CrossRef]
99. Zhong, L.; Chai, N.; Linghu, E.; Li, H.; Yang, J.; Tang, P. A Prospective Study on Contrast-Enhanced Endoscopic Ultrasound for Differential Diagnosis of Pancreatic Cystic Neoplasms. *Dig. Dis. Sci.* **2019**, *64*, 3616–3622. [CrossRef] [PubMed]
100. Ohno, E.; Kawashima, H.; Ishikawa, T.; Iida, T.; Suzuki, H.; Uetsuki, K.; Yashika, J.; Yamada, K.; Yoshikawa, M.; Gibo, N.; et al. Can contrast-enhanced harmonic endoscopic ultrasonography accurately diagnose main pancreatic duct involvement in intraductal papillary mucinous neoplasms? *Pancreatology* **2020**, *20*, 887–894. [CrossRef]
101. Napoleon, B.; Krishna, S.G.; Marco, B.; Carr-Locke, D.; Chang, K.J.; Ginès, À.; Gress, F.G.; Larghi, A.; Oppong, K.W.; Palazzo, L.; et al. Confocal endomicroscopy for evaluation of pancreatic cystic lesions: A systematic review and international Delphi consensus report. *Endosc. Int. Open* **2020**, *8*, E1566–E1581. [CrossRef]

102. Giovannini, M. Needle-based confocal laser endomicroscopy. *Endosc. Ultrasound* **2015**, *4*, 284–288. [CrossRef]
103. Yang, A.; Guo, T.; Xu, T.; Zhang, S.; Lai, Y.; Wu, X.; Wu, D.; Feng, Y.; Jiang, Q.; Wang, Q.; et al. The role of EUS in diagnosing focal autoimmune pancreatitis and differentiating it from pancreatic cancer. *Endosc. Ultrasound* **2021**, *10*, 280–287. [CrossRef]
104. Nista, E.C.; De Lucia, S.S.; Manilla, V.; Schepis, T.; Pellegrino, A.; Ojetti, V.; Pignataro, G.; Verme, L.Z.D.; Franceschi, F.; Gasbarrini, A.; et al. Autoimmune Pancreatitis: From Pathogenesis to Treatment. *Int. J. Mol. Sci.* **2022**, *23*, 12667. [CrossRef]
105. Noguchi, K.; Nakai, Y.; Mizuno, S.; Hirano, K.; Kanai, S.; Suzuki, Y.; Inokuma, A.; Sato, T.; Hakuta, R.; Ishigaki, K.; et al. Role of Endoscopic Ultrasonography-Guided Fine Needle Aspiration/Biopsy in the Diagnosis of Autoimmune Pancreatitis. *Diagnostics* **2020**, *10*, 954. [CrossRef]
106. Hayashi, H.; Miura, S.; Fujishima, F.; Kuniyoshi, S.; Kume, K.; Kikuta, K.; Hamada, S.; Takikawa, T.; Matsumoto, R.; Ikeda, M.; et al. Utility of Endoscopic Ultrasound-Guided Fine-Needle Aspiration and Biopsy for Histological Diagnosis of Type 2 Autoimmune Pancreatitis. *Diagnostics* **2022**, *12*, 2464. [CrossRef]
107. Ishikawa, T.; Kawashima, H.; Ohno, E.; Mizutani, Y.; Fujishiro, M. Imaging diagnosis of autoimmune pancreatitis using endoscopic ultrasonography. *J. Med. Ultrason.* **2021**, *48*, 543–553. [CrossRef]
108. Hoki, N.; Mizuno, N.; Sawaki, A.; Tajika, M.; Takayama, R.; Shimizu, Y.; Bhatia, V.; Yamao, K. Diagnosis of autoimmune pancreatitis using endoscopic ultrasonography. *J. Gastroenterol.* **2009**, *44*, 154–159. [CrossRef]
109. Hocke, M.; Ignee, A.; Dietrich, C.F. Contrast-enhanced endoscopic ultrasound in the diagnosis of autoimmune pancreatitis. *Endoscopy* **2010**, *43*, 163–165. [CrossRef]
110. Cho, M.K.; Moon, S.-H.; Song, T.J.; Kim, R.E.; Oh, D.W.; Park, D.H.; Lee, S.S.; Seo, D.W.; Lee, S.K.; Kim, M.-H. Contrast-Enhanced Endoscopic Ultrasound for Differentially Diagnosing Autoimmune Pancreatitis and Pancreatic Cancer. *Gut Liver* **2018**, *12*, 591–596. [CrossRef]
111. Dietrich, C.F.; Hirche, T.O.; Ott, M.; Ignee, A. Real-time tissue elastography in the diagnosis of autoimmune pancreatitis. *Endoscopy* **2009**, *41*, 718–720. [CrossRef]
112. De Pretis, N.; Crinò, S.F.; Frulloni, L. The Role of EUS-Guided FNA and FNB in Autoimmune Pancreatitis. *Diagnostics* **2021**, *11*, 1653. [CrossRef]
113. Mizuno, N.; Bhatia, V.; Hosoda, W.; Sawaki, A.; Hoki, N.; Hara, K.; Takagi, T.; Ko, S.B.H.; Yatabe, Y.; Goto, H.; et al. Histological diagnosis of autoimmune pancreatitis using EUS-guided trucut biopsy: A comparison study with EUS-FNA. *J. Gastroenterol.* **2009**, *44*, 742–750. [CrossRef]
114. Facciorusso, A.; Barresi, L.; Cannizzaro, R.; Antonini, F.; Triantafyllou, K.; Tziatzios, G.; Muscatiello, N.; Hart, P.A.; Wani, S. Diagnostic yield of endoscopic ultrasound-guided tissue acquisition in autoimmune pancreatitis: A systematic review and meta-analysis. *Endosc. Int. Open* **2021**, *9*, E66–E75. [CrossRef] [PubMed]
115. Kim, M.-H.; Moon, S.-H.; Kamisawa, T. Major Duodenal Papilla in Autoimmune Pancreatitis. *Dig. Surg.* **2010**, *27*, 110–114. [CrossRef]
116. Takasaki, Y.; Ishii, S.; Fujisawa, T.; Ushio, M.; Takahashi, S.; Yamagata, W.; Ito, K.; Suzuki, A.; Ochiai, K.; Tomishima, K.; et al. Endoscopic Ultrasonography Findings of Early and Suspected Early Chronic Pancreatitis. *Diagnostics* **2020**, *10*, 1018. [CrossRef]
117. Kichler, A.; Jang, S. Chronic Pancreatitis: Epidemiology, Diagnosis, and Management Updates. *Drugs* **2020**, *80*, 1155–1168. [CrossRef]
118. Yamashita, Y.; Ashida, R.; Kitano, M. Imaging of Fibrosis in Chronic Pancreatitis. *Front. Physiol.* **2022**, *12*, 800516. [CrossRef]
119. Ito, T.; Ishiguro, H.; Ohara, H.; Kamisawa, T.; Sakagami, J.; Sata, N.; Takeyama, Y.; Hirota, M.; Miyakawa, H.; Igarashi, H.; et al. Evidence-based clinical practice guidelines for chronic pancreatitis 2015. *J. Gastroenterol.* **2016**, *51*, 85–92. [CrossRef]
120. Whitcomb, D.C.; Shimosegawa, T.; Chari, S.T.; Forsmark, C.E.; Frulloni, L.; Garg, P.; Hegyi, P.; Hirooka, Y.; Irisawa, A.; Ishikawa, T.; et al. International consensus statements on early chronic Pancreatitis. Recommendations from the working group for the international consensus guidelines for chronic pancreatitis in collaboration with The International Association of Pancreatology, American Pancreatic Association, Japan Pancreas Society, PancreasFest Working Group and European Pancreatic Club. *Pancreatology* **2018**, *18*, 516–527. [CrossRef]
121. Catalano, M.F.; Sahai, A.; Levy, M.; Romagnuolo, J.; Wiersema, M.; Brugge, W.; Freeman, M.; Yamao, K.; Canto, M.; Hernandez, L.V. EUS-based criteria for the diagnosis of chronic pancreatitis: The Rosemont classification. *Gastrointest. Endosc.* **2009**, *69*, 1251–1261. [CrossRef]
122. Yamashita, Y.; Tanioka, K.; Kawaji, Y.; Tamura, T.; Nuta, J.; Hatamaru, K.; Itonaga, M.; Yoshida, T.; Ida, Y.; Maekita, T.; et al. Utility of Elastography with Endoscopic Ultrasonography Shear-Wave Measurement for Diagnosing Chronic Pancreatitis. *Gut Liver* **2020**, *14*, 659–664. [CrossRef]
123. Domínguez-Muñoz, J.E.; Lariño-Noia, J.; Alvarez-Castro, A.; Nieto, L.; Lojo, S.; Leal, S.; Iglesia-Garcia, D.; Iglesias-Garcia, J. Endoscopic ultrasound-based multimodal evaluation of the pancreas in patients with suspected early chronic pancreatitis. *United Eur. Gastroenterol. J.* **2020**, *8*, 790–797. [CrossRef] [PubMed]
124. Iglesias-Garcia, J.; Domínguez-Muñoz, J.E.; Castiñeira-Alvariño, M.; Luaces-Regueira, M.; Lariño-Noia, J. Quantitative elastography associated with endoscopic ultrasound for the diagnosis of chronic pancreatitis. *Endoscopy* **2013**, *45*, 781–788. [CrossRef]
125. Le Cosquer, G.; Maulat, C.; Bournet, B.; Cordelier, P.; Buscail, E.; Buscail, L. Pancreatic Cancer in Chronic Pancreatitis: Pathogenesis and Diagnostic Approach. *Cancers* **2023**, *15*, 761. [CrossRef] [PubMed]

126. Tonozuka, R.; Itoi, T.; Nagata, N.; Kojima, H.; Sofuni, A.; Tsuchiya, T.; Ishii, K.; Tanaka, R.; Nagakawa, Y.; Mukai, S. Deep learning analysis for the detection of pancreatic cancer on endosonographic images: A pilot study. *J. Hepato-Biliary-Pancreat. Sci.* **2020**, *28*, 95–104. [CrossRef]
127. Ardengh, J.C.; Lopes, C.V.; Campos, A.D.; De Lima, L.F.P.; Venco, F.; Módena, J.L.P. Endoscopic ultrasound and fine needle aspiration in chronic pancreatitis: Differential diagnosis between pseudotumoral masses and pancreatic cancer. *JOP* **2007**, *8*, 413–421.
128. Bournet, B.; Souque, A.; Senesse, P.; Assenat, E.; Barthet, M.; Lesavre, N.; Aubert, A.; O'Toole, D.; Hammel, P.; Levy, P.; et al. Endoscopic ultrasound-guided fine-needle aspiration biopsy coupled with *KRAS* mutation assay to distinguish pancreatic cancer from pseudotumoral chronic pancreatitis. *Endoscopy* **2009**, *41*, 552–557. [CrossRef]
129. DeWitt, J.M.; Al-Haddad, M.A.; Easler, J.J.; Sherman, S.; Slaven, J.; Gardner, T.B. EUS pancreatic function testing and dynamic pancreatic duct evaluation for the diagnosis of exocrine pancreatic insufficiency and chronic pancreatitis. *Gastrointest. Endosc.* **2020**, *93*, 444–453. [CrossRef]
130. Walsh, T.N.; Rode, J.; Theis, B.A.; Russell, R.C. Minimal change chronic pancreatitis. *Gut* **1992**, *33*, 1566–1571. [CrossRef] [PubMed]
131. Stevens, T.; Monachese, M.; Lee, P.; Harris, K.; Jang, S.; Bhatt, A.; Chahal, P.; Lopez, R. EUS and secretin endoscopic pancreatic function test predict evolution to overt structural changes of chronic pancreatitis in patients with nondiagnostic baseline imaging. *Endosc. Ultrasound* **2021**, *10*, 116. [CrossRef] [PubMed]
132. Albashir, S.; Bronner, M.P.; Parsi, M.A.; Walsh, M.R.; Stevens, T. Endoscopic Ultrasound, Secretin Endoscopic Pancreatic Function Test, and Histology: Correlation in Chronic Pancreatitis. *Am. J. Gastroenterol.* **2010**, *105*, 2498–2503. [CrossRef] [PubMed]
133. Goyal, H.; Sherazi, S.A.A.; Gupta, S.; Perisetti, A.; Achebe, I.; Ali, A.; Tharian, B.; Thosani, N.; Sharma, N.R. Application of artificial intelligence in diagnosis of pancreatic malignancies by endoscopic ultrasound: A systemic review. *Ther. Adv. Gastroenterol.* **2022**, *15*, 17562848221093873. [CrossRef] [PubMed]
134. Dahiya, D.S.; Al-Haddad, M.; Chandan, S.; Gangwani, M.K.; Aziz, M.; Mohan, B.P.; Ramai, D.; Canakis, A.; Bapaye, J.; Sharma, N. Artificial Intelligence in Endoscopic Ultrasound for Pancreatic Cancer: Where Are We Now and What Does the Future Entail? *J. Clin. Med.* **2022**, *11*, 7476. [CrossRef] [PubMed]

Disclaimer/Publisher's Note: The statements, opinions and data contained in all publications are solely those of the individual author(s) and contributor(s) and not of MDPI and/or the editor(s). MDPI and/or the editor(s) disclaim responsibility for any injury to people or property resulting from any ideas, methods, instructions or products referred to in the content.

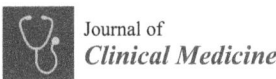

Review

A Comparison of Single Dimension and Volume Measurements in the Risk Stratification of Pancreatic Cystic Lesions

Da Yeon Ryoo [1,†], Bryn Koehler [1,†], Jennifer Rath [2], Zarine K. Shah [2], Wei Chen [3], Ashwini K. Esnakula [3], Phil A. Hart [4] and Somashekar G. Krishna [4,*]

1. Department of Internal Medicine, Ohio State University Wexner Medical Center, Columbus, OH 43210, USA; dayeon.ryoo@osumc.edu (D.Y.R.); bryn.koehler@osumc.edu (B.K.)
2. Department of Radiology, Ohio State University Wexner Medical Center, Columbus, OH 43210, USA; jennifer.rath@osumc.edu (J.R.); zarine.shah@osumc.edu (Z.K.S.)
3. Department of Pathology, Ohio State University Wexner Medical Center, Columbus, OH 43210, USA; wei.chen@osumc.edu (W.C.); ashwini.esnakula@osumc.edu (A.K.E.)
4. Division of Gastroenterology, Department of Internal Medicine, Ohio State University Wexner Medical Center, Columbus, OH 43210, USA; philip.hart@osumc.edu
* Correspondence: somashekar.krishna@osumc.edu
† These authors contributed equally to this work.

Abstract: The incidence of pancreatic cystic lesions (PCLs) has been rising due to improvements in imaging. Of these, intraductal papillary mucinous neoplasms (IPMNs) are the most common and are thought to contribute to almost 20% of pancreatic adenocarcinomas. All major society guidelines for the management of IPMNs use size defined by maximum diameter as the primary determinant of whether surveillance or surgical resection is recommended. However, there is no consensus on how these measurements should be obtained or whether a single imaging modality is superior. Furthermore, the largest diameter may fail to capture the complexity of PCLs, as most are not perfectly spherical. This article reviews current PCL measurement techniques in CT, MRI, and EUS and posits volume as a possible alternative to the largest diameter.

Keywords: pancreatic cancer; pancreatic cystic lesion; IPMN; CT; MRI; MRCP; EUS; maximum diameter; volume

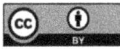

1. Introduction

Despite recent advances in cancer detection and management strategies, pancreatic cancer remains among the deadliest worldwide. In the United States, pancreatic cancer is responsible for 8.2% of all cancer deaths and has an estimated 5-year survival of 11.5 percent [1]. The global incidence is projected to increase to 18.6 per 100,000 by the year 2050, which poses a significant public health burden [2]. There are numerous well-established risk factors for developing pancreatic cancer, including cigarette smoking, family history, age, and male sex. However, due to the lack of effective screening methods, the only populations recommended to undergo any type of screening are those with a significant family history or those with a high-risk genetic screen. For this reason, the effective management of premalignant pancreatic lesions is crucial in both slowing the incidence of cases and improving mortality.

Pancreatic cystic lesions (PCLs) represent a significant portion of premalignant pancreatic lesions and contribute to nearly 20% of pancreatic adenocarcinomas [3]. PCLs are classified as mucinous and non-mucinous. Mucinous PCLs, which include intraductal papillary mucinous neoplasms (IPMNs) and mucinous cystic neoplasms (MCNs), have the potential to progress to pancreatic adenocarcinoma. The surveillance of mucinous PCLs poses a promising opportunity to advance the detection and prevention of pancreatic cancer. Improvements in cross-sectional imaging and its increased utilization in an aging population have contributed to a marked increase in the incidence of PCLs [4]. Due to the heterogeneous nature of these lesions, the challenge lies in accurately classifying them in order to guide management.

Among neoplastic PCLs, IPMNs are the most common. The point prevalence of IPMNs in those above age 60 is ~1 in 100 subjects [5,6]. While many IPMNs are discovered incidentally and are asymptomatic, rarely, they can cause symptoms, including abdominal pain, pancreatitis, and jaundice. They also have a significant malignant potential, with a mean malignancy rate of 61% in main-duct IPMNs (MD-IPMNs) when the duct diameter is $\geq$10 mm and a malignancy rate of 25.5% in branch-duct IPMNs (BD-IPMNs) when the cyst diameter is $\geq$4 cm [7]. Specifically, the risk of malignant transformation of BD-IPMNs is 18–25% at 3–4 cm and >25% at $\geq$4 cm diameter [8,9].

The early detection of high-risk BD-IPMNs is crucial, as the 5-year survival after the surgical resection of IPMNs with invasive cancers ranges from 31 to 60%, compared to 90 to 100% in noninvasive IPMNs [10]. Unfortunately, there are significant limitations in the imaging methods used to identify and risk-stratify BD-IPMNs. Guidelines from multiple professional societies use PCL size to assess the risk of malignant transformation to determine the appropriate surveillance or intervention [9,11–16]. However, these guidelines are difficult to apply since various imaging modalities, including computed tomography (CT) scan, magnetic resonance imaging (MRI)/magnetic resonance cholangiopancreatography (MRCP), and endoscopic ultrasound (EUS), often provide discordant measurements. Therefore, consensus regarding optimal imaging modality and best practices in collecting measurements is needed to ensure that BD-IPMNs are appropriately managed.

2. Current Guidelines Regarding Pancreatic Cystic Lesion Measurement

There are five sets of guidelines from major societies regarding the management of PCLs. Each set of guidelines seeks to establish high-risk features summarized in Table 1 that should prompt closer follow-up or surgical evaluation. While these features vary, PCL size is the one factor uniformly cited by all guidelines. The American College of Gastroenterology (ACG), the American College of Radiology (ACR), the American Gastrointestinal Association (AGA), and the International Association of Pancreatology (IAP) established a diameter of at least 3 cm as indicative of increased risk for advanced neoplasia, whereas the European evidence-based guidelines use a cutoff of 4 cm in diameter. Some of these guidelines, specifically the European and IAP/Fukuoka guidelines, provide management recommendations for specific types of PCLs, whereas the ACG and AGA guidelines offer general strategies for PCL surveillance and management regardless of subtype. The revised 2017 IAP/Fukuoka guidelines are commonly used as they provide specific operative criteria for MD- and BD-IMPNs. According to IAP/Fukuoka guidelines, high-risk stigmata are defined as obstructive jaundice, main pancreatic duct >10 mm, and enhancing mural nodule >5 mm. Surgical resection is strongly recommended for both MD- and BD-IPMNs with any high-risk stigmata. Size-guided surveillance imaging is recommended for BD-IPMNs that are <3 cm and without other worrisome or high-risk features [9].

Despite the consistent use of PCL size as one of the primary determinants of surveillance and management recommendations for BD-IPMNs, there is inconsistent evidence to support this. The two major considerations in cyst measurement are baseline size and incremental growth, where a rate of growth greater than 5 mm every 2 years is regarded as a worrisome feature [9]. However, the consistent implementation of these recommendations is impaired by insufficient consensus on imaging protocols and measurement techniques. The ACR guidelines are the only ones to specifically discuss CT and MRI protocols. Therefore, this article seeks to clarify how PCL measurements are obtained across imaging modalities and determine whether there are discrepancies to be considered in establishing management guidelines.

Table 1. Summary of available pancreatic cyst management guidelines and their characterizations of high-risk pancreatic cysts.

Society		High-Risk Features That May Prompt Surgical Referral
American College of Gastroenterology (ACG) guidelines [15]	High-risk features	Tumor-related jaundice Acute pancreatitis Elevated CA 19-9 with no benign cause present Mural nodule or solid component Main pancreatic duct (PD) > 5 mm Change in main PD caliber with upstream atrophy Size > 3 cm Increase in size > 3 mm/year High-grade dysplasia or invasive malignancy
American College of Radiology (ACR) guidelines [14]	Worrisome features	Cyst diameter ≥ 3 cm Thickened or enhancing cyst wall Non-enhancing mural nodule Main PD ≥ 7 mm
	High-risk stigmata	Tumor-related jaundice Enhancing mural nodule Main PD ≥ 10 mm without obstruction Cytology with high-grade dysplasia or invasive malignancy
American Gastrointestinal Association (AGA) guidelines [13]	Positive features	Size ≥ 3 cm Dilated main PD Solid component Concerning cytology
European evidence-based guidelines [16]	Absolute indications	Cytology with high-grade dysplasia or invasive malignancy Solid mass Tumor-related jaundice Enhancing mural nodule ≥ 5 mm Main PD ≥ 10 mm
	Relative indications	Growth rate ≥ 5 mm/year CA 19-9 ≥ 37 U/mL Main PD 5–9.9 mm Cyst diameter ≥ 4 cm New-onset diabetes or acute pancreatitis Enhancing mural nodule < 5 mm
International Association of Pancreatology (IAP)/Fukuoka guidelines [9]	Worrisome features	Cyst diameter ≥ 3 cm Thickened or enhancing cyst wall Enhancing mural nodule < 5 mm Main PD 5–6 mm Lymphadenopathy Abrupt change in caliber of PD with distal pancreatic atrophy Cyst growth rate ≥ 5 mm/2 years Elevated CA 19-9
	High-risk stigmata	Enhancing mural nodule > 5 mm Main PD ≥ 10 mm Tumor-related jaundice

3. Methods of Measuring PCL Size

3.1. CT, MRI, and EUS

As noted in most of the PCL management guidelines, the three most common imaging modalities for detecting and diagnosing pancreatic cysts are CT, MRI, and EUS. Each modality comes with its own risks and benefits. While MRI can provide the high contrast definition of soft tissue without exposing patients to radiation, it is more time-consuming and expensive than CT [17]. CT is more widely available and time efficient, but it exposes patients to repeated doses of radiation throughout the pancreatic cyst surveillance period. EUS provides the high-resolution imaging of pancreatic cysts with the option to utilize fine needle aspiration (FNA) during the procedure to further assist with the diagnosis of the cyst. However, it is by far the most invasive method of the three [17]. In this review, several studies that measured PCLs were assessed to investigate the differences in imaging modality and size measurement methodology. To account for recent advances in imaging technologies, only studies conducted within the past 15 years were reviewed.

3.2. Maximum Diameter—Variation between Imaging Modalities

Du et al. compared the difference in cyst size measurement and cyst characteristic appearance across CT, MRI, and EUS; (n = 68). They used cyst diameter as the definition of cyst size. While there were no major discrepancies in size, EUS was superior in identifying specific characteristics, such as intracystic nodules, wall thickness, and septations [18]. Similarly, Boos et al. compared incidental pancreatic cyst size measurement (defined by maximal diameter) between CT and MRI and reported a mean absolute size discrepancy of 2.1 ± 1.8 mm (n = 267; median 1.5 mm, range 0–9 mm). This study also determined that the larger the cyst size, the larger the absolute size discrepancy between the imaging modalities [19]. Moreover, CT did not correctly identify incidental PCLs by rate of 22% when compared to MRI.

3.3. Maximum Diameter—Imaging vs. Histopathology

Lee et al. assessed the PCLs of patients who had all CT, MRI, and EUS images taken within three months prior to surgical resection (n = 34). The authors measured the maximum dimension of the pancreatic cyst in two axes—cross-sectional and coronal—in all three imaging modalities. The larger of the two measurements was selected to define cyst size in the analysis. Of the three imaging modalities, EUS had the widest range of 95% limits of agreement (−17.43 to +23.87) and very good reliability with an intraclass correlation coefficient of 0.84 (95% CI 0.58–0.94) for mucinous lesions. EUS was specifically found to underestimate the size of PCLs located in the pancreatic tail when compared to CT and MRI [20]. The authors concluded that EUS findings should be interpreted with caution, particularly when the lesion is located in the tail of the pancreas and is relatively large in size.

Maimone et al. compared the cyst size measurements of 175 patients who underwent some combination of CT, MRI, and EUS imaging prior to surgical resection. They defined cyst size as the single largest cyst diameter. The median size differences between each combination of imaging modalities were: 4 mm (0–25 mm) between EUS and CT, 4 mm (0–17 mm) between EUS and MRI, and 3 mm (2–20 mm) between CT and MRI. Histopathologic data from resection were then compared to 12 EUS, 13 CT, and 8 MRI measurements. The median size differences were: 9.5 mm (0–20 mm) between EUS and pathology, 5 mm (0–21 mm) between CT and pathology, and 5.5 mm (2–44 mm) between MRI and pathology [21]. In this study, the authors noted that there was significant variation in the size estimates of PCLs when assessed using different imaging modalities. Therefore, they recommended the use of a single imaging modality for surveillance to ensure consistency in size measurements.

Two additional studies also compared PCL size data obtained from imaging to surgically resected pathology specimens. Leeds et al. compared the maximum diameters of cysts measured with CT and EUS to the measurements of surgically resected pathology specimens in 70 patients. Measurements included maximum diameter in the axial, sagittal, and coronal planes. There were no significant differences found between measurements obtained via either imaging modality when compared to pathology [22]. Huynh et al. similarly used a small sample size of 57 IPMNs (3 MD, 41 BD, 13 mixed) to compare the three imaging modalities on the strength of their size measurement correlation to the pathological cyst size. Each of the three imaging modalities was used to measure the maximum long-axis cyst diameter, which was later compared to the post-operative pathological cyst maximum diameter. Unlike Leeds et al., this study revealed that CT and MRI significantly overestimated the IPMN size measurement when compared to pathological cyst measurement, while EUS best predicted the pathological cyst size, especially for those smaller than 3 cm [23]. The authors speculated that the differences in cyst size measurement across different imaging modalities could be attributed to the difference in cyst size in coronal and axial views of CT and MRI as opposed to oblique angle views on EUS. Aside from investigating their hypothesis, the authors additionally commented on the lack of standardized protocol in radiographic and pathological pancreatic cyst size measurement.

3.4. Diameter and Volume Estimation—Imaging vs. Histopathology

Literature evidence from the last decade suggests that the three-dimensional growth pattern of PCLs is uneven and may not be accurately estimated when only one or two dimensions are obtained in imaging studies [24]. Chalian et al. compared PCL volumes obtained from CT imaging to the volume of fluid aspirated during EUS. The CT measurement of cyst volume was measured using (a) software-assisted CT volumetry and (b) spherical and ellipsoid volume calculation formulas (spherical volume = $\pi \times R1^3/6$; ellipsoid volume = $R1 \times R2 \times R3 \times \pi/6$ (R1: longest diameter on axial plane; R2: longest diameter on coronal plane; R3: longest diameter on sagittal plane)) (Figure 1). Whether a cyst was spherical or ellipsoid was determined using an elongation value, 1 − aspect ratio, or 1 − (width/length), where cysts that are spherical had an elongation value closer to 0 and those that were ellipsoid had an elongation value closer to 1. Of the 14 fully aspirated PCLs, the mean aspirated cyst volume was 2.05 ± 1.56 mL. The mean volume measured via CT volumetry was 2.27 ± 1.54 mL, while the ellipsoid volume (formula) yielded a mean volume of 2.94 ± 2.06 mL, and the spherical volume (formula) resulted in a mean volume of 3.78 ± 2.47 mL. Although software-assisted CT volumetry was the most accurate method, the utilization of the ellipsoid volume (formulas) was found to be preferable over the spherical volume (formulas) [25].

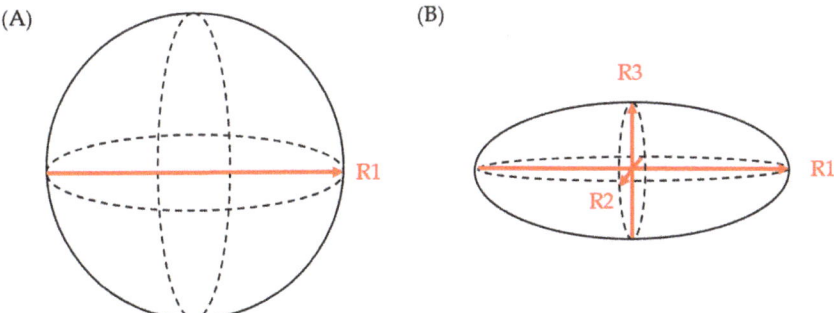

Figure 1. (**A**) spherical volume = $\pi \times R1^3/6$; (**B**) ellipsoid volume = $R1 \times R2 \times R3 \times \pi/6$.

4. Prediction of Advanced Neoplasia in IPMNs—Variation between Imaging Modalities Using Consensus Criteria

Multiple studies have compared the diagnostic accuracy of various imaging modalities (CT, MRI, and EUS) using the IAP/Fukuoka guidelines in predicting advanced neoplasia in IPMNs. In a study of 86 patients with IPMNs, the diagnostic performance of CT and MRI for the prediction of malignant IPMNs was comparable with good inter-modality agreement ($p = 0.43$; $\kappa = 0.70$) [26]. A meta-analysis of 28 studies encompassing 1812 patients with IPMN was conducted to further compare the diagnostic accuracy of multiple imaging modalities. Of the imaging modalities included in the study, PET/CT and MRI/MRCP had the highest overall diagnostic accuracy (area under the curve of summary receiver-operating characteristic curves of 0.92 and 0.87, respectively) and therefore supported the use of either imaging modality interchangeably when assessing the malignant potential of IPMNs [27]. A meta-analysis investigating the difference in diagnostic accuracy for diagnosing malignant PCLs between the three imaging modalities found MRI and CT to have comparable accuracy (sensitivity $p = 0.822$; specificity $p = 0.096$), while EUS showed lesser specificity compared to MRI (75% vs. 80%, $p < 0.05$). This study therefore posits that MRI may be a better imaging tool to guide PCL management than EUS [28].

5. Cyst Size as a Predictor of Advanced Neoplasia

As cited in Table 1, the available guidelines universally cite cyst size ≥ 3 cm as a worrisome feature for advanced pathology and therefore use size as a guide to surveil IPMNs. However, a large study evaluating BD-IPMNs (n = 2258; 36.7% with advanced neoplasia) showed that cyst size (OR 1.024, 95% CI 1.018–1.030), although predictive of advanced neoplasia, had lower odds ratios than main pancreatic duct (MPD) dilation, the presence of mural nodules, and elevation in CA 19-9. However, this study did not specify how the cyst size was defined and measured [29]. The association between cyst size and advanced neoplasia has been corroborated by multiple meta-analyses which also investigated the relationship between various BD-IPMN characteristics and their correlation with malignancy. Again, while cyst size ≥ 3 cm was associated with high-grade dysplasia and malignancy, the odds ratios were significantly lower than those of many other cyst characteristics [30,31]. A retrospective study of 269 patients who underwent the surgical resection of asymptomatic pancreatic cysts showed a remarkable discrepancy between the pathological diagnosis of advanced neoplasia and those expected to be at high risk for neoplasia based on the available guidelines. Of the 269 PCLs, 41 were found to have advanced neoplasia. Of these 41 patients, only 3 met the criteria for resection per AGA guidelines, 22 met the criteria per ACR guidelines, and 30 met the criteria per IAP/Fukuoka guidelines. These findings suggest a lower sensitivity of these guidelines in diagnosing advanced neoplasia. These guidelines were similarly inaccurate for low-grade or benign lesions. Of the 228 patients with low-grade or benign cysts, 27 would have met the criteria for resection per AGA guidelines, 89 for ACR guidelines, and 123 for IAP/Fukuoka guidelines. This correlated to an overall diagnostic accuracy of 49.8% for IAP/Fukuoka, 59.8% for ACR, and 75.8% for AGA guidelines [32]. Yet another study compared one center's resection criteria—symptomatic, suspicious morphologic features through radiography and mucinous characteristics through fluid aspiration—to the size criteria of ≥ 3 cm used by most guidelines. Of the mucinous or cancerous lesions, 73% met the institution's criteria but only 50% were ≥ 3 cm [33].

This inconsistent evidence has prompted some investigators to question whether other criteria might better predict the malignant risk of BD-IPMNs than cyst size. The growth rate has been proposed as a possible alternative. A study of 52 patients with BD-IPMN diagnosed by ERCP or MRI/MRCP had a mean follow-up of 31.2 months to assess for changes in maximum diameter and MPD diameter. Seven of the lesions demonstrated growth on follow-up imaging, and both cyst size > 3 cm and MPD dilatation were associated with an increased likelihood of growth [34]. El Chafic et al. queried whether growth rate may be superior to size at baseline in predicting advanced neoplasia. However, an analysis of 161 patients with BD-IPMN demonstrated that rapid growth, defined as a mean growth rate percentage $\geq 30\%$ per year, was not associated with advanced neoplasia on surgical pathology and did not correlate with other high-risk patient characteristics [35]. Conversely, Ciprani et al. found that, for small PCLs < 15 mm (n = 816), the strongest predictor of malignancy was a growth rate ≥ 2.5 mm per year [36].

Recently, some investigators have evaluated cyst volume as an alternative predictor of malignant risk, as it is proposed to be more accurate for lesions that are not perfectly spherical. For example, a recent radiology guideline paper proposed volumetry as a more objective alternative to diametric size [37]. Studies comparing imaging modalities in other cancers have shown that a small level of growth in the diameter of lesions is associated with a much larger increase in cyst volume. This is true for even perfectly spherical lesions, where a growth of 20% in diameter correlates with a volume increase of 72.8% [38]. Furthermore, volume growth has been shown to be significantly higher in patients who developed worrisome PCL features [39].

6. Cyst Volume Assessment in Other Organs

Multiple imaging modalities, including ultrasound, CT, and MRI, are already being used to assess volume and risk stratify lesions in other solid organs. There is a well-established precedent for this in solid masses. Buerke et al. demonstrated the feasibility and precision of volume assessment of peripheral, abdominal, and thoracic lymph nodes using CT imaging [40]. Subsequently, in a study of primary lung cancers, three reviewers assessed 64 lung tumors on CT scans to compare diametric, areametric, and volumetric measurements. While all three measures had high reproducibility, volumetric measurements were more precise than traditional diametric ones [41]. The accuracy of MRI for solid tumor volume assessment was reinforced by the study of male patients with elevated PSA who underwent radical prostatectomy. MRI tumor volumes were obtained via manual tumor segmentation and compared to histopathologic tumor volumes. Accurate estimates of histopathologic volume were obtained using MRI volumetry, and the accuracy was greater for tumors larger than 0.5 cm^3 [42].

Despite the precedent of solid lesion volumetry with CT and MRI, image-guided volumetry is less frequently used in cystic lesions. Autosomal dominant polycystic kidney disease (ADPKD) is an example where cystic lesion volumes are routinely measured using imaging [43]. Multiple techniques are utilized to obtain total kidney and individual cyst volumes to evaluate disease progression. These range from manual planimetry to semi- or even fully-automated techniques [44]. Manual planimetry has historically been considered the gold standard for ADPKD cyst volume evaluation but is very time-consuming. It requires a reviewer to manually trace the outline of a lesion, calculate the total volume by multiplying all traced areas by axial slice thickness, and then combine slice volumes [44]. Another method of image-guided volume measurement used in ADPKD management is stereology. Areas corresponding to kidney regions are defined with grid points in serial coronal sections of MRI. The areas of cysts or renal parenchyma are then calculated by counting the number of intersections within them and converting this into a pixel count. The renal or cystic volume is then calculated by summing the products of the resulting areas and corresponding slice thickness [44].

The ellipsoid volume formula method (V = length (average of sagittal and coronal lengths) × width × depth × ($\pi/6$)) uses the measurements of longitudinal length, maximum width, and maximum depth from coronal and sagittal MRI slices to calculate volume [45]. The mid-slice method uses a manual tracing on a single middle coronal slice of MRI to calculate area, which is then multiplied by total number of slices, slice thickness, and experimentally defined correction factor to calculate volume [45]. In semi-automated ADPKD cystic volume measurement technique, an algorithm is used to generate a contour using a manually selected reference point in a central slice on MRI [44]. Both CT and MRI have been shown to reliably estimate total kidney and individual cyst volumes in patients with ADPKD [46,47]. These volumes are important for understanding the disease course, as high cyst volumes are negatively associated with renal function, and those with high ratios of cyst volume to total kidney volume have a higher likelihood of requiring dialysis for end-stage renal disease [47,48]. Similar techniques are now being employed in the evaluation of pancreatic cystic lesions.

7. Methods of Volume Assessment for Managing PCLs

Given the lack of evidence that PCL size by the maximum diameter is a reliable tool for determining malignant risk, recent research has focused on PCL volume as a possible alternative for risk assessment. Awe et al. reviewed 195 patients with PCLs at a single center to correlate size, as measured by maximum axial diameter (MAD), and volume. For

MAD measurement, a region of interest (ROI) was drawn in the axial dimension of the CT imaging slice with the largest MAD. Then, a quantitative imaging software platform was used to generate a 3D ROI and edited to exclude vasculature, ducts, surgical hardware, and bowel gas. After a final 3D ROI was generated, the software generated values for MAD, volume, surface area, and sphericity. Results showed that MAD is a poor correlate of volume in smaller cysts (1–3 cm). When there were subsequent CT or MRI images collected over a year later for comparison, MAD changes over that time also correlated poorly with volume changes. Unsurprisingly, these estimates were even less reliable in non-spherical cysts. Therefore, the authors concluded that MAD incompletely captures the complexity of pancreatic cysts [49]. Notably, this study was limited by a lack of pathologic data to correlate cyst characteristics with malignant risk, as most of the patients underwent surveillance without surgical resection.

Similarly, a single-center retrospective study by Pandey et al. evaluated 164 IPMNs on 107 MRI images and compared manual and semi-automatic largest diameter and volume measurements between three radiologists to assess for interobserver reproducibility. All three readers were taught a standard protocol to obtain these measurements. First, each reader measured the largest diameter of the IPMN manually using electronic calipers on both axial T2W and coronal three-dimensional MRCP images on the cross-section with the largest diameter. They then excluded any ductal extension and separated groups of cysts if there was a dividing septum >1 mm thick. This was followed by semi-automatic measurements, which involved the interactive segmentation of the lesion on each slice where the lesion was visible. All measurements were performed using a commonly available commercial Picture Archiving and Communication System (PACS; Carestream Health, Inc., Rochester, NY, USA) software. Of the six measurements collected for each IPMN, the highest interobserver reproducibility was seen for axial manual diameter measurements in cysts $\geq$1.5 cm, while the lowest was seen for coronal manual diameter measurements on cysts measuring <1.5 cm. This overall high interobserver reproducibility was attributed to the standardized measurement protocol taught to the three readers at the beginning of the study. Therefore, the authors concluded that a standardized cyst measurement technique would benefit IPMN follow-up since each follow-up image is often read by different radiologists. Additionally, the semi-automatic method of volume measurement in this study did not rely on the subjective selection of a cyst cross-section with the largest diameter by the reader, suggesting that cyst volume measurement may allow for more a reproducible cyst monitoring mechanism, especially in the absence of a standardized measurement protocol [24].

Pozzi Mucelli et al. assessed 106 patients with a histopathological diagnosis of BD- and mixed-type IPMN with an available preoperative MRI to test the hypothesis that volume could serve as a better predictor of malignancy than size. All MRIs were evaluated on a PACS by two radiologists in consensus reading, with one cyst chosen per patient (the largest or one with the highest suspicion for malignancy). Several IPMN parameters were collected, including a maximum diameter on axial and coronal T2W images, elongation value (defined as 1-(width/length)), maximum MPD diameter, the presence of contrast-enhancing mural nodules, cyst wall thickening $\geq$ 2 mm, growth of >5 mm per year during follow-up, solitary vs. multifocal, location, and volume. Volume was calculated on axial T2W images, on which an ROI was drawn along the edge of the BD-IPMN on multiple levels. The software then automatically calculated the volume. Interestingly, the analysis of these data showed that neither elongation value nor volume were associated with advanced neoplasia. This is despite the confirmation with elongation value data that most of these lesions were not spherical. The only variables in the study which were associated with advanced neoplasia were the presence of contrast-enhancing mural nodules, a diameter of MPD $\geq$ 5 mm, and serum CA 19-9 level > 37 [50].

8. Conclusions

Studies that utilized PCL size as one of the topics of investigation often used the maximum diameter of cysts seen on a 2D imaging modality (MRI, CT, and/or EUS) to define the cyst size. This generalized sizing technique assumes that pancreatic cysts are roughly spherical and that the largest diameter captures the overall size of the cyst. However, this does not reflect the natural variability of PCLs, which can have a multitude of morphological appearances [51]. Therefore, the utilization of maximum diameter on 2D imaging has its shortcomings. Firstly, the maximum diameter depends heavily on the reader's choice of the image plane (axial vs. sagittal vs. coronal) as well as the angle of the images relative to the lesion. Most conventional CT scans and MRIs provide three-plane imaging: coronal, sagittal, and axial. Even if the largest maximum diameter from each of the three views is chosen for the cyst size parameter, there is a chance of overestimating or underestimating the cyst size, depending on the cyst orientation (i.e., the axis of cysts' actual maximal diameter may not be oriented parallel to the image plane) and shape, as shown in Figure 2. EUS offers more freedom in angle of view compared to CT and MRI with a vantage point closer to the cyst of question. However, the view is still limited by the probe's angle of approach to the cyst relative to its orientation and shape. While the maximum cyst diameter has the benefit of being easily measured from any imaging modality, the drawback of this convenience is a lack of standardized protocol for obtaining the measurement. Even the ACG and European guidelines do not comment on the best practices for measuring pancreatic cyst size, despite using it as the primary criteria for the diagnosis, management, and surveillance of pancreatic cysts.

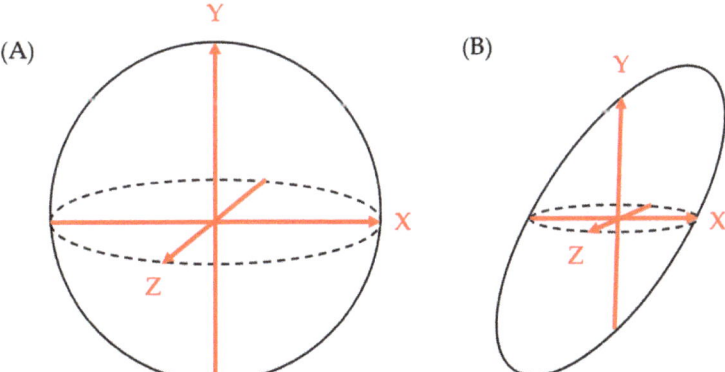

Figure 2. While the maximum length measurements on each of the X-Y-Z axes correlate well to overall spherical shape of figure (**A**), they do not correlate as well to the non-spherical shape of figure (**B**).

The limitations of the maximum diameter measurement on 2D imaging can be somewhat overcome by measuring the cyst's length, height, and width to appropriately capture the three-dimensional volume the cyst occupies rather than merely its maximal length. Such measurements can more accurately evaluate a cyst that does not comply with the spherical assumption. However, the measurements are again restrained by the angle of view available in each imaging modality. The cyst may be oriented in such a way that three perpendicular views are inadequate to estimate an accurate cyst size. While three-axis measurement has the potential to offer improved accuracy by allowing for the calculation of volume, it may be more difficult and time-consuming to obtain and report. Several studies discussed above evaluated the efficacy and reliability of cyst volume measurements, not only in the pancreas but in other organs as well. While one study has suggested the reproducibility of cyst volume measurement using a semi-automatic volume measurement method, another study did not find a strong correlation between cyst volume and the risk of malignancy. Therefore, additional larger studies to evaluate the relationship between cyst volume and malignant risk would provide guidance as to whether developing a uniform system to assess cyst volume would be useful. Given that cyst volume measurement can be relatively reliably reproduced using commercially available PACS software, collecting more data on cyst volume measurement through meta-analysis may prove to be valuable.

The cited references unanimously voice the lack of standardized protocol of cyst size measurement and raise it as a potential threat to accurately monitoring pancreatic cysts. A study has demonstrated that a standardized cyst size measurement method can be taught to radiographic readers with high reproducibility. Such an assessment should be taken into account by entities creating pancreatic cyst diagnosis and management guidelines. The development of a standardized cyst size measurement protocol may become useful to guarantee universal reliability in pancreatic cyst management.

Author Contributions: Conceptualization, S.G.K., D.Y.R. and B.K.; validation, J.R., Z.K.S., W.C., A.K.E., P.A.H. and S.G.K.; investigation, D.Y.R. and B.K.; resources, S.G.K.; writing—original draft preparation, D.Y.R. and B.K.; writing—review and editing, D.Y.R., B.K., W.C., A.K.E., J.R., P.A.H. and S.G.K.; visualization, S.G.K.; supervision, S.G.K. All authors have read and agreed to the published version of the manuscript.

Funding: This research received no external funding.

Informed Consent Statement: Not applicable.

Data Availability Statement: No new data were created or analyzed in this study. Data sharing is not applicable to this article.

Conflicts of Interest: Krishna SG—research grant support (investigator-initiated studies) from Mauna Kea Technologies, Paris, France, and Taewoong Medical, USA.

References

1. National Cancer Institute. *Cancer Stat Facts: Pancreatic Cancer*; NIH National Cancer Institute: Bethesda, MD, USA, 2022.
2. Hu, J.-X.; Zhao, C.-F.; Chen, W.-B.; Liu, Q.-C.; Li, Q.-W.; Lin, Y.-Y.; Gao, F. Pancreatic cancer: A review of epidemiology, trend, and risk factors. *World J. Gastroenterol.* **2021**, *27*, 4298–4321. [CrossRef] [PubMed]
3. Singhi, A.D.; Koay, E.J.; Chari, S.T.; Maitra, A. Early Detection of Pancreatic Cancer: Opportunities and Challenges. *Gastroenterology* **2019**, *156*, 2024–2040. [CrossRef] [PubMed]
4. Buerlein, R.C.; Shami, V.M. Management of pancreatic cysts and guidelines: What the gastroenterologist needs to know. *Ther. Adv. Gastrointest. Endosc.* **2021**, *14*, 26317745211045769. [CrossRef] [PubMed]
5. Ferrone, C.R.; Correa-Gallego, C.; Warshaw, A.L.; Brugge, W.R.; Forcione, D.G.; Thayer, S.P.; Castillo, C.F.-D. Current trends in pancreatic cystic neoplasms. *Arch. Surg.* **2009**, *144*, 448–454. [CrossRef]
6. Reid-Lombardo, K.M.; Sauver, J.S.; Li, Z.; Ahrens, W.A.; Unni, K.K.; Que, F.G. Incidence, prevalence, and management of intraductal papillary mucinous neoplasm in Olmsted County, Minnesota, 1984–2005: A population study. *Pancreas* **2008**, *37*, 139–144. [CrossRef]
7. Machado, N.O.; Al Qadhi, H.; Al Wahibi, K. Intraductal Papillary Mucinous Neoplasm of Pancreas. *North. Am. J. Med. Sci.* **2015**, *7*, 160–175. [CrossRef]
8. Scheiman, J.M.; Hwang, J.H.; Moayyedi, P. American gastroenterological association technical review on the diagnosis and management of asymptomatic neoplastic pancreatic cysts. *Gastroenterology* **2015**, *148*, 824–848.e22. [CrossRef]
9. Tanaka, M.; Fernández-del Castillo, C.; Kamisawa, T.; Jang, J.Y.; Levy, P.; Ohtsuka, T.; Salvia, R.; Shimizu, Y.; Tada, M.; Wolfgang, C.L. Revisions of international consensus Fukuoka guidelines for the management of IPMN of the pancreas. *Pancreatology* **2017**, *17*, 738–753. [CrossRef]
10. Farrell, J.J. Prevalence, Diagnosis and Management of Pancreatic Cystic Neoplasms: Current Status and Future Directions. *Gut Liver* **2015**, *9*, 571–589. [CrossRef]
11. Tanaka, M.; Chari, S.; Adsay, V.; Fernandez-del Castillo, C.; Falconi, M.; Shimizu, M.; Yamaguchi, K.; Yamao, K.; Matsuno, S. International consensus guidelines for management of intraductal papillary mucinous neoplasms and mucinous cystic neoplasms of the pancreas. *Pancreatology* **2006**, *6*, 17–32. [CrossRef]
12. Tanaka, M.; Fernández-del Castillo, C.; Adsay, V.; Chari, S.; Falconi, M.; Jang, J.-Y.; Kimura, W.; Levy, P.; Pitman, M.B.; Schmidt, C.M.; et al. International consensus guidelines 2012 for the management of IPMN and MCN of the pancreas. *Pancreatology* **2012**, *12*, 183–197. [CrossRef] [PubMed]
13. Vege, S.S.; Ziring, B.; Jain, R.; Moayyedi, P.; Adams, M.A.; Dorn, S.D.; Dudley-Brown, S.L.; Flamm, S.L.; Gellad, Z.F.; Gruss, C.B.; et al. American gastroenterological association institute guideline on the diagnosis and management of asymptomatic neoplastic pancreatic cysts. *Gastroenterology* **2015**, *148*, 819–822, quize12-3. [CrossRef]

14. Megibow, A.J.; Baker, M.E.; Morgan, D.E.; Kamel, I.R.; Sahani, D.V.; Newman, E.; Brugge, W.R.; Berland, L.L.; Pandharipande, P.V. Management of Incidental Pancreatic Cysts: A White Paper of the ACR Incidental Findings Committee. *J. Am. Coll. Radiol.* **2017**, *14*, 911–923. [CrossRef]
15. Elta, G.H.; Enestvedt, B.K.; Sauer, B.G.; Lennon, A.M. ACG Clinical Guideline: Diagnosis and Management of Pancreatic Cysts. *Am. J. Gastroenterol.* **2018**, *113*, 464–479. [CrossRef] [PubMed]
16. European Study Group on Cystic Tumours of the Pancreas. European evidence-based guidelines on pancreatic cystic neoplasms. *Gut* **2018**, *67*, 789–804. [CrossRef]
17. Bruenderman, E.; Martin, R.C. A cost analysis of a pancreatic cancer screening protocol in high-risk populations. *Am. J. Surg.* **2015**, *210*, 409–416. [CrossRef]
18. Du, C.; Chai, N.-L.; Linghu, E.-Q.; Li, H.-K.; Sun, L.-H.; Jiang, L.; Wang, X.-D.; Tang, P.; Yang, J. Comparison of endoscopic ultrasound, computed tomography and magnetic resonance imaging in assessment of detailed structures of pancreatic cystic neoplasms. *World J. Gastroenterol.* **2017**, *23*, 3184–3192. [CrossRef]
19. Boos, J.; Brook, A.; Chingkoe, C.M.; Morrison, T.; Mortele, K.; Raptopoulos, V.; Pedrosa, I.; Brook, O.R. MDCT vs. MRI for incidental pancreatic cysts: Measurement variability and impact on clinical management. *Abdom. Radiol.* **2017**, *42*, 521–530. [CrossRef]
20. Lee, Y.S.; Paik, K.-H.; Kim, H.W.; Lee, J.-C.; Kim, J.; Hwang, J.-H. Comparison of Endoscopic Ultrasonography, Computed Tomography, and Magnetic Resonance Imaging for Pancreas Cystic Lesions. *Medicine* **2015**, *94*, e1666. [CrossRef] [PubMed]
21. Maimone, S.; Agrawal, D.; Pollack, M.J.; Wong, R.C.; Willis, J.; Faulx, A.L.; Isenberg, G.A.; Chak, A. Variability in measurements of pancreatic cyst size among EUS, CT, and magnetic resonance imaging modalities. *Gastrointest. Endosc.* **2010**, *71*, 945–950. [CrossRef]
22. Leeds, J.; Nayar, M.; Dawwas, M.; Scott, J.; Anderson, K.; Haugk, B.; Oppong, K. Comparison of endoscopic ultrasound and computed tomography in the assessment of pancreatic cyst size using pathology as the gold standard. *Pancreatology* **2013**, *13*, 263–266. [CrossRef] [PubMed]
23. Huynh, T.; Ali, K.; Vyas, S.; Dezsi, K.; Strickland, D.; Basinski, T.; Chen, D.-T.; Jiang, K.; Centeno, B.; Malafa, M.; et al. Comparison of imaging modalities for measuring the diameter of intraductal papillary mucinous neoplasms of the pancreas. *Pancreatology* **2020**, *20*, 448–453. [CrossRef] [PubMed]
24. Pandey, P.; Pandey, A.; Varzaneh, F.N.; Ghasabeh, M.A.; Fouladi, D.; Khoshpouri, P.; Shao, N.; Zarghampour, M.; Hruban, R.H.; Canto, M.; et al. Are pancreatic IPMN volumes measured on MRI images more reproducible than diameters? An assessment in a large single-institution cohort. *Eur. Radiol.* **2018**, *28*, 2790–2800. [CrossRef]
25. Chalian, H.; Seyal, A.R.; Rezai, P.; Töre, H.G.; Miller, F.H.; Bentrem, D.J.; Yaghmai, V. Pancreatic mucinous cystic neoplasm size using CT volumetry, spherical and ellipsoid formulas: Validation study. *J. Pancreas* **2014**, *15*, 25–32. [CrossRef]
26. Lee, J.E.; Choi, S.-Y.; Min, J.H.; Yi, B.H.; Lee, M.H.; Kim, S.S.; Hwang, J.A.; Kim, J.H. Determining Malignant Potential of Intraductal Papillary Mucinous Neoplasm of the Pancreas: CT versus MRI by Using Revised 2017 International Consensus Guidelines. *Radiology* **2019**, *293*, 134–143. [CrossRef]
27. Liu, H.; Cui, Y.; Shao, J.; Shao, Z.; Su, F.; Li, Y. The diagnostic role of CT, MRI/MRCP, PET/CT, EUS and DWI in the differentiation of benign and malignant IPMN: A meta-analysis. *Clin. Imaging.* **2021**, *72*, 183–193. [CrossRef]
28. Udare, A.; Agarwal, M.; Alabousi, M.; McInnes, M.; Rubino, J.G.; Marcaccio, M.; van der Pol, C.B. Diagnostic Accuracy of MRI for Differentiation of Benign and Malignant Pancreatic Cystic Lesions Compared to CT and Endoscopic Ultrasound: Systematic Review and Meta-analysis. *J. Magn. Reson. Imaging* **2021**, *54*, 1126–1137. [CrossRef] [PubMed]
29. Jang, J.-Y.; Park, T.; Lee, S.; Kim, Y.; Lee, S.Y.; Kim, S.-W.; Kim, S.-C.; Song, K.-B.; Yamamoto, M.; Hatori, T.; et al. Proposed Nomogram Predicting the Individual Risk of Malignancy in the Patients with Branch Duct Type Intraductal Papillary Mucinous Neoplasms of the Pancreas. *Ann. Surg.* **2017**, *266*, 1062–1068. [CrossRef]
30. Zhao, W.; Liu, S.; Cong, L.; Zhao, Y. Imaging Features for Predicting High-Grade Dysplasia or Malignancy in Branch Duct Type Intraductal Papillary Mucinous Neoplasm of the Pancreas: A Systematic Review and Meta-Analysis. *Ann. Surg. Oncol.* **2022**, *29*, 1297–1312. [CrossRef]
31. Kwon, W.; Han, Y.; Byun, Y.; Kang, J.S.; Choi, Y.J.; Kim, H.; Jang, J.-Y. Predictive Features of Malignancy in Branch Duct Type Intraductal Papillary Mucinous Neoplasm of the Pancreas: A Meta-Analysis. *Cancers* **2020**, *12*, 2618. [CrossRef]
32. Xu, M.-M.; Yin, S.; Siddiqui, A.A.; Salem, R.R.; Schrope, B.; Sethi, A.; Poneros, J.M.; Gress, F.G.; Genkinger, J.M.; Do, C.; et al. Comparison of the diagnostic accuracy of three current guidelines for the evaluation of asymptomatic pancreatic cystic neoplasms. *Medicine* **2017**, *96*, e7900. [CrossRef]
33. Walsh, R.M.; Vogt, D.P.; Henderson, J.M.; Hirose, K.; Mason, T.; Bencsath, K.; Hammel, J.; Brown, N. Management of suspected pancreatic cystic neoplasms based on cyst size. *Surgery* **2008**, *144*, 677–684. [CrossRef]
34. Guarise, A.; Faccioli, N.; Ferrari, M.; Salvia, R.; Mucelli, R.P.; Morana, G.; Megibow, A.J. Evaluation of serial changes of pancreatic branch duct intraductal papillary mucinous neoplasms by follow-up with magnetic resonance imaging. *Cancer Imaging.* **2008**, *8*, 220–228. [CrossRef]
35. El Chafic, A.; El Hajj, I.I.; DeWitt, J.; Schmidt, C.M.; Siddiqui, A.; Sherman, S.; Aggarwal, A.; Al-Haddad, M. Does cyst growth predict malignancy in branch duct intraductal papillary mucinous neoplasms? Results of a large multicenter experience. *Dig. Liver Dis.* **2018**, *50*, 961–968. [CrossRef]

36. Ciprani, D.; Weniger, M.; Qadan, M.; Hank, T.; Horick, N.; Harrison, J.; Marchegiani, G.; Andrianello, S.; Pandharipande, P.; Ferrone, C.; et al. Risk of malignancy in small pancreatic cysts decreases over time. *Pancreatology* **2020**, *20*, 1213–1217. [CrossRef] [PubMed]
37. Hecht, E.M.; Khatri, G.; Morgan, D.; Kang, S.; Bhosale, P.R.; Francis, I.R.; Gandhi, N.S.; Hough, D.M.; Huang, C.; Luk, L.; et al. Intraductal papillary mucinous neoplasm (IPMN) of the pancreas: Recommendations for Standardized Imaging and Reporting from the Society of Abdominal Radiology IPMN disease focused panel. *Abdom. Radiol.* **2021**, *46*, 1586–1606. [CrossRef]
38. Goldmacher, G.V.; Conklin, J. The use of tumour volumetrics to assess response to therapy in anticancer clinical trials. *Br. J. Clin. Pharmacol.* **2012**, *73*, 846–854. [CrossRef]
39. Innocenti, T.; Danti, G.; Lynch, E.N.; Dragoni, G.; Gottin, M.; Fedeli, F.; Palatresi, D.; Biagini, M.R.; Milani, S.; Miele, V.; et al. Higher volume growth rate is associated with development of worrisome features in patients with branch duct-intraductal papillary mucinous neoplasms. *World J. Clin. Cases.* **2022**, *10*, 5667–5679. [CrossRef] [PubMed]
40. Buerke, B.; Puesken, M.; Müter, S.; Weckesser, M.; Gerss, J.; Heindel, W.; Wessling, J. Measurement accuracy and reproducibility of semiautomated metric and volumetric lymph node analysis in MDCT. *AJR Am. J. Roentgenol.* **2010**, *195*, 979–985. [CrossRef]
41. Frenette, A.; Morrell, J.; Bjella, K.; Fogarty, E.; Beal, J.; Chaudhary, V. Do Diametric Measurements Provide Sufficient and Reliable Tumor Assessment? An Evaluation of Diametric, Areametric, and Volumetric Variability of Lung Lesion Measurements on Computerized Tomography Scans. *J. Oncol.* **2015**, *2015*, 632943. [CrossRef] [PubMed]
42. Turkbey, B.; Mani, H.; Aras, O.; Rastinehad, A.R.; Shah, V.; Bernardo, M.; Pohida, T.; Daar, D.; Benjamin, C.; McKinney, Y.L.; et al. Correlation of magnetic resonance imaging tumor volume with histopathology. *J. Urol.* **2012**, *188*, 1157–1163. [CrossRef] [PubMed]
43. Grantham, J.J.; Torres, V.E.; Chapman, A.B.; Guay-Woodford, L.M.; Bae, K.T.; King, B.F.; Wetzel, L.H.; Baumgarten, D.A.; Kenney, P.J.; Harris, P.C.; et al. Volume progression in polycystic kidney disease. *N. Engl. J. Med.* **2006**, *354*, 2122–2130. [CrossRef]
44. Magistroni, R.; Corsi, C.; Martí, T.; Torra, R. A Review of the Imaging Techniques for Measuring Kidney and Cyst Volume in Establishing Autosomal Dominant Polycystic Kidney Disease Progression. *Am. J. Nephrol.* **2018**, *48*, 67–78. [CrossRef]
45. Sharma, K.; Caroli, A.; Van Quach, L.; Petzold, K.; Bozzetto, M.; Serra, A.L.; Remuzzi, G.; Remuzzi, A. Kidney volume measurement methods for clinical studies on autosomal dominant polycystic kidney disease. *PLoS ONE* **2017**, *12*, e0178488. [CrossRef]
46. Bae, K.T.; Tao, C.; Wang, J.; Kaya, D.; Wu, Z.; Bae, J.T.; Chapman, A.B.; Torres, V.E.; Grantham, J.J.; Mrug, M.; et al. Novel approach to estimate kidney and cyst volumes using mid-slice magnetic resonance images in polycystic kidney disease. *Am. J. Nephrol.* **2013**, *38*, 333–341. [CrossRef]
47. King, B.F.; Reed, J.E.; Bergstralh, E.J.; Sheedy, P.F.; Torres, V.E. Quantification and longitudinal trends of kidney, renal cyst, and renal parenchyma volumes in autosomal dominant polycystic kidney disease. *J. Am. Soc. Nephrol.* **2000**, *11*, 1505–1511. [CrossRef]
48. Sise, C.; Kusaka, M.; Wetzel, L.H.; Winklhofer, F.; Cowley, B.D.; Cook, L.T.; Gordon, M.; Grantham, J.J. Volumetric determination of progression in autosomal dominant polycystic kidney disease by computed tomography. *Kidney Int.* **2000**, *58*, 2492–2501. [CrossRef]
49. Awe, A.M.; Rendell, V.R.; Lubner, M.G.; Weber, S.; Winslow, E.R. Pancreatic cyst characterization: Maximum axial diameter does not measure up. *HPB* **2021**, *23*, 1105–1112. [CrossRef] [PubMed]
50. Mucelli, R.M.P.; Moro, C.F.; Del Chiaro, M.; Valente, R.; Blomqvist, L.; Papanikolaou, N.; Löhr, J.-M.; Kartalis, N. Branch-duct intraductal papillary mucinous neoplasm (IPMN): Are cyst volumetry and other novel imaging features able to improve malignancy prediction compared to well-established resection criteria? *Eur. Radiol.* **2022**, *32*, 5144–5155. [CrossRef]
51. Aghaei Lasboo, A.; Rezai, P.; Yaghmai, V. Morphological analysis of pancreatic cystic masses. *Acad. Radiol.* **2010**, *17*, 348–351. [CrossRef] [PubMed]

Disclaimer/Publisher's Note: The statements, opinions and data contained in all publications are solely those of the individual author(s) and contributor(s) and not of MDPI and/or the editor(s). MDPI and/or the editor(s) disclaim responsibility for any injury to people or property resulting from any ideas, methods, instructions or products referred to in the content.

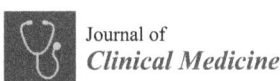

Article

Endoscopic Ultrasound-Guided Botox Injection for Refractory Anal Fissure

Navkiran Randhawa [1,*], Ahamed Khalyfa [2], Rida Aslam [3], M. Christopher Roebuck [4], Mahnoor Inam [5] and Kamran Ayub [6,*]

1. Department of Internal Medicine, Pacific Northwest University of Health Sciences, Yakima, WA 98901, USA
2. Department of Internal Medicine, A.T. Still University, Kirksville, MO 63501, USA
3. Department of Gastroenterology, Franciscan Health Olympia Fields, Olympia Fields, IL 60461, USA
4. Rx Economics, Hunt Valley, MD 21031, USA
5. Southwest Gastroenterology, Oak Lawn, IL 60453, USA
6. Silver Cross Hospital, New Lenox, IL 60451, USA
* Correspondence: randhnk@gmail.com (N.R.); kamranayub@icloud.com (K.A.)

Abstract: Background: Anal fissures cause severe pain and can be difficult to treat. Medical therapy is initially used, followed by sigmoidoscopy-guided botox injections if the medical therapy is not successful. With this technique, however, it is not clear whether botox is injected into the muscle layer or submucosa. Aim: To evaluate the efficacy of EUS-guided botox injection directly into the internal sphincter. Methods: Consecutive patients with chronic anal fissure refractory to conventional endoscopic botulinum toxin type A injection were enrolled in the study. EUS was performed using a linear array echoendoscope, and a 25 G needle was used to inject botox. All patients were followed up at one- and two-month intervals. Results: Eight patients with chronic anal fissures were included in the study. Six patients had an excellent response to botox at the two-month interval using a visual analog pain scale, while one patient had a moderate response with a pain score reduction of 40%. One patient had no response. No complications were noted. An improvement in visual analog scale (pre-score > post-score) was statistically significant at the $p < 0.01$ level. Conclusion: EUS-guided botox injection into the internal sphincter appears to be a promising technique for patients with refractory anal fissure with pain.

Keywords: EUS; botox; anal fissure; endoscopy

1. Introduction

Anal fissures are a well-known disease worldwide. In the United States, approximately 235,000 new cases of anal fissures are diagnosed each year, while in Italy it is the second most common cause of proctologist visits [1,2]. Anal fissure symptoms cause patients significant distress and reduce their quality of life substantially [3]. Although the etiology of anal fissures is controversial, hypertonia of the internal anal sphincter (IAS) has been recognized as a key player in the pathogenesis of the disease. Persistent IAS ischemia and ulceration can lead to severe complications including perianal fistulas, anorectal abscess formation, and anal incontinence [4,5].

Thus, treatment for anal fissures is aimed at reducing IAS spasms to relieve pain, decrease ischemia and promote the healing of ulcers. Acute anal fissures are commonly managed by conservative medical treatment, while chronic anal fissures are refractory to such treatment. Surgical treatment, such as sphincterotomy, is commonly required for the treatment of chronic anal fissures or abscesses, providing symptomatic relief [6,7]. However, this procedure requires sphincter injury and has been associated with permanent complications ranging from incontinence of gas in up to 45% of patients to stool incontinence in up to 22% [8,9].

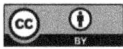

Due to such surgical complications, reversible relaxation of the IAS through botulinum toxin type A (BTX) injection has become a common treatment [10]. The injection of type A botulinum neurotoxin produces a constant reduction in maximum resting pressure of IAS and acts like a chemical sphincterotomy. The effect lasts for a few months, giving time for the fissure to heal. Despite being clinically beneficial and causing minimal side effects, achieving proper placement is difficult due to the small target involved [11–13]. Ultrasonography has been utilized for direct visual guidance in prior research papers. In 1997, Hofmann et al. reported the first endoscopic ultrasound (EUS)-guided injection of BTX directly into the lower esophageal sphincter muscle as a treatment of achalasia. This treatment proved to be more effective than endoscopic BTX injection without visualization of the direct tissue layers. Our paper similarly explores the utilization of EUS-guided BTX injection directly into the sphincter muscle to treat anal fissures. Our aim is to evaluate the efficacy and safety of EUS-guided BTX injection directly into the internal sphincter in patients with chronic anal fissure refractory to conventional endoscopic botox injection.

2. Materials and Methods

2.1. Study Patients

Consecutive symptomatic adults with chronic anal fissure refractory to conventional endoscopic four-quadrant BTX injection were enrolled in the study. Refractory was defined by patient's who failed prior medication and endoscopic botox treatment without the guidance of an endoscopic ultrasound. The inclusion criteria were as follows: (i) evidence of induration in the anal canal, (ii) persistent symptoms of post-defecation/nocturnal pain or bleeding for over 3 months, (iii) failed previous endoscopic injection.

The exclusion criteria included: acute anal fissure, anal fissure secondary to underlying pathology, known sensitivity to BTX, or patients who were unable to consent to the procedure.

The study protocol was approved by the Institutional Review Board.

2.2. Operative Technique

EUS was performed using a linear array echoendoscope (Figures 1–3). Eighty units of type A botulinum neurotoxin was diluted in 2 cc of isotonic saline. An echoendoscope was introduced into the anal canal. The internal sphincter was identified sonographically and a 25-gauge needle was introduced into the internal sphincter. Then, 0.5 cc of saline-containing 20IU BTX was injected into the internal sphincter. The needle was withdrawn, the scope was rotated 90 degrees and the second injection was given. This process was repeated for a total of 4 times giving 0.5 cc per quadrant. Conscious sedation or MAC anesthesia was used for the procedure.

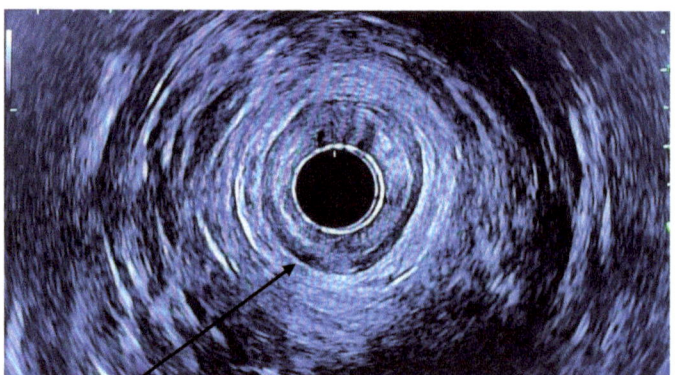

Figure 1. Radial EUS with arrow pointing to IAS.

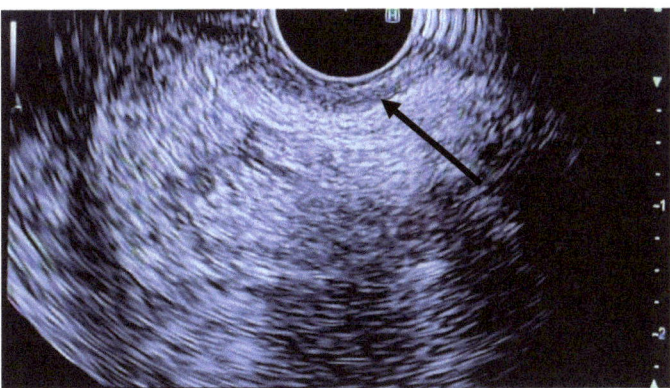

Figure 2. Linear EUS with arrow pointing to IAS.

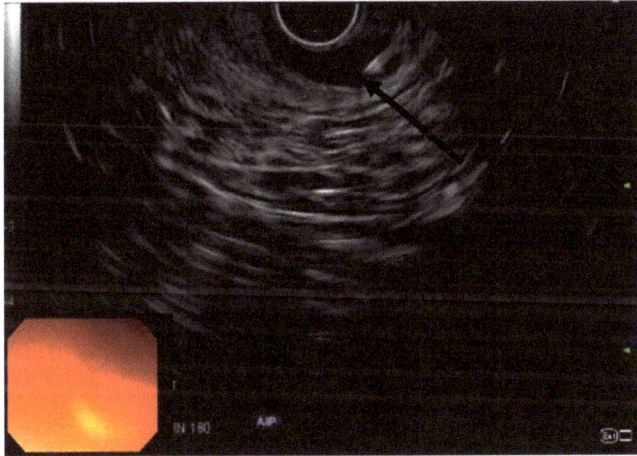

Figure 3. Linear EUS with arrow pointing to the needle injecting the IAS with expansion of the IAS due to the injection.

2.3. Clinical Care and Follow-Up

All patients were followed up at 1- and 2-month intervals by telephone or in person. The patients were asked to determine their pain level by using a 10-point visual analog pain scale. This was compared to the pain score at baseline.

2.4. Statistical Analysis

All statistical analyses were performed using Excel. All results were expressed as the mean +/− standard deviation, and differences between pre- and post-visual analogs were determined via a paired t-test. p-values of less than 0.05 were considered to be statistically significant.

3. Results

Twelve consecutive patients were assessed for eligibility; of these, four patients did not meet the inclusion criteria. Three patients were unable to consent or refused to consent to participate in the study, and one patient had an acute fissure (not chronic) and superimposed hemorrhoids.

All patients reported severe post-defecation pain. All patients had evidence of a posterior anal fissure from a digital rectal exam and colonoscopy.

We offered EUS-guided BTX injections into the IAS to all patients who presented with anal fissure pain for over 3 months that had been refractory to prior endoscopic BTX treatments. A total of eight patients with prior flexible sigmoidoscopy with BTX injection were included in the study. The outcome was defined as excellent if there was a 50% or greater decrease in the visual analog pain score. Six patients had an excellent response to BTX at the two-month interval using the visual analog pain scale. One patient had a moderate response with a pain score reduction of 40%. One patient, on chronic narcotic treatment, had no response (Table 1). Opioid addiction and opioid-induced hyperalgesia is suspected to explain one patient's lack of response to chronic opioid therapy. No complications, including incontinence, were reported by the patients after the EUS-guided BTX injection of the internal anal sphincter. The mean pre-treatment visual analog scale score was 9.75, whereas the post-treatment score at week 4 was 5, and 3.8 at week 8. The improvement in this score (pre-score versus post-score) was statistically significant at the $p < 0.01$ level.

Table 1. Study patients.

Patients	Age (y)/Sex	Initial Visual Analog Pain Score	Prior Failed Therapy	Visual Analog Pain Scale Improvement 1 Month after Procedure	Visual Analog Pain Scale Improvement 2 Months after Procedure	Final Outcome
1	22/M	10	Medication + Endoscopic botulinum toxin (BTX)	5	3	Excellent Response
2	33/M	10	Medication + Endoscopic BTX	4	3	Excellent Response
3	48/F	10	Medication + Endoscopic BTX	3	3	Excellent Response
4	61/F	10	Medication + Endoscopic BTX	4	2	Excellent Response
5	42/F	9	Medication + Endoscopic BTX	4	2	Excellent Response
6	60/M	9	Medication + Endoscopic BTX	4	2	Excellent Response
7	40/F	10	Medication + Endoscopic BTX	6	6	Moderate Response
8	48/M **	10	Medication + Endoscopic BTX	10	10	No response

** Patient was on narcotic pain medications from an outside clinic. Excellent response = 50% or greater decrease in the visual analog pain score. Moderate response = pain score reduction of 40%. No response = 0% change in pain score.

4. Discussion

Current therapies for anal fissure include pharmacotherapy, flexible sigmoidoscopy-guided BTX injection and surgical myotomy. In a prior study, Brisinda et al. compared a conservative treatment of 0.2% glyceryl trinitrate ointment to botulinum toxin in patients. This study revealed a 96% healing rate in the botulinum toxin group, compared with 60% in the glyceryl trinitrate group [12]. Thus, medical therapy alone with topical agents including nitrates can be relatively ineffective for chronic anal fissures [14]. On the other hand, surgical myotomy has the potential to offer long-term benefits, but it carries the risk of complications [15]. Alternative treatments are needed for patients with comorbidities or advanced age. The injection of BTX into the IAS has been shown to treat refractory anal fissure with good outcomes [10]. Maria et al. in their study found the local injection of botulinum toxin into the IAS to be a promising approach to the treatment of anal fissures [10]. However, this procedure when completed blindly can be technically challenging, as it relies on the endoscopist's tactile sense for the proper placement of the needle into the IAS. Cagri et al. further described the efficacy and safety of endoanal ultrasound (EAUS)-guided botulinum toxin in the treatment of chronic anal fissure [16]. The study revealed that the efficacy rate was higher in the EAUS group, but these results were not statistically significant.

In this pilot case series, we examined the utility of EUS-guided BTX injection into the IAS under direct visualization in patients with anal fissures refractory to medications and endoscopic therapies. Consecutive patients in our study who underwent EUS-guided BTX injection had excellent responses with a reduction in pain score with no complications. Furthermore, a statistically significant improvement in the visual analog scale was seen.

While, to our knowledge, our study is the first case series to report on EUS-guided botulinum injection for refractory anal fissures, we recognize several limitations. First, patients' inclusion and response assessment was based on some subjective criteria which are difficult to quantify and, therefore, might potentially introduce bias into our results. Second, the sample size was small, and thus our results may not be generalizable or applicable to larger populations. In addition, because our sample size was small, we cannot exclude the presence of selection bias in our study. Finally, the follow-up time was short and, therefore, no firm conclusions can be drawn from our results on long-term outcomes of this procedure and related complications. Furthermore, large multicenter studies will be needed to address these limitations.

5. Conclusions

In summary, EUS-guided BTX injection is a promising technique for patients with anal fissure refractory to medical therapy and appears to be superior to endoscopic BTX injection without ultrasound guidance. More studies need to be conducted to confirm the efficacy of this approach.

Author Contributions: Conceptualization, N.R., A.K., R.A. and K.A.; methodology, N.R., A.K., R.A. and K.A.; software, M.C.R.; validation, K.A.; formal analysis, M.C.R.; investigation, N.R., A.K., R.A. and K.A.; resources, N.R., A.K., R.A. and K.A.; data curation, N.R., A.K., R.A. and K.A.; writing—original draft preparation, N.R., A.K., R.A. and K.A.; writing—review and editing, N.R., A.K., R.A., M.I. and K.A.; visualization, N.R., A.K., R.A. and K.A.; supervision, K.A.; project administration, N.R. and R.A.; funding acquisition, none. All authors have read and agreed to the published version of the manuscript.

Funding: This research received no external funding.

Institutional Review Board Statement: Not applicable.

Informed Consent Statement: Informed consent was obtained from all subjects involved in the study.

Data Availability Statement: Not applicable.

Conflicts of Interest: The authors declare no conflict of interest.

References

1. Madalinski, M.H. Identifying the best therapy for chronic anal fissure. *World J. Gastrointest. Pharmacol. Ther.* **2011**, *2*, 9–16. [CrossRef] [PubMed]
2. Nelson, R.L.; Abcarian, H.; Davis, F.G.; Persky, V. Prevalence of benign anorectal disease in a randomly selected population. *Dis. Colon Rectum* **1995**, *38*, 341–344. [CrossRef] [PubMed]
3. Griffin, N.; Acheson, A.G.; Tung, P.; Sheard, C.; Glazebrook, C.; Scholefield, J.H. Quality of life in patients with chronic anal fissure. *Colorectal Dis.* **2004**, *6*, 39–44. [CrossRef] [PubMed]
4. Carter, D.; Dickman, R. The Role of Botox in Colorectal Disorders. *Curr. Treat. Options Gastroenterol.* **2018**, *16*, 541–547. [CrossRef] [PubMed]
5. Dat, A.; Chin, M.; Skinner, S.; Farmer, C.; Wale, R.; Carne, P.; Bell, S.; Warrier, S.K. Botulinum toxin therapy for chronic anal fissures: Where are we at currently? *ANZ J. Surg.* **2017**, *87*, E70–E73. [CrossRef] [PubMed]
6. Garg, P.; Kaur, B.; Yagnik, V.D.; Dawka, S. A New Anatomical Pathway of Spread of Pus/Sepsis in Anal Fistulas Discovered on MRI and Its Clinical Implications. *Clin. Exp. Gastroenterol.* **2021**, *14*, 397–404. [CrossRef] [PubMed]
7. Pietroletti, R.; Ciarrocchi, A.; Lely, L.; Rizza, V. Results of surgical treatment in chronic anal fissure complicated by abscess or fistula in a retrospective cohort of patients. *Eur. PMC* **2021**, *74*, 179–183. [CrossRef] [PubMed]

8. Oh, C.; Divino, C.M.; Steinhagen, R.M. Anal fissure. 20-year experience. *Dis. Colon Rectum* **1995**, *38*, 378–382. [CrossRef] [PubMed]
9. Trindade, A.J.; Hirten, R.; Greenberg, R.E.; Sejpal, D.V. EUS-guided botulinum toxin injection of the internal anal sphincter in anorectal outlet obstruction. *Am. J. Gastroenterol.* **2014**, *109*, 1293–1294. [CrossRef] [PubMed]
10. Maria, G.; Brisinda, G.; Bentivoglio, A.R.; Cassetta, E.; Gui, D.; Albanese, A. Influence of botulinum toxin site of injections on healing rate in patients with chronic anal fissure. *Am. J. Surg.* **2000**, *179*, 46–50. [CrossRef]
11. Brisinda, G.; Maria, G.; Sganga, G.; Bentivoglio, A.R.; Albanese, A.; Castagneto, M. Effectiveness of higher doses of botulinum toxin to induce healing in patients with chronic anal fissures. *Surgery* **2002**, *131*, 179–184. [CrossRef] [PubMed]
12. Brisinda, G.; Cadeddu, F.; Brandara, F.; Brisinda, D.; Maria, G. Treating chronic anal fissure with botulinum neurotoxin. *Nat. Clin. Pract. Gastroenterol. Hepatol.* **2004**, *1*, 82–89. [CrossRef] [PubMed]
13. Brisinda, G.; Maria, G.; Bentivoglio, A.R.; Cassetta, E.; Gui, D.; Albanese, A. A comparison of injections of botulinum toxin and topical nitroglycerin ointment for the treatment of chronic anal fissure. *N. Engl. J. Med.* **1999**, *341*, 65–69. [CrossRef] [PubMed]
14. Maria, G.; Cassetta, E.; Gui, D.; Brisinda, G.; Bentivoglio, A.R.; Albanese, A. A comparison of botulinum toxin and saline for the treatment of chronic anal fissure. *N. Engl. J. Med.* **1998**, *338*, 217–220. [CrossRef]
15. Hoffman, B.J.; Knapple, W.L.; Bhutani, M.S.; Verne, G.N.; Hawes, R.H. Treatment of achalasia by injection of botulinum toxin under endoscopic ultrasound guidance. *Gastrointest. Endosc.* **1997**, *45*, 77–79. [CrossRef]
16. Akalin, Ç.; Yavuzarslan, A.B.; Akyol, C. Efficacy and Safety of Endoanal Ultrasound-Guided Botulinum Toxin in Chronic Anal Fissure. *Am. Surg.* **2021**, 31348211034750. [CrossRef] [PubMed]

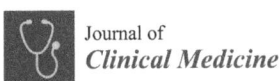

Article

Reduction of Lams-Related Adverse Events with Accumulating Experience in a Large-Volume Tertiary Referral Center

Sebastian Stefanovic [1,2], Helena Degroote [1] and Pieter Hindryckx [1,*]

1. Department of Gastroenterology, University Hospital of Ghent, Corneel Heymanslaan 10, 1K12-IE, 9000 Ghent, Belgium
2. Diagnostic Center Bled, Pod Skalo 4, 4260 Bled, Slovenia
* Correspondence: pieter.hindryckx@uzgent.be; Tel.: +32-(0)9-332-2371

Abstract: Background and aims: Lumen-apposing metal stents (LAMSs) are increasingly used both for on- and off-label indications. We continuously adapt our step-by-step protocol to optimize the safe deployment of LAMSs for the different indications. The aim of this study was to evaluate the impact of this approach over time. Methods: We conducted a single-center study on consecutive patients who underwent LAMS placement for on- and off-label indications between June 2020 and June 2022. Endpoints included technical success, clinical success and adverse event rates. We compared the results with our previously published early experience with LAMSs (N = 61), between March 2018 and May 2020. Results: This cohort consisted of 168 LAMSs in 153 patients. Almost half of them (47.6%) were placed for off-label indications (gastro-enterostomy, temporary access to the excluded stomach in patients with previous gastric bypass, drainage of postsurgical collections, stenting of short refractory gastrointestinal strictures). While the technical and clinical success rates were similar to those in our previously published cohort (97% and 93.5% versus 93.4% and 88.5%, respectively), the adverse event rate dropped from 21.3% to 8.9%. Conclusions: Our results demonstrate the impact of a learning curve in LAMS placement, with a clinically relevant drop in LAMS-related adverse events over time.

Keywords: EUS; LAMS; interventional EUS; adverse events; guideline

1. Introduction

Lumen-apposing metal stents (LAMSs) were first approved by the FDA in 2013 for drainage of peripancreatic collections [1–3], but their use quickly expanded to manage complicated situations that were previously referred to interventional radiology and/or surgery.

Currently, the use of LAMSs is also approved for gallbladder drainage in nonsurgical candidates and bile duct drainage in cases of failed endoscopic retrograde cholangiopancreatography (ERCP) and/or malignant distal biliary obstruction. Off-label indications include the creation of a luminal anastomosis (e.g., to alleviate gastric outlet obstruction in cases of duodenal obstruction or to create temporary access to the excluded stomach for endoscopy in gastric bypass patients), the drainage of postsurgical collections and the management of short refractory gastrointestinal strictures [3,4].

Although the clinical benefit of LAMSs may be substantial for many patients, one should be aware of potential (serious) adverse events related to LAMS procedures. We have previously reported an adverse event of 21.3%. Choi et al. [5] recently published similar results in the largest cohort study to date.

As for any other endoscopic intervention, three criteria should be fulfilled to minimize the adverse event rate and related morbidity: First, one should be fully aware of the potential complications of the procedure (what can happen?). Second, one should know the strategies to maximally prevent these complications (how to prevent it from happening?). Finally, one should be able to manage the complications in the appropriate way (do I have a plan B if it happens?).

The recent publication of expert consensus guidelines for interventional endoscopic ultrasound is very helpful in this regard, but data on young and evolving endoscopic techniques, such as LAMS placement, remain scarce and make large cohort studies of particular value.

The aim of our study was to assess the impact of a learning curve in LAMS placement in terms of technical success, clinical success and adverse event rate.

2. Methods

2.1. Study Design/Population

This was a retrospective single-center cohort study of consecutive patients who underwent LAMS placement (Hot AXIOS stent, Boston Scientific Corporation, Natick, MA, USA) at our tertiary referral center between June 2020 and June 2022. The study was reviewed and approved by the institutional ethical review board (reference: ONZ-2022-0179).

Patients were divided into categories: A: drainage of peripancreatic collections, B: biliary drainage (CBD), C: gallbladder drainage (GBD), D: gastroenteric anastomosis, E: temporary gastric access for endoscopy (GATE), F: treatment of refractory gastrointestinal (GI) strictures and G: miscellaneous, other indications.

2.2. Data Collection and Analysis

Using the electronic medical records and our prospectively collected database (for internal quality monitoring), we collected data on patient demographics, indications, technical and clinical success rates and adverse events of all LAMS procedures performed at our department during the period of interest.

Technical success was defined as the successful deployment of the LAMS in the desired position.

Clinical success was defined based on a previously published manuscript regarding the use of LAMSs [6]. For refractory anastomotic strictures, we used the following definition: normal oral intake for the anticipated period of stenting (12 weeks).

The severity of adverse events was graded based on the newly published American Society for Gastrointestinal Endoscopy AGREE classification [7]. Adverse events were recorded based on retrospective EMR reviews.

All obtained results were compared with those from our previously published cohort [6]. This historical cohort included all consecutive cases since the introduction of LAMSs in the University Hospital of Ghent, Belgium, all performed by PH who had no previous experience with LAMSs (except for training in models). The current cohort includes all consecutive patients after this historical cohort. All cases were performed by PH or HDG in direct supervision of PH. Data analysis was performed with SPSS 25 statistical software (IBM, Chicago, IL, USA). Proportions were compared using the chi-square test for 2 × 2 tables. A 2-sided p value < 0.5 was considered statistically significant.

3. Results

3.1. Indications

We included 168 procedures performed in 153 patients. Fifteen patients had received more than one LAMS placement for different indications. The patient characteristics are provided in Table 1.

Table 1. Baseline characteristics of patients.

Characteristic	Values n, (%)
No. of patients	153
No. of procedures	168
Median age, y, IQR	62.8 [49.9–72.9]
Sex, M: F	93 (57.4): 69 (42.6)

Table 1. Cont.

Characteristic	Values n, (%)
ASA score	II 96 (59.3) III 66 (40.7)
ECOG PS score	I 22 (13.6) II 88 (54.3) III 51 (31.5) IV 1 (0.6)

IQR—interquartile range, ASA—American Society of Anesthesiology Score, ECOG PS—performance status.

Eighty-eight procedures (52.4%) were performed for on-label indications, and seventy-eight (47.6%) were performed for off-label indications. The numbers for each indication can be found in Table 2. A comparison with the previously published cohort can be found in Supplementary Table S1.

Table 2. Procedural details of patients undergoing LAMS placement.

Indication (N = 168)	Number of Procedures	Location	Technical Success	Clinical Success	Adverse Events	Underlying Malignancy
PFC	N = 40		38 (95.0)	35 (87.5)	2 (5.0)	0 (0)
- Pseudocyst	7 (17.5)		7 (100)	7 (100)	0 (0.0)	0 (0)
- WON	33 (82.5)		31 (93.9)	28 (84.8)	2 (6.1)	0 (0)
GE	N = 35	GG = 4 (11.4)	33 (94.3)	33 (94.3)	3 (8.6)	24 (68.6)
- Benign GOO	11 (31.4)	GJ = 31 (88.6)	11 (100)	11 (100)	0 (0.0)	0 (0.0)
- Malignant GOO	24 (68.6)		22 (91.7)	22 (91.7)	3 (12.5)	24 (100)
EUS-BD	N = 21		21 (100)	20 (95.2)	2 (9.5)	17 (81.0)
EUS-GBD	N = 27		27 (100)	27 (100)	5 (18.5)	17 (63.0)
GATE	N = 25		25 (100)	25 (100)	1 (4.0)	1 (4.0)
Treatment of refractory GI strictures	N = 6	Esophagus 5 (83.3) Pyloric Channel 1 (16.7)	6 (100)	4 (66.7)	0 (0)	0 (0)
Miscellaneous	N = 12		11 (91.7)	11 (91.7)	3 (25.0)	1 (8.3)

PFC—peripancreatic fluid collections, GE—gastroenterostomy, EUS-BD—endoscopic ultrasound guided biliary drainage, EUS-GBD—endoscopic ultrasound guided gallbladder drainage, GATE—temporary access for endoscopic procedures, GI—gastrointestinal.

3.2. Technical Success

The technical success rate in our current cohort was higher (163/168; 97%; Table 3) but not significantly different from our historical cohort (57/61; 93.4%; $p = 0.22$). Procedure outcomes of LAMS placement for the different on- and off-label indications can be found in Table 2.

Table 3. Outcomes overall. Graded according to the AGREE classification [7].

Characteristic, N = 168	Values N, (%)
Technical success	163/168 (97.0)
Clinical success	157/168 (93.5)
Adverse events	17 (10.1)
1	0 (0)
2	1 (0.1)
3a	15 (8.9)
3b	1 (0.6)

Table 3. Cont.

Characteristic, N = 168	Values N, (%)
4a	0 (0)
4b	0 (0)
5	0 (0)

In five patients, LAMS deployment was either not possible (too long a distance between the GI lumen and the target, N = 2, both in the EUS-GE group) or considered unsafe (due to poor visualization, N = 2, both in the PFC group). One misplacement occurred in a patient with known metastatic rectal carcinoma who needed drainage of a pararectal abscess.

3.3. Clinical Success Rate

The clinical success rate in our current cohort was higher (157/168; 93.5%, Table 3) but not significantly different from our historical cohort (54/61; 88.5%; $p = 0.21$).

Clinical failures included the five patients with technical failures described above. The remaining six cases included three patients with peripancreatic fluid collections, one patient with malignant distal biliary obstruction and two patients with refractory esophageal strictures.

3.4. Adverse Events

The adverse event rate was significantly lower (15/168; 8.9%, Table 2) than that in our historical cohort (13/56; 21.3%; $p = 0.01$) (Table 4). We performed a comparative subanalysis between the current and the historical cohort for the two most frequent LAMS indications (PFC and CBD), clearly demonstrating a caseload-dependent reduction in adverse events (Figure 1A,B). All AEs were categorized based on the AGREE criteria and are described below [7].

Table 4. Complications, management and outcome for respective LAMS indications.

Indication	Adverse Event Based on AGREE [7]	Frequency	Description of Event	Management	Outcome
PFC	1	0			
	2	0			
	3a	2	Bleeding (N = 2)	Endoscopy (N = 2)	Resolved (N = 2)
	3b	0			
	4a	0			
	4b	0			
	5	0			
GE	1	0			
	2	0			
	3a	3	Colono-enteral fistula (N = 1) Ulcers at the level of jejunum (N = 1) Bleeding (N = 1)	Endoscopy (N = 3)	Resolved (N = 3)
	3b	0			
	4a	0			
	4b	0			
	5	0			
CBD	1	0	Overgrowth of AXIOS with tumor tissue (N = 1) Bleeding requiring bicap and transfusion (N = 1) Ascending cholangitis (N = 1) Uncertainty about position of distal flange (N = 1)	Endoscopy (N = 4)	Resolved (N = 4)
	2	0			
	3a	4			
	3b	0			
	4a	0			
	4b	0			
	5	0			

Table 4. Cont.

Indication	Adverse Event Based on AGREE [7]	Frequency	Description of Event	Management	Outcome
GBD	1	0	Bleeding (N = 2)	Medical treatment (N = 1) Endoscopy (N = 1)	Resolved (N = 2)
	2	1			
	3a	1			
	3b	0			
	4a	0			
	4b	0			
	5	0			
GATE	1	0	Dislocation of LAMS (N = 1)	Surgery (N = 1)	Resolved (N = 1)
	2	0			
	3a	0			
	3b	1			
	4a	0			
	4b	0			
	5	0			
Miscellaneous	1	0	Aberrant LAMS position (N = 1) Leakage of collection fluid into peritoneum (N = 1) LAMS migration (N = 1)	Medical treatment (N = 2) Endoscopy (N = 1)	Resolved (N = 1) Non-resolved (N = 1)
	2	0			
	3a	3			
	3b	0			
	4a	0			
	4b	0			
	5	0			

LAMS—lumen apposing metal stent, PFC—peripancreatic fluid collections, GE—gastroenterostomy, EUS BD—endoscopic ultrasound guided biliary drainage, EUS GBD—endoscopic ultrasound guided gallbladder drainage, GATE—temporary access for endoscopic procedures, GI—gastrointestinal.

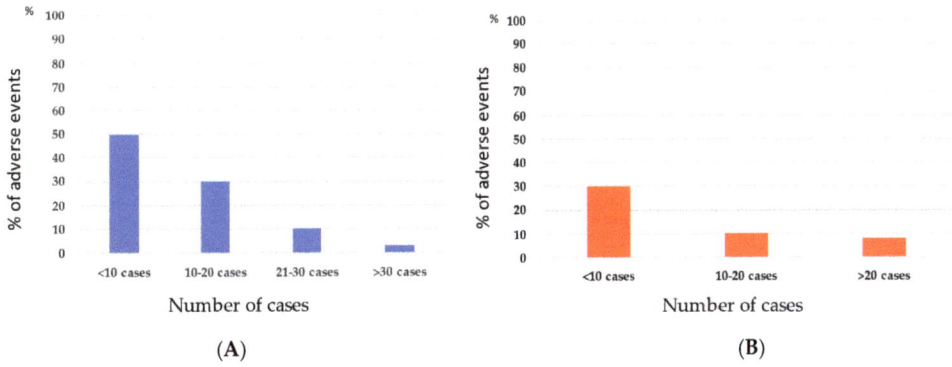

Figure 1. Caseload-dependent reduction in adverse events in EUS drainage of PFCs and CBD. Caseload-dependent reduction in AEs in EUS drainage of PFCs (**A**) and bile duct drainage (**B**) based on a combined subanalysis of the current cohort and a previously published historical cohort [6]. AE—adverse events, EUS—endoscopic ultrasound, PFC—peripancreatic fluid collection, CBD—common bile duct.

3.4.1. Grade II AEs

One grade II adverse event was seen in the choledochoduodenostomy (CDS) (Group D). The patient showed symptoms of postprocedural gastrointestinal bleeding with melena. However, despite using imaging diagnostics, we were unable to identify the cause of the bleeding (EGD, colonoscopy and CTA). The patient's progress was uneventful following conservative treatment and fluid resuscitation.

3.4.2. Grade III AEs

A total of 15 IIIa adverse events occurred. Five patients (two in the walled-off necrosis (WON) group, two in the CDS group and one in the EUS-GE group) had postprocedural gastrointestinal bleeding needing endoscopic intervention. One patient in the CDS group required a blood transfusion in addition to endoscopic care.

The LAMS had to be removed or endoscopically replaced in eight patients either due to tumor overgrowth (N = 2), enterocolonic fistula (N = 1), air and fluid leaks (N = 1), stent migration (N = 3) or ascending cholangitis (N = 1).

One of the most serious adverse events was observed in a patient who had a rectal abscess from metastatic rectal malignancy. A subsequent CT scan revealed that the distal flange had been deployed into the muscle tissue as a result of low visibility. The LAMS was removed, but the fistula was not closed because of poor bowel preparation. Due to the patient's complex surgical history and his poor prognosis, conservative management was initiated after multidisciplinary discussion. Although the patient did not die from this adverse event, postprocedural chronic pain persisted until his death.

3.4.3. Grade IIIb AEs

One patient experienced a grade IIIb AE that necessitated surgery. The patient with a history of gastric bypass underwent LAMS gastro-gastrostomy to perform ERCP (common bile duct stone). Although the interval between LAMS placement and ERCP was only 8 days, LAMS dislocation during ERCP led to a perforation. The defect was successfully closed from the stomach pouch with an over-the-scope, but the patient developed signs of peritonitis, necessitating laparoscopic surgery with a smooth recovery afterward.

There were no grade I, IVa, IVb, or grade V AEs in our cohort.

4. Discussion

The results of our cohort clearly demonstrate the impact of a learning curve on the outcome of LAMS procedures. Over time, we observed only a slight (non-significant) increase in technical and clinical success rates but a significant and relevant drop in the adverse event rate.

Our general safety measures across all indications to prevent bleeding and misplacement of the LAMS include preprocedural cross-sectional imaging, the use of Doppler imaging, measurement of the distance between the gastrointestinal (GI) tract lumen and the target, taking time to find the best scope position, the immediate removal of the electrocautery cable once the target has been penetrated with the catheter and the use of the appropriate LAMS diameter.

The use of LAMSs was first authorized for peripancreatic fluid collections. Most of the data regarding the use of LAMSs come from this indication [1,8–14]. Our technical (95.0%) and clinical (87.5%) success rates were in line with recently published data [8,9].

We observed a notable drop in LAMS-related adverse events for this indication, from 33% in our previous cohort to 5% in the current cohort. Similar to our observations, Facciorusso et al. [10] found that adverse events decrease with increasing caseload. Over time, we took the following measures to achieve this low adverse event rate: a systematic use of periprocedural antibiotics, the use of broad diameter stents (preferably 20 mm) in case of WON, the use of double pigtail catheters inside the LAMS lumen to protect patency by preventing complete blockage of the lumen by food or necrotic tissue and early follow-up imaging (after 1–2 weeks in case of pseudocysts and 3–4 weeks in case of WON) to check for resolution of the collection and to ensure timely removal of the LAMS with or without replacement by pigtail catheters. The latter is important to avoid severe bleeding resulting from erosion of the PFC wall by the LAMS and in line with previous recommendations [9,11–15]. A recent study published by Najar et al., however, found no increase in adverse events if the LAMS was removed after more than four weeks [16].

Choledochoduodenostomy is the second approved indication for LAMS in patients with failed ERCP and/or malignant distal biliary obstruction. The benefit over percutaneous biliary drainage (PTBD) in this indication has now been clearly demonstrated [17]. While ERCP remains the procedure of choice for the management of obstructive biliary drainage, a potential paradigm shift toward first-line choledochoduodenostomy has been claimed in the context of inoperable malignant distal biliary obstruction and is currently under further investigation in the ELEMENT trial [18].

One of the most important messages is that one should be trained in small-space LAMS placement before proceeding with this indication since the consequences of misplacement are severe [6]. We now use a guidewire for bile ducts < 14 mm (introduced after freehand introduction of the LAMS catheter into the bile duct) to allow for a rescue intervention (covered self-expanding metal stent (SEMS) placement) in case of misplacement.

LAMS misplacement and persistent or recurrent cholestasis (20%) was also a major issue in the Choi et al. [5] group. This was due to biliary food impaction. Our personal experience is that it can be avoided by always using a 6 × 8 mm LAMS size independent of the bile duct diameter. This issue of the unavailability of narrower stents in the USA and subsequent adverse events related to food impaction was also noted in the meta-analysis by Peng et al. [19] In this regard, one ongoing RCT investigates the added value of a pigtail inside the lumen of a small-to-medium size LAMS (BAMPI trial) [20].

LAMSs are approved for gallbladder drainage in nonoperative candidates and should be preferred over percutaneous drainage if expertise is available [21–24]. In our cohort, we noted a high technical and clinical success rate with low rates of AEs.

We believe that the transduodenal route should be preferred over the transgastric route since the risk of migration is much lower. Early migration of the LAMS (<1 week after placement) might lead to gastric perforation and biliary peritonitis that can only be resolved with surgery in a high-risk population. In addition, one should be aware of the risk of pyloric obstruction by the proximal flange of the LAMS if the gastric route is chosen. Finally, as in our own experience, future cholecystectomy is not hampered by the presence of a cholecystoduodenostomy.

In the absence of gallbladder stones, we place an 8/8 or 10/10 stent, sufficient for adequate drainage in our series. A larger diameter LAMS (15/10) is preferred in cases with stones present. We recommend a double pigtail inside the lumen of the LAMS, especially in a case with stones, to preserve the LAMS patency.

EUS-guided gastroenterostomy (EUS-GE) to alleviate gastric outlet obstruction is a promising but off-label indication for LAMSs. Retrospective studies and our personal experience suggest that EUS-GE is safe, provides better functional results than duodenal stenting and is associated with a quicker recovery and a shorter hospital stay compared to surgery [25–27]. While different techniques of EUS-GE exist [27–30], we only use the direct anterograde method. Technical and clinical success rates were high (94.3%), which is in agreement with the available data [28,29].

Stent maldeployment might have serious consequences in cases of a jejunal perforation that, in most cases, will not be accessible for endoscopic closure. Accidental deployment in the colon instead of the jejunum is another potential hazard. Careful selection of the best position, adequate distension of the jejunal loop with colored saline, a test puncture in case the jejunal filling catheter cannot be seen with EUS, the use of antispasmodics and short-term apnea are all helpful to minimize the risk of maldeployment.

To maximize the functional results of EUS-GE, we always use a 20 mm LAMS for this indication. We dilate the lumen up to 18 mm after deployment and clipping of the LAMS to hasten the time to normal oral dietary intake, but further data to support this approach are lacking [30].

According to Jovani et al., 25 procedures can be considered as the threshold to achieve proficiency in EUS-GE [31].

Twenty-five patients in our cohort had LAMSs placed for temporary endoscopic access (GATE) due to the need for other endoscopic procedures (ERCP). We noted 100% technical and clinical success rates. These results are better than those available in the literature [32,33].

Based on one serious adverse event in our institution and similar to Wang et al. [32], we now use a 20 mm LAMS if possible and delay ERCP for at least 2 weeks after placement if possible. If there is a need for emergency ERCP, we fix the LAMS with an over-the-scope stent fix clip (OTSC) and leave a guidewire in the excluded stomach upon withdrawal of the duodenoscope to allow for a rescue procedure (covered stent placement) in case of dislocation. We have only performed three of these one-step cases, all without complications.

We sometimes use LAMSs for refractory anastomotic strictures to minimize the risk of stent migration and stent-related inflammation. However, our experience is too limited to provide any recommendations for this indication. The potential use of LAMSs for short gastrointestinal strictures has previously been proposed by others [34].

Our study has some limitations. It was performed in a single high-volume tertiary academic referral center. All procedures were performed by two expert endoscopists with extensive experience in EUS and ERCP (HDG and PH). Outcomes may vary according to local expertise. One other limitation of the study was the use of only one LAMS type (Hot AXIOS). Our results might not be fully applicable to other LAMSs on the market. Although our study was retrospective, the data were carefully recorded, and there are no missing data.

In summary, our study demonstrates the most important impact of a learning curve in LAMS placement is a significant drop in complications over time due to protocol optimization. Expert consensus guidelines on the safe deployment of LAMSs for the different indications are crucial to validate our recommendations and reduce the overall risk of LAMS-related adverse events in the broader community.

Supplementary Materials: The following supporting information can be downloaded at: https://www.mdpi.com/article/10.3390/jcm12031037/s1, Table S1. A comparison of number of procedures, technical and clinical success and adverse events between the previously published cohort and current cohort.

Author Contributions: S.S. and P.H. have been involved in data acquisition, analysis, literature review and writing the manuscript; H.D. and P.H. conceived the idea of the manuscript and performed the final revision of the manuscript. All authors have read and agreed to the published version of the manuscript.

Funding: This research received no external funding.

Institutional Review Board Statement: The study was reviewed and approved by the institutional ethical review board (reference: ONZ-2022-0179) and conducted with accordance with the Declaration of Helsinki.

Informed Consent Statement: No written informed consent was obtained because of the retrospective study design and all patients were treated by the authors of the manuscript.

Data Availability Statement: Data supporting reported results was generated with the use of electronic medical records. The data presented in this study are available on request from the corresponding author.

Conflicts of Interest: S.S. and H.D. have no conflict of interests. P.H.: Consultant and speaker for Boston Scientific, FujiFilm, MedWork and Viatris.

References

1. Shah, R.J.; Shah, J.N.; Waxman, I.; Kowalski, T.E.; Sanchez-Yague, A.; Nieto, J.; Brauer, B.C.; Gaidhane, M.; Kahaleh, M. Safety and efficacy of endoscopic ultrasound-guided drainage of pancreatic fluid collections with lumen-apposing covered self-expanding metal stents. *Clin. Gastroenterol. Hepatol.* **2015**, *13*, 747–752. [CrossRef] [PubMed]
2. Siddiqui, A.A.; Adler, D.G.; Nieto, J.; Shah, J.N.; Binmoeller, K.F.; Kane, S.; Yan, L.; Laique, S.N.; Kowalski, T.; Loren, D.E.; et al. EUS-guided drainage of peripancreatic fluid collections and necrosis by using a novel lumen-apposing stent: A large retrospective, multicenter U.S. experience (with videos). *Gastrointest. Endosc.* **2016**, *83*, 699–707. [CrossRef] [PubMed]
3. Sahar, N.; Kozarek, R.; Kanji, Z.; Ross, A.S.; Gluck, M.; Gan, S.I.; Larsen, M.; Irani, S. Do lumen-apposing metal stents (LAMS) improve treatment outcomes of walled-off pancreatic necrosis over plastic stents using dual-modality drainage? *Endosc. Int. Open* **2017**, *5*, E1052–E1059. [CrossRef] [PubMed]

4. Li, J.; Basseri, H.; Donnellan, F.; Harris, A. Lumen-apposing metals stents in advanced endoscopic ultrasound-guided interventions: Novel applications, potential complications and radiologic assessment. *Abdom. Radiol.* **2021**, *46*, 776–791. [CrossRef] [PubMed]
5. Choi, J.H.; Kozarek, R.A.; Larsen, M.C.; Ross, A.S.; Law, J.K.; Krishnamoorthi, R.; Irani, S. Effectiveness and safety of lumen-apposing metal stents in endoscopic interventions for off-label indications. *Dig. Dis. Sci.* **2021**, *67*, 2327–2336. [CrossRef]
6. Hindryckx, P.; Degroote, H. Lumen-apposing metal stents for approved and off-label indications: A single-centre experience. *Surg. Endosc.* **2020**, *35*, 6013–6020. [CrossRef]
7. Nass, K.J.; Zwager, L.W.; van der Vlugt, M.; Dekker, E.; Bossuyt, P.M.M.; Ravindran, S.; Thomas-Gibson, S.; Fockens, P. Novel classification for adverse events in GI endoscopy: The AGREE classification. *Gastrointest. Endosc.* **2022**, *95*, 1078–1085.e8. [CrossRef]
8. Mohan, B.; Jayaraj, M.; Asokkumar, R.; Shakhatreh, M.; Pahal, P.; Ponnada, S.; Navaneethan, U.; Adler, D.G. Lumen apposing metal stents in drainage of pancreatic walled-off necrosis, are they any better than plastic stents? A systematic review and meta-analysis of studies published since the revised Atlanta classification of pancreatic fluid collections. *Endosc. Ultrasound.* **2019**, *8*, 82–90.
9. Bang, J.Y.; Varadarajulu, S. Lumen-apposing metal stents for endoscopic ultrasound-guided drainage of pancreatic fluid collections. *Tech. Innov. Gastrointest. Endosc.* **2020**, *22*, 14–18. [CrossRef]
10. Facciorusso, A.; Amato, A.; Crinò, S.F.; Sinagra, E.; Maida, M.; Fugazza, A.; Binda, C.; Coluccio, C.; Repici, A.; Anderloni, A.; et al. Definition of a hospital volume threshold to optimize outcomes after drainage of pancreatic fluid collections with lumen-apposing metal stents: A nationwide cohort study. *Gastrointest. Endosc.* **2022**, *95*, 1158–1172. [CrossRef]
11. Bang, J.Y.; Hawes, R.H.; Varadarajulu, S. Lumen-apposing metal stent placement for drainage of pancreatic fluid collections: Predictors of adverse events. *Gut* **2020**, *69*, 1379–1381. [CrossRef]
12. Bang, J.Y.; Hasan, M.; Navaneethan, U.; Hawes, R.; Varadarajulu, S. Lumen-apposing metal stents (LAMS) for pancreatic fluid collection (PFC) drainage: May not be business as usual. *Gut* **2016**, *66*, 2054–2056. [CrossRef]
13. Siddiqui, A.A.; Kowalski, T.E.; Loren, D.E.; Khalid, A.; Soomro, A.; Mazhar, S.M.; Isby, L.; Kahaleh, M.; Karia, K.; Yoo, J.; et al. Fully covered self-expanding metal stents versus lumen-apposing fully covered self-expanding metal stent versus plastic stents for endoscopic drainage of pancreatic walled-off necrosis: Clinical outcomes and success. *Gastrointest. Endosc.* **2017**, *85*, 758–765. [CrossRef] [PubMed]
14. Zeissig, S.; Sulk, S.; Brueckner, S.; Matthes, K.; Hohmann, M.; Reichel, S.; Ellrichmann, M.; Arlt, A.; Will, U.; Hampe, J. Severe bleeding is a rare event in patients receiving lumen-apposing metal stents for the drainage of pancreatic fluid collections. *Gut* **2018**, *68*, 945–946. [CrossRef] [PubMed]
15. Kumta, N.A.; Tyberg, A.; Bhagat, V.H.; Siddiqui, A.A.; Kowalski, T.E.; Loren, D.E.; Desai, A.P.; Sarkisian, A.M.; Brown, E.G.; Karia, K.; et al. EUS-guided drainage of pancreatic fluid collections using lumen apposing metal stents: An international, multicenter experience. *Dig. Liver Dis.* **2019**, *51*, 1557–1561. [CrossRef]
16. Nayar, M.; Leeds, J.S.; Oppong, K.; UK & Ireland LAMS Collaborative. Lumen-apposing metal stents for drainage of pancreatic fluid collections: Does timing of removal matter? *Gut* **2022**, *71*, 850–853. [CrossRef] [PubMed]
17. Ginestet, C.; Sanglier, F.; Hummel, V.; Rouchaud, A.; Legros, R.; Lepetit, H.; Dahan, M.; Carrier, P.; Loustaud-Ratti, V.; Sautereau, D.; et al. EUS-guided biliary drainage with electrocautery-enhanced lumen-apposing metal stent placement should replace PTBD after ERCP failure in patients with distal tumoral biliary obstruction: A large real-life study. *Surg. Endosc.* **2021**, *36*, 3365–3373. [CrossRef] [PubMed]
18. Chen, Y.-I.; Callichurn, K.; Chatterjee, A.; Desilets, E.; Fergal, D.; Forbes, N.; Gan, I.; Kenshil, S.; Khashab, M.A.; Kunda, R.; et al. ELEMENT TRIAL: Study protocol for a randomized controlled trial on endoscopic ultrasound-guided biliary drainage of first intent with a lumen-apposing metal stent vs. endoscopic retrograde cholangio-pancreatography in the management of malignant distal biliary obstruction. *Trials* **2019**, *20*, 696.
19. Peng, Z.; Li, S.; Tang, Y.; Wei, W.; Pi, R.; Liang, X.; Wan, Y.; Liu, H. Efficacy and safety of EUS-guided choledochoduodenostomy using electrocautery-enhanced lumen-apposing metal stents (ECE-LAMS) in the treatment of biliary obstruction: A systematic review and meta-analysis. *Can. J. Gastroenterol. Hepatol.* **2021**, *2021*, 6696950. [CrossRef]
20. Garcia-Sumalla, A.; Loras, C.; Sanchiz, V.; Sanz, R.P.; Vazquez-Sequeiros, E.; Aparicio, J.R.; de la Serna-Higuera, C.; Luna-Rodriguez, D.; Andujar, X.; Capilla, M.; et al. Multicenter study of lumen-apposing metal stents with or without pigtail in endoscopic ultrasound-guided biliary drainage for malignant obstruction—BAMPI TRIAL: An open-label, randomized controlled trial protocol. *Trials* **2022**, *23*, 181. [CrossRef]
21. Manta, R.; Mutignani, M.; Galloro, G.; Conigliaro, R.; Zullo, A. Endoscopic ultrasound-guided gallbladder drainage for acute cholecystitis with a lumen-apposing metal stent: A systematic review of case series. *Eur. J. Gastroenterol. Hepatol.* **2018**, *30*, 695–698. [CrossRef]
22. David, Y.N.; Kakked, G.; Dixon, R.E.; Confer, B.; Shah, R.N.; Khara, H.S.; Diehl, D.L.; Krafft, M.R.; Shah-Khan, S.M.; Nasr, J.Y.; et al. Su1260 endoscopic ultrasound guided gallbladder drainage (EUS-GBD) with lumen apposing metal stents (lams) in patients with acute cholecystitis has excellent long-term outcomes: A large, multicenter us study. *Gastrointest. Endosc.* **2020**, *91*, AB298–AB299. [CrossRef]

23. Siddiqui, A.; Kunda, R.; Tyberg, A.; Arain, M.A.; Noor, A.; Mumtaz, T.; Iqbal, U.; Loren, D.E.; Kowalski, T.E.; Adler, D.G.; et al. Three-way comparative study of endoscopic ultrasound-guided transmural gallbladder drainage using lumen-apposing metal stents versus endoscopic transpapillary drainage versus percutaneous cholecystostomy for gallbladder drainage in high-risk surgical patients with acute cholecystitis: Clinical outcomes and success in an International, Multicenter Study. *Surg. Endosc.* **2018**, *33*, 1260–1270.
24. Van der Merwe, S.W.; van Wanrooij, R.L.J.; Bronswijk, M.; Everett, S.; Lakhtakia, S.; Rimbas, M.; Hucl, T.; Kunda, R.; Badaoui, A.; Law, R.; et al. Therapeutic endoscopic ultrasound: European Society of Gastrointestinal Endoscopy (ESGE) Guideline. *Endoscopy* **2021**, *54*, 185–205. [CrossRef]
25. Perez-Miranda, M.; Tyberg, A.; Sharaiha, R.Z.; Toscano, E.; Gaidhane, M.; Desai, A.P.; Kumta, N.A.; Nieto, J.; Barthet, M.; Shah, R.; et al. EUS-guided gastrojejunostomy versus laparoscopic gastrojejunostomy: An international collaborative study. *J. Clin. Gastroenterol.* **2017**, *51*, 896–899. [CrossRef] [PubMed]
26. Stefanovic, S.; Draganov, P.V.; Yang, D. Endoscopic ultrasound guided gastrojejunostomy for gastric outlet obstruction. *World J. Gastrointest. Surg.* **2021**, *13*, 620–632. [CrossRef]
27. Irani, S.; Itoi, T.; Baron, T.H.; Khashab, M. EUS-guided gastroenterostomy: Techniques from East to West. *VideoGIE* **2019**, *5*, 48–50. [CrossRef]
28. McCarty, T.R.; Garg, R.; Thompson, C.C.; Rustagi, T. Efficacy and safety of EUS-guided gastroenterostomy for benign and malignant gastric outlet obstruction: A systematic review and meta-analysis. *Endosc. Int. Open* **2019**, *7*, E1474–E1482. [CrossRef]
29. Mangiavillano, B.; Repici, A. EUS-guided gastro-enteral anastomosis for the treatment of gastric outlet obstruction: Is the end of the enteral stent? *Expert Rev. Gastroenterol. Hepatol.* **2022**, *16*, 587–589. [CrossRef]
30. Sobani, Z.A.; Paleti, S.; Rustagi, T. Endoscopic ultrasound-guided gastroenterostomy using large-diameter (20 mm) lumen apposing metal stent (LLAMS). *Endosc. Int. Open* **2021**, *9*, E895–E900. [CrossRef]
31. Jovani, M.; Ichkhanian, Y.; Parsa, N.; Singh, S.; Gutierrez, O.I.B.; Keane, M.G.; Al Ghamdi, S.S.; Ngamruengphong, S.; Kumbhari, V.; Khashab, M.A. Assessment of the learning curve for EUS-guided gastroenterostomy for a single operator. *Gastrointest. Endosc.* **2021**, *93*, 1088–1093. [CrossRef]
32. Wang, T.J.; Thompson, C.C.; Ryou, M. Gastric access temporary for endoscopy (GATE): A proposed algorithm for EUS-directed transgastric ERCP in gastric bypass patients. *Surg. Endosc.* **2019**, *33*, 2024–2033. [CrossRef]
33. Wang, T.J.; Thompson, C.C.; Ryou, M. An international, multicenter, comparative trial of EUS-guided gastrogastrostomy-assisted ERCP versus enteroscopy-assisted ERCP in patients with Roux-en-Y gastric bypass anatomy. *Gastrointest. Endosc.* **2018**, *88*, 486–494.
34. Mahmoud, T.; Beran, A.; Bazerbachi, F.; Matar, R.; Jaruvongvanich, V.; Razzak, F.A.; Abboud, D.M.; Vargas, E.J.; Martin, J.A.; Kellogg, T.A.; et al. Lumen-apposing metal stents for the treatment of benign gastrointestinal tract strictures: A single-center experience and proposed treatment algorithm. *Surg. Endosc.* **2022**, 1–10. [CrossRef]

Disclaimer/Publisher's Note: The statements, opinions and data contained in all publications are solely those of the individual author(s) and contributor(s) and not of MDPI and/or the editor(s). MDPI and/or the editor(s) disclaim responsibility for any injury to people or property resulting from any ideas, methods, instructions or products referred to in the content.

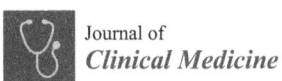

Article

The Efficacy and Safety of EUS-Guided Gallbladder Drainage as a Bridge to Surgery for Patients with Acute Cholecystitis

Ken Ishii [1], Yuji Fujita [1,*], Eisuke Suzuki [1], Yuji Koyama [1], Seitaro Tsujino [1], Atsuki Nagao [2], Kunihiro Hosono [3], Takuma Teratani [1], Kensuke Kubota [3] and Atsushi Nakajima [3]

1. Department of Hepato-Biliary-Pancreatic Medicine, NTT Tokyo Medical Center, 5-9-22 Higashi-Gotanda, Shinagawa-ku, Tokyo 141-8625, Japan; meitokuso@yahoo.co.jp (K.I.)
2. Department of Surgery, NTT Tokyo Medical Center, Tokyo 141-8625, Japan
3. Department of Gastroenterology and Hepatology, Yokohama City University School of Medicine, Yokohama 236-0004, Japan
* Correspondence: yufuji5395@gmail.com; Tel.: +81-3448-6111; Fax: +81-3448-6071

Abstract: Background and Aim: This study aimed to compare the efficacy and safety of endoscopic ultrasound-guided gallbladder drainage and percutaneous transhepatic gallbladder drainage as a bridge to surgery in patients with acute cholecystitis unfit for urgent cholecystectomy. Methods: This retrospective study included 46 patients who underwent cholecystectomy following endoscopic ultrasound-guided gallbladder drainage (EUS-GBD) or percutaneous transhepatic gallbladder drainage (PTGBD) for acute cholecystitis in NTT Tokyo Medical Center. We surveyed 35 patients as the EUS-GBD group and 11 patients as the PTGBD group, and compared the rate of technical success of the cholecystectomy and periprocedural adverse events. A 7-F, 10-cm double pigtail plastic stent was used for ultrasound-guided gallbladder drainage. Results: The rate of technical success of cholecystectomy was 100% in both groups. Regarding postsurgical adverse events, no significant difference was noted between the two groups (EUS-GBD group, 11.4%, vs. PTGBD group, 9.0%; $p = 0.472$). Conclusions: EUS-GBD as a BTS seems to be an alternative for patients with AC because it can ensure lower adverse events. On the other hand, there are two major limitations in this study—the sample size is small and there is a risk of selection bias.

Keywords: EUS drainage; acute cholecystitis; bridge to surgery

1. Introduction

Cholecystectomy is the curative treatment for acute cholecystitis (AC). Early cholecystectomy is mandatory for AC; however, emergency cholecystectomy for AC is associated with high morbidity (20–30%) and mortality (6–30%) rates in patients with significant co-morbidities [1–3]. As a result, some surgeons prefer non-surgical procedures as makeshift treatments, such as antibiotic administration with/without percutaneous/endoscopic drainage, as an alternative to emergent cholecystectomy. However, elective surgery may lead to several complications, including empyema, gangrene, perforation, pericholecystitis with abscess formation, peritonitis, and sepsis [4,5]. Emergent surgery may not be safe and practical in patients with high surgical risk [6]. Percutaneous transhepatic gallbladder drainage (PTGBD) has been performed as a bridge for delayed surgical treatment in vulnerable patients with high surgical risk. The presence of a drainage tube may increase the risk of an adverse event during surgery by 16.2% to 25% [7–9]. Recently, endoscopic ultrasound-guided gallbladder drainage (EUS-GBD) has gained attention as a treatment for internal drainage of the gallbladder in high-risk patients [10–18]. Although PTGBD followed by late laparoscopic cholecystectomy for high-risk patients has been accepted as the standard procedure [19–21], there are limitations of PTGBD, such as inconvenience for patients and risk of its dislocation. However, there are no reports on alternatives to PTGBD focusing on the bridge to surgery (BTS). Thus, the present study aimed to validate the efficacy and safety of EUS-GBD as a BTS in patients with AC who are considered unfit for urgent cholecystectomy.

2. Materials and Methods

2.1. Study Design

This was a retrospective study conducted between April 2016 and July 2021. This study protocol was approved by the Institutional Review Board (ID18-313) of our institute. The study was investigator-initiated and conducted according to the ethical principles of the Declaration of Helsinki. Written informed consent was obtained from all patients.

2.2. Patients

Patients with a diagnosis of AC admitted to our institute between April 2016 and July 2021 were retrospectively identified. The diagnosis of AC was made using a combination of patient history, physical examination, laboratory analysis, and imaging (abdominal ultrasonography, computed tomography, and magnetic resonance imaging), and based on the Tokyo Guideline 2018 [22]. Patients with common bile duct stones were excluded because they had concurrent cholangitis. Patients were divided into two groups: one group who underwent cholecystectomy following EUS-GBD during the period from April 2019 to June 2021, and another group who underwent cholecystectomy following PTGBD during the period from April 2016 to June 2018.

2.3. Procedures

2.3.1. EUS-GBD

EUS-GBD was performed by endoscopists who had performed over 500 interventional-EUS procedures and over 500 therapeutic ERCP procedures. Endoscopists used an oblique-viewing, curved-linear array echoendoscope (GF-UCT260 or GF-UCT240; Olympus Medical Systems, Tokyo, Japan) and a dedicated processor (ME-1/2; Olympus Medical Systems). The gallbladder was depicted by ultrasound imaging from the duodenal bulb or gastric antrum and punctured using a 19-gauge fine aspiration needle (EZ Shot 3 Plus; Olympus Medical Systems). Thereafter, a 0.025-inch guidewire (VisiGlide2; Olympus Medical Systems) was inserted into the gallbladder lumen, and the tract was dilated using a 4-mm balloon catheter with a tapered tip (REN; Kaneka Corporation, Tokyo, Japan). Finally, a 7-Fr 10-cm double-pigtail plastic stent (DPPS) (Through & Pass DP; Gadelius Medical K.K, Tokyo, Japan) was placed in the gallbladder through the duodenal bulb or gastric antrum (Figure 1). The inclusion criteria were: obvious cholecystitis identified by the presence of gallstones, no gallbladder perforation, and the provision of written informed consent.

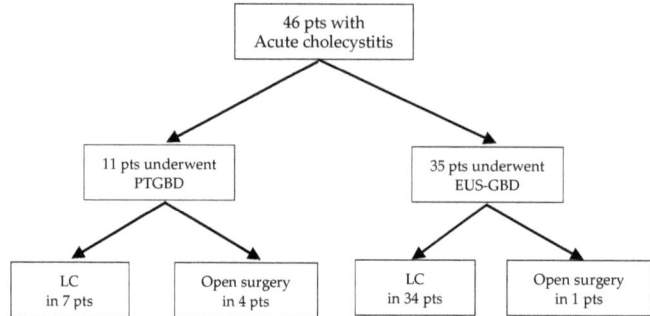

Figure 1. Result of analyzed patients (pts) with acute cholecystitis.

2.3.2. PTGBD

PTGBD was performed under local anesthesia by trained interventional radiologists in the interventional suite. A transhepatic route was used in all patients, and a 7-Fr pigtail drainage catheter (Hanako Medical Co., Ltd., Saitama, Japan) was placed between the seventh or eighth intercostal space under combined sonographic and fluoroscopic guidance.

2.4. Follow-Up

All patients underwent plain abdominal radiography and laboratory tests the day after the procedure and leading up to the surgery. Oral diet was started when clinical symptoms improved without any severe adverse events. DPPS was kept in place without periodical exchange until the surgery.

2.5. Laparoscopic Cholecystectomy

Laparoscopic cholecystectomy was performed for eligible patients at least 1 month after EUS-GBD. The previous day before the surgery, the DPPS was endoscopically removed. The surgery was performed under general anesthesia using a standard four-trocar technique. Surgeons identified the enterocholecysto fistula, which was then immediately cut using a stapler. If the laparoscopic surgery was difficult to complete, conversion to open cholecystectomy was performed at the operator's discretion. All laparoscopic cholecystectomy procedures were performed by one hepatobiliary pancreatic surgeon who had previously performed more than 500 laparoscopic cholecystectomies.

Difficult laparoscopic cholecystectomy (DLC) was defined as a procedure with an operative time $\geq$ 3 h, bleeding volume $\geq$ 300 mL common bile duct injury, partial cholecystectomy, the need for a second surgeon, and/or conversion to open surgery [22].

2.6. Outcomes

The primary outcome was technical success of the cholecystectomy after EUS-GBD. Technical success was defined as successful gallbladder removal during cholecystectomy without complications. Clinical success was defined as clinical improvement (resolution of fever, decrease in white blood cell count, and resolution of pain and tenderness) within 72 h after the procedure. The secondary outcome was periprocedural adverse events including prolonged surgical time after cholecystectomy.

2.7. Statistical Analysis

Data are summarized as mean $\pm$ standard deviation for continuous data and as frequency and percentages for categorical data. For continuous data, characteristics and outcomes of the two groups were compared using the student's t-test or Mann–Whitney U test based on the viability of the normality assumption. The Chi-squared or Fisher's exact test was used to compare the two groups with regard to categorical characteristics and outcomes. The level of significance was set at a two-sided p-value < 0.05. Statistical analysis was performed using BellCurve for Excel (Social Survey Research Information Co., Ltd., Tokyo, Japan).

3. Results

3.1. Patient Characteristics

In this period, 46 patients were included in this study (Figure 1): 35 patients underwent EUS-GBD (62.9% male; average age, 69.2 $\pm$ 13.4 years) and 11 patients underwent PTGBD (90.9% male; average age, 72.4 $\pm$ 12.2 years), followed by cholecystectomy. No statistical differences were found in age, sex, or body mass index between the two groups (Table 1). The etiology of cholecystitis was gallstone disease ($n = 35$, 100%) in the EUS-GBD group and gallstone disease ($n = 10$, 81.8%), acalculous disease ($n = 1$, 9.1%), and gallbladder cancer ($n = 1$, 9.1%) in the PTGBD group ($p = 0.005$). No significant differences were noted regarding baseline diseases, advanced cancers ($p = 0.721$), cerebrovascular disorder ($p = 0.912$), or cardiopulmonary disease ($p = 0.886$) between the two groups. The severities for cholecystitis were moderate ($n = 33$, 94.3%) and severe ($n = 2$, 5.7%) in the EUS-GBD group and moderate ($n = 11$, 100%) in the PTGBD group. Cholecystectomy was proposed for all patients at the initial diagnosis for AC; however, if the surgeons, endoscopists, and radiologists regarded these patients as unsuitable surgical candidates, either EUS-GBD or PTGBD was performed.

Table 1. Patient characteristics.

Variable	EUS-GBD (n = 35)	PTGBD (n = 11)	p Value
Age (years)	69.2 ± 13.4 (34–88)	72.4 ± 12.2 (44–82)	0.900
Sex (male/female)	22/13	10/1	0.052
BMI	24.2 ± 3.8 (15–32.8)	22.9 ± 2.6 (18.9–25.8)	0.286
Etiology of cholecystitis			
Gallstone	35 (100)	9 (81.8)	0.005
Acalculous	0	1 (9.0)	
Gallbladder cancer	0	1 (9.0)	
Underlying conditions			
Baseline disease			
Advanced cancer	6 (17.1)	3 (27.3)	0.721
Cerebrovascular disorder	2 (5.7)	1 (9.1)	0.912
Cardiopulmonary disease	8 (22.9)	2 (18.2)	0.886
ASA-PS I	5 (14.3)	1 (9.0)	0.445
ASA-PS II	28 (80.0)	6 (54.5)	0.094
ASA-PS III	2 (57.1)	3 (27.3)	0.272
ASA-PS IV	0	1 (9.0)	
Severity of cholecystitis (based on Tokyo guideline 2018)			
Moderate	33 (94.3)	11 (100)	0.201
Severe	2 (5.7)	0	

Numbers are shown in number (%) or average ± SD (range); EUS-GBD, endoscopic ultrasound-guided gallbladder drainage; PTGBD, percutaneous transhepatic gallbladder drainage; BMI, body mass index; ASA-PS, American Society of Anesthesiologists physical status; SD, standard deviation.

3.2. Primary Outcome

Clinical success of gallbladder drainage was achieved in 100% of patients in the EUS-GBD group and 81.8% of patients in the PTGBD group; two patients in the PTGBD group exhibited catheter dislodgement. No significant difference was observed regarding the duration from drainage to cholecystectomy between the two groups ($p = 0.512$).

Technical success of cholecystectomy was achieved in 100% of patients in both groups (Table 2). All patients in the EUS-GBD group underwent laparoscopic cholecystectomy, and only one (2.9%) patient required conversion to open surgery. In the PTGBD group, eight patients (72.7%) underwent laparoscopic cholecystectomy, three patients (27.3%) underwent open cholecystectomy, and one patient (12.5%) required conversion to open cholecystectomy. The number of patients who required conversion was not statistically different between the two groups ($p = 0.400$). No significant differences were noted regarding operation time ($p = 0.707$), estimated blood loss ($p = 0.493$), or duration from operation to discharge ($p = 0.541$) between the two groups.

Table 2. Comparison of drainage procedure outcomes.

Variable	EUS-GBD (n = 35)	PTGBD (n = 11)	p Value
Technical success of gallbladder drainage	35 (100)	11 (100)	
Clinical success of gallbladder drainage	35 (100)	9 (81.8)	0.005
Procedure time (min)	25.1 ± 9.2 (13–52)	No record	
Time from drainage to cholecystectomy (days)	86.7 ± 113.7 (29–632)	62.0 ± 87.8 (7–308)	0.512
Technical success of cholecystectomy	35 (100)	11 (100)	
Type of cholecystectomy			
Laparoscopic	35 (100)	8 (72.7)	0.002
Open	0	3 (27.3)	

Table 2. Cont.

Variable	EUS-GBD (n = 35)	PTGBD (n = 11)	p Value
Laparoscopic converted to open	1 (2.9)	1 (12.5)	0.4
Operating time (min)	171.9 ± 71.7 (46–368)	182.0 ± 53.5 (110–302)	0.707
Estimated blood loss (ml)	75.5 ± 99.5 (5–400)	103.2 ± 130.8 (10–440)	0.493
Time from operation to discharge (days)	5.4 ± 2.5 (3–14)	6.5 ± 2.8 (3–13)	0.541

Numbers are shown as number (%) or average ± SD (range); EUS-GBD, endoscopic ultrasound-guided gallbladder drainage; PTGBD, percutaneous transhepatic gallbladder drainage; SD, standard deviation.

3.3. Secondary Outcome

Postsurgical adverse events were observed in four patients (11.4%) in the EUS-GBD group and in one patient (9.0%) in the PTGBD group; no significant differences were found between the two groups ($p = 0.472$) (Table 3). In the EUS-GBD group, four patients suffered from abscesses that were managed by adjusting the position of the drain placed at the time of cholecystectomy. In the PTGBD group, the single adverse event was postoperative heart failure, managed with medication.

Table 3. Comparison of adverse events.

Variable	EUS-GBD (n = 35)	PTGBD (n = 11)	p Value
Post procedural adverse events	6 (17.1)	3 (27.2)	0.361
Types of adverse events			
Recurrent cholecystitis	0	1 (9.0)	0.035
Drain dislodging	0	2 (18.2)	0.005
Peritonitis	6 (17.1)	0	0.071
Patients requiring repeat procedure	0	0	
Postsurgical adverse events	4 (11.4)	1 (9.0)	0.472
Recurrent biliary events	0	0	
Abscess	4 (11.4)	0	0.418

Numbers are shown as number (%) or average ± SD (range); EUS-GBD, endoscopic ultrasound-guided gallbladder drainage; PTGBD, percutaneous transhepatic gallbladder drainage; SD, standard deviation.

4. Discussion

This paper indicated that EUS-GBD could be an alternative to PTGBD as a BTS. Ryu's meta-analysis and systematic review reported EUS-GBD was comparable with PTGBD regarding clinical success, with less reintervention and readmission, for acute cholecystitis with high surgical risk [23]. However, postprocedural adverse events, which could be conservatively managed, occurred in 6 of 35 patients (17.1%) in the EUS-GBD group; controllable peritonitis occurred in all patients. As bile leak reportedly occurs in one in eight (12.5%) patients with DPPS [24], the rate of bile leak in this study (17.1%) was relatively high. Although a 4-mm balloon catheter was used in all patients in our study, a high rate of bile leak may have occurred due to the use of this catheter, and leakage after the dilation procedure was convertibly countered. On the other hand, postprocedural adverse events occurred in 3 of 11 patients (27.2%) in the PTGBD group, and 2 of these patients exhibited drain dislodging. Bile leak peritonitis can be treated conservatively with antibiotics, but drain dislodging is a serious adverse event. This suggests that EUS-GBD is an acceptable method for BTS in terms of adverse events. In the PTGBD group, one patient had gallbladder cancer as the etiology of acute cholecystitis. The length of time from operating to discharge for this patient was 5 days. In addition, this patient did not require conversion to open. Therefore, in our report, gallbladder cancer was not affected by length of time from operating to discharge and conversion to open.

Moreover, concerning difficult LC (DLC), the rate of DLCs was relatively high compared to a previous paper [25] (45.7% vs. 26.3%). In other reports, 3 of 12 (25%) patients and 2 of 23 (9%) patients required conversion to open cholecystectomy [26,27]; in our study, only 1 of 35 (2.9%) patients required conversion. Thus, LC led EUS-GBD could be endured when it comes to patients with DLC.

Jang et al. [27] reported rates of conversion to open cholecystectomy after EUS-GBD had an adverse effect on laparoscopic cholecystectomy and showed that EUS-GBD did not cause severe inflammation or adhesion to surrounding gallbladder tissue; however, this study only included surgical candidates, and cholecystectomy was performed after a median of 5 days after EUS-GBD. In our study, cholecystectomy was performed as elective surgery based on the results of Altieri et al. [28], who revealed that a duration of ≤8 weeks ($n = 1211$) was associated with a higher overall rate of complications.

A well-timed LC 8 weeks after EUS-GBD would be preferable, since the inflammation would be ameliorated, ensuring better surgical outcomes [28]. In our study, the duration from drainage to cholecystectomy in the EUS-GBD group was 86.7 days; this was >8 weeks and longer than the duration in the PTGBD group. However, in the report by Altieri et al., the average time to cholecystectomy was 203 days in the >8 weeks group [28]. Therefore, the rate of DLC in our study could be lower if the waiting period for the surgery was lowered. All patients in our study demonstrated moderate or mild adhesions and fibrosis during surgery; nevertheless, surgery was performed safely, and despite the presence of adhesions and fibrosis, only one patient required conversion to open cholecystectomy. This also indicated that the inflammation due to EUS-GBD can be a surmountable event for experienced laparoscopic surgeons. The EUS-GBD group showed moderate and mild adhesions and fibrosis in all of the patients, yet despite these adhesions and fibrosis, as far as we can observe, there are no long-term postoperative complications such as upper gastrointestinal obstruction in the two groups.

Adverse events (AEs) due to drainage present an independent risk for postsurgical adverse events. In our study, peritonitis and drain dislodging were the most common postprocedural AEs, with bile leak closely related to these events. Bile leak may make cholecystectomy difficult due to the severe adhesion around the gallbladder and enterocholecysto fistula; thus, to minimize the risk of bile leak in EUS-GBD, lumen-apposing metal stent (LAMS) is used. EUS-GBD using LAMS is becoming a widely accepted therapeutic approach for gallbladder drainage with high clinical and technical success rates and low rates of adverse events, as shown by several studies [29]; however, it is only covered by insurance for pancreatic pseudocyst and walled-off necrosis in Japan. Therefore, although plastic stents were used in the EUS-GBD group in our study, it may be that LAMS provides more safety during the procedure [29].

In one previous report, AC had clinical particularities in aged patients with an increased rate of postoperative complications [30]. We obtained the same result in our study. In an aging society, PTGBD is a routine procedure; however, dislocation would be critical for patients with AC. Indeed, drain migration is reported in 0.3–12% of patients [1,31–34]; besides, EUS-GBD in our study resulted in few cases of drain migration. Therefore, EUS-GBD will be safer and more reliable in the future. EUS-GBD would be more patient-friendly than the PTGBD without dislocation and inconvenience.

A review conducted by Lee et al. [35] revealed that nine patients demonstrated rapid clinical improvement within 72 h after EUS-GBD. Elective laparoscopic cholecystectomy was eventually performed in seven patients and was successful in six patients, and transduodenal cholecystostomy was converted to open cholecystectomy in one patient (14.3%) without complication. The rate of technical success of cholecystectomy was 100% in the report of both Lee et al. and our own report, whereas the rates of conversion to open cholecystectomy were 14.3% and 2.9%; thus, both studies demonstrate that LC following EUS-GBD was safe.

This study had some limitations. First, this was a retrospective study. Doctors' treatment preferences may have resulted in a bias. The decision to PTGBD or EUS drainage was made at the discretion of the surgeons, endoscopists, and radiologists, and it may have led to a selection bias. Furthermore, due to the characteristics of our hospital in this study, the proportion of patients with underlying medical conditions was high, so the population may be slightly different from the usual acute cholecystitis patients. This may limit the generalizability of the study.

Second, the sample size of PTGBD patients included was small. In Ryu's meta-analysis and systematic review, reported EUS-GBD was associated with fewer adverse events than PTGBD [23]. However, in our study, post procedural adverse events were observed in six patients (17.1%) in the EUS-GBD group and in three patients (27.2%) in the PTGBD group; no significant differences were found between the two groups ($p = 0.472$). However, no significant difference is seen, although that does not mean there are no differences between EUS-GBD and PTGBD. Hence, randomized controlled trials or non-inferiority trials with more patients should be planned to prove the present results.

Third, our study was conducted by only one expert hepatobiliary pancreatic surgeon; therefore, it may not be valid to generalize our results across other centers, as the surgeons may have varying levels of clinical experience and familiarity with cholecystectomy for high-risk patients with acute cholecystitis. Hence, larger prospective studies are required to confirm our results. Third, since LAMS cannot be used for EUS-GBD in Japan, we hope that a global study using LAMS will be conducted in the future.

In conclusion, this paper indicated that EUS-GBD could be an alternative to PTGBD as a BTS. However, further studies are needed to confirm this.

Author Contributions: Conceptualization, Y.F.; methodology, Y.K.; software, E.S.; validation, S.T.; formal analysis, Y.K.; investigation, Y.F.; resources, Y.F.; data curation, Y.K.; writing—original draft preparation, K.I.; writing—review and editing, K.I.; visualization, A.N. (Atsuki Nagao); supervision, K.H.; project administration, T.T.; funding acquisition, A.N. (Atsushi Nakajima) and K.K. All authors have read and agreed to the published version of the manuscript.

Funding: This research received no external funding.

Institutional Review Board Statement: This was a retrospective study conducted between April 2016 and July 2021. This study protocol was approved by the Institutional Review Board (ID18-313 in January 2016) of our institute. The study was investigator-initiated and conducted according to the ethical principles of the Declaration of Helsinki.

Informed Consent Statement: Written informed consent has been obtained from the patients to publish this paper.

Data Availability Statement: Not applicable.

Conflicts of Interest: The authors declare no conflict of interest.

References

1. Glenn, F. Cholecystostomy in the high risk patient with biliary tract disease. *Ann. Surg.* **1977**, *185*, 185–191. [CrossRef] [PubMed]
2. Margiotta, S.J., Jr.; Willis, I.H.; Wallack, M.K. Cholecystectomy in the elderly. *Am. Surg.* **1988**, *54*, 34–39. [CrossRef] [PubMed]
3. Edlund, G.; Ljungdahl, M. Acute cholecystitis in the elderly. *Am. J. Surg.* **1990**, *159*, 414–416. [CrossRef]
4. Lai, P.B.S.; Kwong, K.H.; Leung, K.L.; Kwok, S.P.Y.; Chan, A.C.W.; Chung, S.C.S.; Lau, W.Y. Randomized trial of early versus delayed laparoscopic cholecystectomy for acute cholecystitis. *Br. J. Surg.* **1998**, *85*, 764–767. [CrossRef] [PubMed]
5. Weigelt, J.A.; Norcross, J.F.; Aurbakken, C.M. Cholecystectomy after tube cholecystostomy. *Am. J. Surg.* **1983**, *146*, 723–726. [CrossRef]
6. De Geus, T.; Moriarty, H.K.; Waters, P.S.; O'Reilly, M.K.; Lawler, L.; Geoghegan, T.; Conneely, J.; McEntee, G.; Farrelly, C. Outcomes of patients treated with upfront cholecystostomy for severe acute cholecystitis. *Surg. Laparosc. Endosc. Percutan. Tech.* **2020**, *30*, 79–84. [CrossRef]
7. Kortram, K.; de Vries Reilingh, T.S.; Wiezer, M.J.; van Ramshorst, B.; Boerma, D. Percutaneous drainage for acute calculous cholecystitis. *Surg. Endosc.* **2011**, *25*, 3642–3646. [CrossRef]
8. Winbladh, A.; Gullstrand, P.; Svanvik, J.; Sandström, P. Systematic review of cholecystostomy as a treatment option in acute cholecystitis. *HPB* **2009**, *11*, 183–193. [CrossRef]
9. McGillicuddy, E.A.; Schuster, K.M.; Barre, K.; Suarez, L.; Hall, M.R.; Kaml, G.J.; Davis, K.A.; Longo, W.E. Non-operative management of acute cholecystitis in the elderly. *Br. J. Surg.* **2012**, *99*, 1254–1261. [CrossRef]
10. Tyberg, A.; Saumoy, M.; Sequeiros, E.V.; Giovannini, M.; Artifon, E.; Teoh, A.; Nieto, J.; Desai, A.; Kumta, N.A.; Gaidhane, M.; et al. EUS-guided versus percutaneous gallbladder drainage: Isn't it time to convert? *J. Clin. Gastroenterol.* **2018**, *52*, 79–84. [CrossRef]
11. Irani, S.; Ngamruengphong, S.; Teoh, A.; Will, U.; Nieto, J.; Abu Dayyeh, B.K.; Gan, S.I.; Larsen, M.; Yip, H.C.; Topazian, M.D.; et al. Similar efficacies of endoscopic ultrasound gallbladder drainage with a lumen-apposing metal stent versus percutaneous transhepatic gallbladder drainage for acute cholecystitis. *Clin. Gastroenterol. Hepatol.* **2017**, *15*, 738–745. [CrossRef]

12. Teoh, A.Y.B.; Serna, C.; Penas, I.; Chong, C.C.N.; Perez-Miranda, M.; Ng, E.K.W.; Lau, J.Y.W. Endoscopic ultrasound-guided gallbladder drainage reduces adverse events compared with percutaneous cholecystostomy in patients who are unfit for cholecystectomy. *Endoscopy* **2017**, *49*, 130–138. [CrossRef]
13. Choi, J.H.; Kim, H.W.; Lee, J.-C.; Paik, K.-H.; Seong, N.J.; Yoon, C.J.; Hwang, J.-H.; Kim, J. Percutaneous transhepatic versus EUS-guided gallbladder drainage for malignant cystic duct obstruction. *Gastrointest. Endosc.* **2017**, *85*, 357–364. [CrossRef]
14. Dollhopf, M.; Larghi, A.; Will, U.; Rimbaș, M.; Anderloni, A.; Sanchez-Yague, A.; Teoh, A.Y.B.; Kunda, R. EUS-guided gallbladder drainage in patients with acute cholecystitis and high surgical risk using an electrocautery-enhanced lumen-apposing metal stent device. *Gastrointest. Endosc.* **2017**, *86*, 636–643. [CrossRef] [PubMed]
15. Choi, J.H.; Lee, S.S.; Choi, J.H.; Park, D.H.; Seo, D.W.; Lee, S.K.; Kim, M.H. Long-term outcomes after endoscopic ultrasonography-guided gallbladder drainage for acute cholecystitis. *Endoscopy* **2014**, *46*, 656–661. [CrossRef]
16. de la Serna-Higuera, C.; Pérez-Miranda, M.; Gil-Simón, P.; Ruiz-Zorrilla, R.; Diez-Redondo, P.; Alcaide, N.; Val, L.S.-D.; Nuñez-Rodriguez, H. EUS-guided transenteric gallbladder drainage with a new fistula-forming, lumen-apposing metal stent. *Gastrointest. Endosc.* **2013**, *77*, 303–308. [CrossRef]
17. Kamata, K.; Takenaka, M.; Kitano, M.; Omoto, S.; Miyata, T.; Minaga, K.; Yamao, K.; Imai, H.; Sakurai, T.; Watanabe, T.; et al. Endoscopic ultrasound-guided gallbladder drainage for acute cholecystitis: Long-term outcomes after removal of a self-expandable metal stent. *World J. Gastroenterol.* **2017**, *23*, 661–667. [CrossRef] [PubMed]
18. Chan, S.M.; Teoh, A.Y.B.; Yip, H.C.; Wong, V.W.Y.; Chiu, P.W.Y.; Ng, E.K.W. Feasibility of per-oral cholecystoscopy and advanced gallbladder interventions after EUS-guided gallbladder stenting (with video). *Gastrointest. Endosc.* **2017**, *85*, 1225–1232. [CrossRef] [PubMed]
19. McKay, A.; Abulfaraj, M.; Lipschitz, J. Short- and long-term outcomes following percutaneous cholecystostomy for acute cholecystitis in high-risk patients. *Surg. Endosc.* **2012**, *26*, 1343–1351. [CrossRef] [PubMed]
20. Akyürek, N.; Salman, B.; Yüksel, O.; Tezcaner, T.; İrkörücü, O.; Yücel, C.; Oktar, S.; Tatlicioğlu, E. Management of acute calculous cholecystitis in high-risk patients: Percutaneous cholecystotomy followed by early laparoscopic cholecystectomy. *Surg. Laparosc. Endosc. Percutan. Tech.* **2005**, *15*, 315–320. [CrossRef]
21. Patterson, E.J.; McLoughlin, R.F.; Mathieson, J.R.; Cooperberg, P.L.; MacFarlane, J.K. An alternative approach to acute cholecystitis. Percutaneous cholecystostomy and interval laparoscopic cholecystectomy. *Surg. Endosc.* **1996**, *10*, 1185–1188. [CrossRef]
22. Kiriyama, S.; Kozaka, K.; Takada, T.; Strasberg, S.M.; Pitt, H.A.; Gabata, T.; Hata, J.; Liau, K.-H.; Miura, F.; Horiguchi, A.; et al. Tokyo Guidelines 2018, diagnostic criteria and severity grading of acute cholangitis (with videos). *J. Hepatobiliary Pancreat. Sci.* **2018**, *25*, 17–30. [CrossRef]
23. Lyu, Y.; Li, T.; Wang, B.; Cheng, Y.; Chen, L.; Zhao, S. Ultrasound-Guided Gallbladder Drainage Versus Percutaneous Transhepatic Gallbladder Drainage for Acute Cholecystitis with High Surgical Risk: An Up-to-Date Meta-Analysis and Systematic Review. *J. Laparoendosc. Adv. Surg. Tech. A* **2021**, *11*, 1232–1240. [CrossRef]
24. Song, T.J.; Park, D.H.; Eum, J.B.; Moon, S.-H.; Lee, S.S.; Seo, D.W.; Lee, S.K.; Kim, M.-H. EUS-guided cholecystoenterostomy with single-step placement of a 7F double-pigtail plastic stent in patients who are unsuitable for cholecystectomy: A pilot study (with video). *Gastrointest. Endosc.* **2010**, *71*, 634–640. [CrossRef] [PubMed]
25. Maehira, H.; Kawasaki, M.; Itoh, A.; Ogawa, M.; Mizumura, N.; Toyoda, S.; Okumura, S.; Kameyama, M. Prediction of difficult laparoscopic cholecystectomy for acute cholecystitis. *J. Surg. Res.* **2017**, *216*, 143–148. [CrossRef] [PubMed]
26. Matsubara, S.; Isayama, H.; Nakai, Y.; Kawakubo, K.; Yamamoto, N.; Saito, K.; Saito, T.; Takahara, N.; Mizuno, S.; Kogure, H.; et al. Endoscopic ultrasound-guided gallbladder drainage with a combined internal and external drainage tubes for acute cholecystitis. *J. Gastroenterol. Hepatol.* **2020**, *35*, 1821–1827. [CrossRef]
27. Jang, J.W.; Lee, S.S.; Song, T.J.; Hyun, Y.S.; Park, D.H.; Seo, D.; Lee, S.; Kim, M.; Yun, S. Endoscopic ultrasound-guided transmural and percutaneous transhepatic gallbladder drainage are comparable for acute cholecystitis. *Gastroenterology* **2012**, *142*, 805–811. [CrossRef] [PubMed]
28. Altieri, M.S.; Yang, J.; Yin, D.; Brunt, L.M.; Talamini, M.A.; Pryor, A.D. Early cholecystectomy (≤ 8 weeks) following percutaneous cholecystostomy tube placement is associated with higher morbidity. *Surg. Endosc.* **2020**, *34*, 3057–3063. [CrossRef]
29. Zain, A.; Christina, L.; Tarun, R. Endoscopic Ultrasound-Guided Gallbladdar Drainage. *Dig. Dis. Sci.* **2021**, *66*, 2154–2161.
30. Serban, D.; Socea, B.; Balasescu, S.; Badiu, C.; Tudor, C.; Dascalu, A.; Vancea, G.; Spataru, R.; Sabau, A.; Sabau, D.; et al. Safety of laparoscopic cholecystectomy for acute cholecystitis in the elderly: A multivariate analysis of risk factors for intra and postoperative complications. *Medicina* **2021**, *57*, 230. [CrossRef]
31. Kiviniemi, H.; Mäkelä, J.T.; Autio, R.; Tikkakoski, T.; Leinonen, S.; Siniluoto, T.; Perälä, J.; Päivänsalo, M.; Merikanto, J. Percutaneous cholecystostomy in acute cholecystitis in high-risk patients: An analysis of 69 patients. *Int. Surg.* **1998**, *83*, 299–302.
32. Sugiyama, M.; Tokuhara, M.; Atomi, Y. Is percutaneous cholecystostomy the optimal treatment for acute cholecystitis in the very elderly? *World J. Surg.* **1998**, *22*, 459–463. [CrossRef] [PubMed]
33. Ito, K.; Fujita, N.; Noda, Y.; Kobayashi, G.; Kimura, K.; Sugawara, T.; Horaguchi, J. Percutaneous cholecystostomy versus gallbladder aspiration for acute cholecystitis: A prospective randomized controlled trial. *AJR Am. J. Roentgenol.* **2004**, *183*, 193–196. [CrossRef] [PubMed]

34. Hatzidakis, A.A.; Prassopoulos, P.; Petinarakis, I.; Sanidas, E.; Chrysos, E.; Chalkiadakis, G.; Tsiftsis, D.; Gourtsoyiannis, N.C. Acute cholecystitis in high-risk patients: Percutaneous cholecystostomy vs. conservative treatment. *Eur. Radiol.* **2002**, *12*, 1778–1784. [CrossRef]
35. Lee, S.S.; Park, D.H.; Hwang, C.Y.; Ahn, C.-S.; Lee, T.Y.; Seo, D.-W.; Lee, S.K.; Kim, M.-W. EUS-guided transmural cholecystostomy as rescue management for acute cholecystitis in elderly or high-risk patients: A prospective feasibility study. *Gastrointest. Endosc.* **2007**, *66*, 1008–1012. [CrossRef] [PubMed]

Disclaimer/Publisher's Note: The statements, opinions and data contained in all publications are solely those of the individual author(s) and contributor(s) and not of MDPI and/or the editor(s). MDPI and/or the editor(s) disclaim responsibility for any injury to people or property resulting from any ideas, methods, instructions or products referred to in the content.

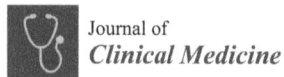

Article

Secondary Tumors of the Pancreas: A Multicenter Analysis of Clinicopathological and Endosonographic Features

Marco Spadaccini [1,2], Maria Cristina Conti Bellocchi [3], Benedetto Mangiavillano [4], Alberto Fantin [5], Daoud Rahal [6], Erminia Manfrin [3], Francesca Gavazzi [7], Silvia Bozzarelli [8], Stefano Francesco Crinò [3], Maria Terrin [1,2], Milena Di Leo [9], Cristiana Bonifacio [10], Antonio Facciorusso [11], Stefano Realdon [5], Chiara Cristofori [5], Francesco Auriemma [4], Alessandro Fugazza [1], Luca Frulloni [3], Cesare Hassan [1,2], Alessandro Repici [1,2] and Silvia Carrara [1,*]

1. Endoscopic Unit, Department of Gastroenterology, IRCCS Humanitas Research Hospital, Via Manzoni 56, 20089 Milan, Italy; marcospadaccini9@gmail.com (M.S.)
2. Department of Biomedical Sciences, Humanitas University, Via Manzoni 113, 20089 Milan, Italy
3. Gastroenterology and Digestive Endoscopy Unit, The Pancreas Institute, G.B. Rossi University Hospital, 37134 Verona, Italy
4. Digestive Endoscopy Unit, Division of Gastroenterology, Humanitas Mater Domini, 21053 Castellanza, Italy
5. Gastroenterology Unit, Istituto Oncologico Veneto IOV-IRCCS, 35128 Padova, Italy
6. Department of Pathology, IRCCS Humanitas Research Hospital, Via Manzoni 56, 20089 Milan, Italy
7. Pancreatic Surgery Unit, IRCCS Humanitas Research Hospital, Via Manzoni 56, 20089 Milan, Italy
8. Medical Oncology and Hematology Unit, Humanitas Cancer Center, IRCCS Humanitas Research Hospital, Via Manzoni 56, 20089 Milan, Italy
9. Digestive Endoscopy Unit, Division of Gastroenterology, San Paolo Hospital, 20090 Milan, Italy
10. Department of Radiology, IRCCS Humanitas Research Hospital, Via Manzoni 56, 20089 Milan, Italy
11. Gastroenterology Unit, Department of Surgical and Medical Sciences, University of Foggia, 71122 Foggia, Italy
* Correspondence: silvia.carrara@humanitas.it; Tel.: +39-(0)282247288

Abstract: Many tumors may secondarily involve the pancreas; however, only retrospective autopic and surgical series are available. We retrospectively collected data from all consecutive patients with histologically confirmed secondary tumors of the pancreas referred to five Italian centers between 2010 and 2021. We described clinical and pathological features, therapeutic approach and treatment outcomes. EUS characteristics of the lesions and the tissue acquisition procedures (needle, passages, histology) were recorded. A total of 116 patients (males/females 69/47; mean age 66.7) with 236 histologically confirmed pancreatic metastases were included; kidney was the most common primary site. EUS was performed to confirm the diagnosis in 205 lesions which presented as predominantly solitary (59), hypoechoic (95) and hypervascular (60), with a heterogeneous ($n = 54$) pattern and well-defined borders ($n = 52$). EUS-guided tissue acquisition was performed in 94 patients with an overall accuracy of 97.9%. Histological evaluation was possible in 88.3% of patients, obtaining final diagnosis in all cases. When cytology alone was performed, the final diagnosis was obtained in 83.3% of cases. A total of 67 patients underwent chemo/radiation therapy, and surgery was attempted in 45 (38.8%) patients. Pancreatic metastases are a possible event in the natural history of solid tumors, even long after the diagnosis of the primary site. EUS-guided fine needle biopsy may be suggested to implement the differential diagnosis.

Keywords: pancreas; cancer; oncology; surgery; metastasis

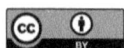

1. Introduction

Many extrapancreatic tumors may secondarily involve the pancreas, with an incidence ranging from 3% to 12% [1,2] and a broad spectrum of both clinicopathological features and outcomes. Knowledge is still lacking about the molecular pathways and the anatomical reasons supporting the behavior of some of the most common tumors associated with pancreatic metastasis, such as renal cell carcinoma and melanoma [3,4].

Most evidence is based on retrospective analysis of autopsies and surgical series, due to the high incidence (around one-third of secondary pancreatic tumors) of lesions clinically mistaken as primary pancreatic tumors before surgical resection [1]. For these reasons, those series could not provide data on how to improve accuracy during the diagnostic work-up.

Considering the morbidity (and mortality) related to pancreatic surgery, pancreatic resections should be performed only when they are clinically indicated. As a matter of fact, among other challenges, in the differential diagnosis of a pancreatic mass, the possibility of a metastatic lesion should always be considered. In this regard, accurate oncological anamnesis, extensive background knowledge of malignancies possibly involving the pancreas through metastasis and a precise imaging-based diagnosis of a pancreatic mass, particularly in a patient with concomitant or previous history of extra-pancreatic cancer, are mandatory. However, even if fundamental in raising the suspicion, clinical, epidemiological and radiological data are often useless in distinguishing between primary pancreatic cancer and metastases.

As a consequence, the role of endoscopic ultrasound (EUS) in the diagnostic work-up of pancreatic masses has already been demonstrated and the EUS-guided tissue acquisition is of paramount importance for obtaining a reliable diagnosis [5], even if no data are available about the role of core needles for histology (over cytology) assessment.

The aim of this study was to describe clinical, endosonographic and pathological features of secondary tumors of the pancreas, along with their therapeutic approach and related outcomes.

2. Materials and Methods

2.1. Patients

A retrospective review of prospectively maintained databases of EUS procedures was carried out to identify all patients referred to the Endoscopic Units of five Italian centers (Humanitas Bergamo, Castellanza, and Rozzano; Policlinico GB Rossi Verona; Istituto Oncologico Veneto, Castelfranco Veneto) between April 2010 and April 2021. Data from patients with a histologically confirmed diagnosis of secondary pancreatic tumors were retrieved for the study analysis. Furthermore, we performed a chart revision of all patients who underwent pancreatic resections for secondary pancreatic malignancies in the five centers during the same timeframe.

Patients with locally advanced non-pancreatic primary tumors that involved the pancreas by direct extension (e.g., pancreatic infiltration by left kidney cancer) were excluded.

Demographic and clinical characteristics were collected. In particular, the time of recurrence was defined as the time (in months) between the first radiographic remission of the primary neoplasia and the histological diagnosis of metastasis into the pancreatic parenchyma. Treatment and outcome data were collected as well.

The study was conducted according to the Declaration of Helsinki and approved by the institutional review board (IRB) of the coordinating center (Humanitas Research Center, Rozzano). All the patients gave their consent to the procedures and to the research purposes. The study protocol was registered at Clinicaltrial.gov (NCT02855151).

2.2. Endoscopic Ultrasound Procedures

The Olympus GF-UCT180 series linear array echoendoscope (Olympus Europa SE & CO. KG, Hamburg, Germany) in combination with the new EU-ME2 echoprocessor (Olympus SE & CO. KG, Hamburg, Germany) or Pentax EG-3870UTK linear echoendoscope (Pentax Medical, Hamburg, Germany) in combination with a Hitachi ultrasound machine were used.

Fine-flow (Pentax) or H-Flow (Olympus) were used to enhance the micro-vascularization of the masses: when a mass is kept very close to the tip, this modality shows high resolution details of the vascular pattern of the lesion. To define the vascular pattern of the lesion, contrast-enhanced EUS with intravenous contrast agent administration (Sonovue™, Bracco Imaging, Milan, Italy) was performed, as per centers' shared protocol since 2015.

For each patient, EUS characteristics of the lesions were collected: size, location, number of focal masses, echotexture and vascularization.

Adverse events were recorded. Eloubeidi et al. [6] defined an adverse event as any deviation from the expected clinical course during or after EUS, related to the procedure.

EUS-guided tissue acquisition was performed with 22-gauge, 25-gauge or 19-gauge needles (Expect™ Slimline, Acquire™, Boston Scientific, Boston, MA, USA; Beacon bnx®, SharkCore Needle™, Medtronic, Newton, MA, USA), chosen at the discretion of the endosonographers. The biopsies were performed combining the fanning technique and the slow-pull technique [7,8]. In general, especially for hypervascularized lesions, no suction was applied, in order to reduce the contamination of the specimen with blood.

At each pass, if a micro-fragment or "worm-like" material was observed, it was placed in a container of 10% neutral buffered formalin fixative for the final histological examination and immunohistochemistry (IHC) staining. If drop-like material was obtained, it was smeared between 2 glass slides, fixed with ethanol and stained with a Papanicolaou stain for cytological analysis.

The therapeutic path was always decided through multidisciplinary team (MDT) discussion involving endoscopists, surgeons, oncologists, radiation oncologists and radiologists. The surgical methodology is reported in the Appendix A.

2.3. Pathological Evaluation of EUS and Surgical Specimens

After 24 h fixation in 10% buffered formalin, all the biopsy specimens were stained with haematoxylin and eosin (H&E) and the slides were evaluated by expert pathologists specialized in Hepato-Bilio-Pancreatic disease. Ancillary analysis such as immunohistochemistry (IHC) staining was performed if the pathologist deemed it was necessary to better define the histological diagnosis and grading and in the case of hormone-secreting tumors.

The surgical specimens were observed by the pathologist and a gross description was made: size, site and number of lesions were recorded in the pathological report.

2.4. Statistical Analysis

Data were entered into an Excel spreadsheet (Microsoft Excel 2010; Microsoft Corporation, Redmond, WA, USA). All continuous variables were described as mean and standard deviation, while dichotomous variables were reported as percentage. Statistical analysis was performed using SPSS version 17 (SPSS Inc., Chicago, IL, USA).

3. Results

3.1. Baseline Characteristics

A total of 116 patients (male/female: 69/47; mean age: 66.7 ± 10.1 years—range: 26–86 years) with 236 histologically confirmed pancreatic metastases were included in the analysis (Figure 1).

Lesion distribution was relatively even among pancreatic head, uncinated process, neck, body and tail, and the mean lesion size was 25.4 ± 15.2 mm, ranging from 2.7 to 90.0 mm (Table 1).

Table 1. Baseline characteristics. * 79 lesions >20 mm, 110 lesions 10–20 mm, 47 lesions < 10 mm.

Patients (n)	116
Male (n)	69
Mean age (years)	66.7 ± 10.1
Primary tumor (n)	
Kidney	75
Colon	9
Breast	7
Lung	7
Melanoma	7
Fibro-leiomyosarcoma	3
Ovarian cancer	3
Liver cancer	2
Merkel cell tumor	1
Thyroid cancer	1
Non-Hodgkin lymphoma	1
Diagnostic timing (n)	
Synchronous	7
Metachronous	109
Symptoms (n)	
Asymptomatic	94
Jaundice	9
Pancreatic-like pain	7
Weight loss	3
Anemia	2
Asthenia	1
Lesions (n)	236
Mean size (mm) *	25.4 ± 15.2
Location	
Head	57
Uncinated process	43
Neck	37
Body	50
Tail	49

The most common primary neoplastic site was the kidney (75 cases), with all of the histology types being clear cell renal carcinoma. In 40 out of 75 cases (53.3%), the pancreas was the unique metastatic site. The other most common primary sites were the colon ($n = 9$), breast ($n = 7$), lung ($n = 7$) and melanoma ($n = 7$). In addition, there were three cases of fibro-leiomyosarcoma, three of ovarian cancer, two of liver cancer and one case of Merkel cell tumor, thyroid cancer and non-Hodgkin lymphoma. In most of the non-kidney cancers (37/41, 90.2%), the pancreas was not the only metastatic site.

In seven cases, the lesions were found during the initial staging work-up. Among the other 109 patients, pancreatic metastases were diagnosed after a mean time of 97.8 ± 79.4 months, with nearly two-thirds of cases ($n = 70$, 60.3%) having a latency interval of at least 5 years. Of note, no cases of lung metastasis were found after more than two years from the initial diagnosis. In most of the cases ($n = 94$), the lesions were asymptomatic, which were incidental findings during the staging/follow-up. Nine lesions caused jaundice and pancreatic-like pain was reported in seven cases. Further, weight loss, anemia and asthenia were reported by a minority of patients ($n = 6$).

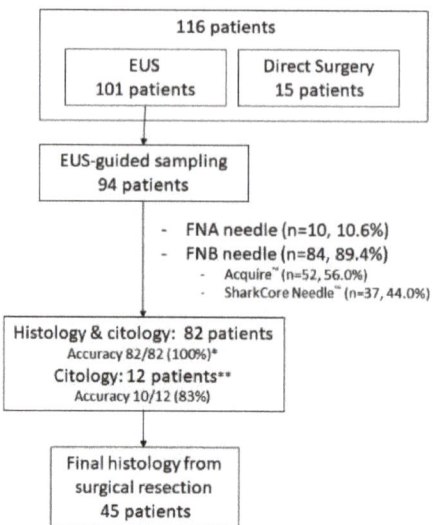

Figure 1. Study flowchart. * histology only accuracy 81/82 (98.8%), cytology only accuracy 73/82 (89.0%); ** no core obtained, but material adequate for cytological diagnosis.

3.2. EUS Characteristics

In 101 patients, an EUS was performed in order to confirm the diagnosis of 205 pancreatic lesions with a mean size of 23.8 ± 15.3 mm, ranging from 2.7 to 73.0 mm. In most of the cases, they were solitary ($n = 59$), hypoechoic ($n = 95$) lesions, with a heterogeneous ($n = 54$) pattern and well-defined borders ($n = 52$) (Figure 2).

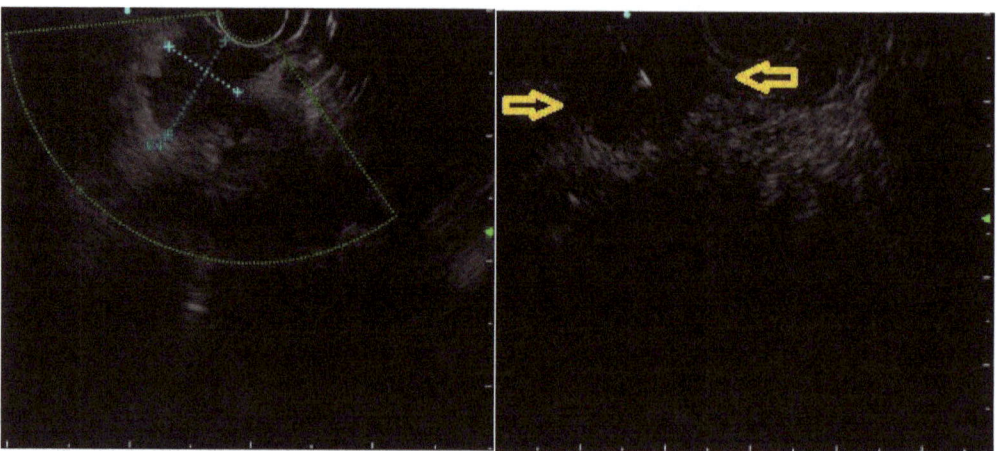

Figure 2. Breast cancer metastasis to pancreas. Yellow arrows point at margins' irregularity.

The vascular evaluation showed 60 hypervascular lesions, with a heterogeneous vascular pattern in 32 cases. EUS features per histology type are reported in Table 2 for main histology types.

EUS-guided fine needle sampling was successfully performed in 94 patients with an overall diagnostic yield of 97.9% (92/94) after an average number of 2.4 ± 1.3 needle passes (range: 1–4). In 82 out of 94 cases (88.3%), the presence of a "worm-like" core also allowed a histologic evaluation after formalin fixation, and the final diagnosis was obtained in all cases. In 9 of the 82 patients (11.0%) with availability of both cytological and histological specimens, the cytology alone had failed in reaching the diagnosis. Conversely, among the 12 cases in which no tissue core was retrieved because of the drop-like or bloody aspect of the material obtained, the final diagnosis was enabled by cytology assessment in 10 out of 12 cases (83.3%).

Table 2. EUS features per histology type. Less than 3 patients with fibro-leiomyosarcoma, ovarian cancer, liver and thyroid cancer, Merkel cell tumor and non-Hodgkin lymphoma underwent EUS.

Histology (n)	Echogenicity	Echogenicity (Pattern)	Vascularization	Vascularization (Pattern)	Borders
Kidney (63)	Hypo = 59 Iso = 2 Hyper = 2	Homo = 32 Etero = 31	Hypo = 3 Hyper = 60	Homo = 46 Etero = 17	Regular = 50 Irregular = 13
Colon (8)	Hypo = 8 Iso = 8 Hyper = 8	Homo = 1 Etero = 7	Hypo = 6 Hyper = 2	Homo = 6 Etero = 2	Regular = 6 Irregular = 2
Lung (7)	Hypo = 6 Iso = 0 Hyper = 1	Homo = 1 Etero = 6	Hypo = 6 Hyper = 6	Homo = 3 Etero = 4	Regular = 1 Irregular = 2
Breast (6)	Hypo = 6 Iso = 0 Hyper = 0	Homo = 1 Etero = 5	Hypo = 6 Hyper = 0	Homo = 3 Etero = 3	Regular = 3 Irregular = 3
Melanoma (6)	Hypo = 6 Iso = 0 Hyper = 0	Homo = 5 Etero = 1	Hypo = 4 Hyper = 2	Homo = 3 Etero = 3	Regular = 2 Irregular = 4

Immunostaining studies were performed on 78 out of 82 formalin-fixed histology samples (95.1%) and on 9 out of 33 cytology samples (27.3%).

3.3. Treatment and Outcomes

Sixty-five patients underwent chemotherapy and two patients underwent radiation therapy. In 45 patients (38.8%), the surgical approach was attempted (see surgical outcomes in Appendix A).

A total of 90 patients were followed up for a mean time of 25.3 ± 21.1 months and 16 of them died during the follow-up period (4 deaths due to unrelated causes). Among those still alive, 43 out of 74 patients were free from disease after a mean follow-up time of 24.9 ± 8.4 months. Eighteen patients were lost at follow-up.

4. Discussion

Most pancreatic lesions are primary neoplasms, and of these more than 90% are pancreatic ductal adenocarcinomas, but the pancreatic parenchyma may also be a site of metastases from other primary sites. As a matter of fact, secondary tumors of the pancreas can have an incidence rate ranging from 3% to 12% [2]. In particular, some tumors seem to favor the pancreas, and the biological mechanisms that sustain this interaction between the circulating tumor cells and the host organ have yet to be fully explained [9]. Thus, in a patient with a previous history of cancer and a new diagnosis of a pancreatic mass, determining whether the pancreatic lesion is a primary or secondary tumor is necessary in order to plan the best treatment. This is even more relevant considering the possible long interval time between primary tumor and metastasis diagnoses, ruling out any possibility of identifying any sort of "safe zone". Indeed, in our series, secondary pancreatic tumors occurred after a mean period of more than 8 years, after the clinical and/or radiological remission of the primary tumor, with a maximum period of 17 years. Our findings corroborate the long time between the diagnosis and management of the primary tumor and the evidence of pancreatic metastasis, with a maximum latency period ranging from 14 months to 22 years [10] described in the literature. As a result, secondary tumors are often not the first hypothesis during an initial evaluation of the pancreatic masses. This is why, when a secondary neoplasm is suspected, a thoroughly detailed clinical history is of paramount importance in order to orient the diagnosis through adequate imaging and EUS-guided sampling, planning the right panel of immunohistochemical staining.

In the literature, the most common cancers with metastases to the pancreas include lung cancer, renal cell cancer, colon cancer, melanoma, sarcoma and breast cancer [11], but haematological malignancy metastases have also been described [12]. We described a prevalence of the kidney as the primary site of pancreatic secondary tumors, as described in previous studies [13–18]. However, an autopsy study from Japan reported gastric adenocarcinoma as the most common primary site [11], while in previous clinical series, more than a quarter of metastases to the pancreas had originated from the lung [1,19]. The different incidence in the primary site may be due to population-based differences, in particular for the Japanese study [11], but also to the patients analyzed (case series vs autopsy cases) and to a different prognosis of the primary neoplasm over time.

Symptoms of pancreatic secondary tumors are often absent and therefore they are identified during the initial work-up of the primary tumor or during routine surveillance after its resection. We reported 80% of asymptomatic patients as described in other series [14,20]. Unfortunately, when secondary tumors cause symptoms, they are similar to those reported for primary pancreatic cancer, such as abdominal pain and jaundice [21]. The similar clinical presentation and the long interval from primary neoplasm treatment make it difficult to differentiate the clinical diagnosis between primary pancreatic tumor and pancreatic metastasis.

Moreover, in half of our cases, the patients had only one pancreatic mass. In these cases, the distribution of metastases did not help to distinguish secondary tumors from primary pancreatic cancer, as stated in previous studies [5,13]. However, other series have reported the pancreatic head as the favored site of secondary tumors [22,23]. In this scenario, the role of EUS has become fundamental in order to reach a final diagnosis and choose the best treatment option for the patient. Noninvasive cross-sectional imaging (multidetector computed tomography and magnetic resonance imaging) can provide a general assessment of malignancy potential and resectability, and the presence of lymphadenopathy and/or of distant metastases [24]. However, the radiologic distinction between a primary and secondary pancreatic neoplasm is often limited, although enhanced computed tomography scans and magnetic resonance imaging may be contributory, especially if contrast medium is used [25–27].

The most prevalent EUS characteristics in our series were a heterogeneous hypoechoic pattern without cystic component and with well-defined borders. Our experience confirmed data from the literature, where the more common EUS characteristic of secondary pancreatic neoplasms are hypoechoic, hypervascular and masses with well-defined borders [14,20,28]. However, it also appeared clear that the endosonographic aspect of secondary pancreatic lesions alone fails to reliably distinguish among the different histologies and primary pancreatic cancer, with only kidney carcinoma having a stable EUS pattern (hypoechoic, hypervascular lesions with well-defined borders; Figure 3).

This underlines, on the one hand, the importance of always considering the possibility of looking at a pancreatic metastasis irrespective from the EUS specific patterns, and on the other hand, the option of EUS-guided sampling appears as an unmatched opportunity for pancreatic lesion diagnosis. As a matter of fact, even in our series, tissue acquisition is usually necessary to reach the final pathological diagnosis and to assess the site of origin of the mass. EUS biopsy is a safe, effective and efficient diagnostic tool in the evaluation of pancreatic masses. Cytopathological specimens, and more recently core biopsies, may be obtained with high sensitivity (75–98%), specificity (71–100%), positive predictive value (96–100%), negative predictive value (33–85%) and accuracy (79–98%) in the diagnosis of pancreatic cancer as compared to other modalities [29]. In agreement with the pathologist, a biopsy fragment should always be processed in a way that guarantees the better preservation of cells and tissues and reduces the risk to lose material, independently from the caliber and geometry of the needle used. In this regard, the main finding of our study is to highlight a potential benefit of using fine-needle biopsy (EUS-FNB) for its higher diagnostic yield and a higher possibility of immunohistochemical-based tests when compared to cytology, suggesting the choice of dedicated needles for adequate samples. FNB needles may therefore be preferred over FNA needles when available. Conversely, the relevance of both Rapid On-Site Evaluation (ROSE) and Macroscopic On-Site Evaluation (MOSE) in the case of suspected pancreatic metastasis needs to be assessed in further studies.

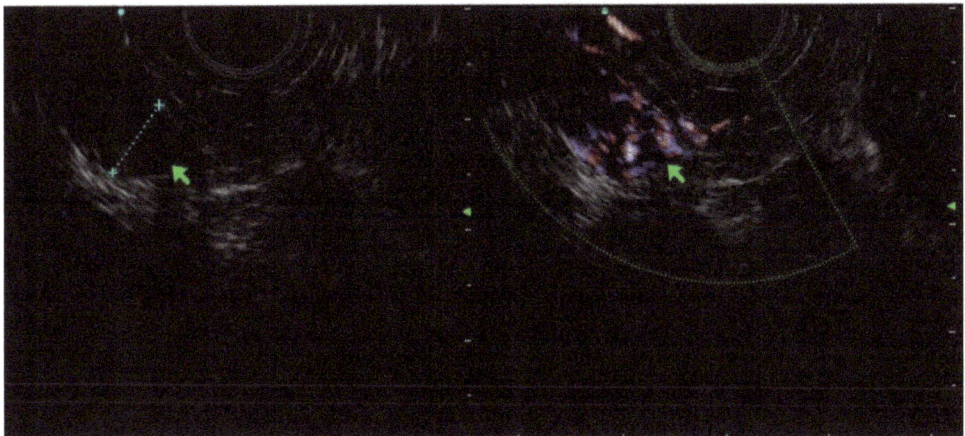

Figure 3. Renal cancer metastasis to pancreas. Green arrows point at margins' irregularity.

Our study is limited by a few drawbacks. First, the retrospective design prevents us from drawing unbiased conclusions. As a matter of fact, possible confounders in terms of lesion heterogeneity, clinical management and EUS protocol across the different centers cannot be ruled out. However, this large cohort represents one of the most comprehensive points of view on this underestimated issue. Secondly, we could report EUS data of only 205 among the 236 lesions (86.9%), since some of the lesions were directly referred to surgery after CT scan. In our opinion, such sharing of real-life data is aimed at increasing awareness of this issue. Interestingly, reports of pancreatic metastasis have been increasing in recent years [3], probably due to better accuracy of diagnostic examination and to the improvement in neoplastic disease outcomes with longer follow-up. In the near future, this may allow for the undertaking of a multicenter-based prospective effort in order to confirm the need for tissue sampling, and the superiority of EUS-FNB over fine-needle aspiration, in attempting to assess the optimal modality for an EUS-based approach. Moreover, another limitation of our study is that it failed in providing any hint about the reason why the pancreas is such a common site for specific tumor metastases, even if we may consider this beyond the purpose of this study. This topic has been diffusely investigated by previous studies; however, knowledge is still scarce, even for some of the most common tumors associated with pancreatic metastasis [3,4]. In particular, different mechanisms of occurrence of metastasis in renal cell cancer have been proposed; the exclusive pancreatic involvement we observed in several cases is difficult to reconcile with a systemic haematogenous seeding, especially when considering the small amount of blood flowing through the 120–180 g of pancreatic tissue. However, previous population-based studies attributed only little if any role to a local mechanism (i.e., lymphogenic or venous) [9], and further studies are still needed.

5. Conclusions

Metastases to the pancreas are a possible occurrence in the natural history of various solid tumors even long time after primary tumor diagnosis. EUS-guided tissue acquisition with fine-needle biopsy needles may be suggested to implement ancillary studies necessary for differential diagnosis.

Author Contributions: Conceptualization, M.S. and S.C.; formal analysis, M.S. and A.F. (Antonio Facciorusso); investigation, M.S., M.C.C.B., B.M., A.F. (Alberto Fantin), D.R., E.M., F.G., S.B., M.T., S.F.C., M.D.L., C.B., S.R., C.C., F.A., A.F. (Alessandro Fugazza) and S.C.; supervision, L.F., C.H. and A.R.; writing—original draft, M.S. and S.C. All authors have read and agreed to the published version of the manuscript.

Funding: This research received no external funding.

Institutional Review Board Statement: The study was conducted in accordance with the Declaration of Helsinki, and approved by the Institutional Review Board (IRB) of the coordinating center (Humanitas Research Center, Rozzano, Italy). The study protocol was registered at Clinicaltrial.gov (NCT02855151).

Informed Consent Statement: Informed consent was obtained from all subjects involved in the study.

Data Availability Statement: The data are available upon request from the corresponding author.

Acknowledgments: We acknowledge Elena Finati and Rosangela Nicoletti for their support in data collection and patients' follow up.

Conflicts of Interest: The authors declare no conflict of interest.

Appendix A. Surgical Procedures

Surgical interventions included total pancreatectomy, pancreaticoduodenectomy, distal pancreatectomy and enucleation. Demolition of the surgical specimen in total pancreatectomy was performed "en-bloc" to allow an accurate pathological examination. Reconstruction, when necessary, was realized with antecholic gastrojejunostomy. Pancreaticoduodenectomy was performed by end-to-side double-layer pancreaticojejunostomy, when duct-to-mucosa was possible. End-to-side hepaticojejunostomy was carried out 10–15 cm distal to the pancreatic anastomosis. A pylorus preservation procedure was usually performed, and an end-to-side ante-colic duodenojejunostomy was realized 30 cm distal to the biliary-enteric anastomosis. Distal pancreatectomy was usually performed according to radical antegrade modular pancreatosplenectomy (RAMPS) technique [9]. During surgical pancreatic enucleation, US was performed to confirm enough distance between lesion and Wirsung duct ($\geq$3 mm).

Post-operative morbidity, mortality (death within 30 days after day of hospital discharge), reintervention and readmission rates were evaluated. Post-operative complications, including pancreatic, biliary, duodenal/gastric and lymphatic fistulas, abdominal abscess, delayed gastric emptying (DGE), wound infection and post-pancreatectomy haemorrhage (PPH) were graded according to the Clavien–Dindo Classification [10]. Post-operative pancreatic fistula (POPF), PPH and DGE were defined according to the International Study Group for Pancreatic Surgery recommendations [11–13].

References

1. Adsay, N.V.; Andea, A.; Basturk, O.; Kilinc, N.; Nassar, H.; Cheng, J.D. Secondary tumors of the pancreas: An analysis of a surgical and autopsy database and review of the literature. *Virchows Arch. Int. J. Pathol.* **2004**, *444*, 527–535. [CrossRef] [PubMed]
2. David, O.; Green, L.; Reddy, V.; Kluskens, L.; Bitterman, P.; Attal, H.; Prinz, R.; Gattuso, P. Pancreatic masses: A multi-institutional study of 364 fine-needle aspiration biopsies with histopathologic correlation. *Diagn. Cytopathol.* **1998**, *19*, 423–427. [CrossRef]
3. Zerbi, A.; Pecorelli, N. Pancreatic metastases: An increasing clinical entity. *World J. Gastrointest. Surg.* **2010**, *2*, 255–259. [CrossRef] [PubMed]
4. Sperti, C.; Pozza, G.; Brazzale, A.R.; Buratin, A.; Moletta, L.; Beltrame, V.; Valmasoni, M. Metastatic tumors to the pancreas: A systematic review and meta-analysis. *Minerva Chir.* **2016**, *71*, 337. [PubMed]
5. DeWitt, J.; Jowell, P.; Leblanc, J.; McHenry, L.; McGreevy, K.; Cramer, H.; Volmar, K.; Sherman, S.; Gress, F. EUS-guided FNA of pancreatic metastases: A multicenter experience. *Gastrointest. Endosc.* **2005**, *61*, 689–696. [CrossRef] [PubMed]

6. Eloubeidi, M.A.; Gress, F.G.; Savides, T.J.; Wiersema, M.J.; Kochman, M.L.; Ahmad, N.A.; Ginsberg, G.G.; Erickson, R.A.; Dewitt, J.; Van Dam, J.; et al. Acute pancreatitis after EUS-guided FNA of solid pancreatic masses: A pooled analysis from EUS centers in the United States. *Gastrointest. Endosc.* **2004**, *60*, 385–389. [CrossRef] [PubMed]
7. Facciorusso, A.; Crinò, S.F.; Ramai, D.; Madhu, D.; Fugazza, A.; Carrara, S.; Spadaccini, M.; Mangiavillano, B.; Gkolfakis, P.; Mohan, B.P.; et al. Comparative Diagnostic Performance of Different Techniques for Endoscopic Ultrasound-Guided Fine-Needle Biopsy of Solid Pancreatic Masses: A Network Meta-analysis. *Gastrointest. Endosc.* **2023**, *in press*. [CrossRef]
8. Polkowski, M.; Jenssen, C.; Kaye, P.; Carrara, S.; Deprez, P.; Gines, A.; Fernández-Esparrach, G.; Eisendrath, P.; Aithal, G.P.; Arcidiacono, P.; et al. Technical aspects of endoscopic ultrasound (EUS)-guided sampling in gastroenterology: European Society of Gastrointestinal Endoscopy (ESGE) Technical Guideline—March 2017. *Endoscopy* **2017**, *49*, 989–1006. [CrossRef]
9. Sellner, F.; Thalhammer, S.; Klimpfinger, M. Tumour Evolution and Seed and Soil Mechanism in Pancreatic Metastases of Renal Cell Carcinoma. *Cancers* **2021**, *16*, 1342. [CrossRef]
10. Z'Graggen, K.; Fernandez-del Castillo, C.; Rattner, D.W.; Sigala, H.; Warshaw, A.L. Metastases to the pancreas and their surgical extirpation. *Arch. Surg.* **1998**, *133*, 413–417. [CrossRef]
11. Nakamura, E.; Shimizu, M.; Itoh, T.; Manabe, T. Secondary tumors of the pancreas: Clinicopathological study of 103 autopsy cases of Japanese patients. *Pathol. Int.* **2001**, *51*, 686–690. [CrossRef] [PubMed]
12. Tan, C.H.; Tamm, E.P.; Marcal, L.; Balachandran, A.; Charnsangavej, C.; Vikram, R.; Bhosale, P. Imaging features of hematogenous metastases to the pancreas: Pictorial essay. *Cancer Imaging Off. Publ. Int. Cancer Imaging Soc.* **2011**, *11*, 9–15. [CrossRef] [PubMed]
13. Waters, L.; Si, Q.; Caraway, N.; Mody, D.; Staerkel, G.; Sneige, N. Secondary tumors of the pancreas diagnosed by endoscopic ultrasound-guided fine-needle aspiration: A 10-year experience. *Diagn. Cytopathol.* **2014**, *42*, 738–743. [CrossRef] [PubMed]
14. El Hajj, I.I.; LeBlanc, J.K.; Sherman, S.; Al-Haddad, M.A.; Cote, G.A.; McHenry, L.; DeWitt, J.M. Endoscopic ultrasound-guided biopsy of pancreatic metastases: A large single-center experience. *Pancreas* **2013**, *42*, 524–530. [CrossRef] [PubMed]
15. Konstantinidis, I.T.; Dursun, A.; Zheng, H.; Wargo, J.A.; Thayer, S.P.; Fernandez-del Castillo, C.; Warshaw, A.L.; Ferrone, C.R. Metastatic tumors in the pancreas in the modern era. *J. Am. Coll. Surg.* **2010**, *211*, 749–753. [CrossRef]
16. Masetti, M.; Zanini, N.; Martuzzi, F.; Fabbri, C.; Mastrangelo, L.; Landolfo, G.; Fornelli, A.; Burzi, M.; Vezzelli, E.; Jovine, E. Analysis of prognostic factors in metastatic tumors of the pancreas: A single-center experience and review of the literature. *Pancreas* **2010**, *39*, 135–143. [CrossRef]
17. Layfield, L.J.; Hirschowitz, S.L.; Adler, D.G. Metastatic disease to the pancreas documented by endoscopic ultrasound guided fine-needle aspiration: A seven-year experience. *Diagn. Cytopathol.* **2012**, *40*, 228–233. [CrossRef]
18. Reddy, S.; Edil, B.H.; Cameron, J.L.; Pawlik, T.M.; Herman, J.M.; Gilson, M.M.; Campbell, K.A.; Schulick, R.D.; Ahuja, N.; Wolfgang, C.L. Pancreatic resection of isolated metastases from nonpancreatic primary cancers. *Ann. Surg. Oncol.* **2008**, *15*, 3199–3206. [CrossRef]
19. Benning, T.L.; Silverman, J.F.; Berns, L.A.; Geisinger, K.R. Fine needle aspiration of metastatic and hematologic malignancies clinically mimicking pancreatic carcinoma. *Acta Cytol.* **1992**, *36*, 471–476.
20. Ardengh, J.C.; Lopes, C.V.; Kemp, R.; Venco, F.; de Lima-Filho, E.R.; dos Santos, J.S. Accuracy of endoscopic ultrasound-guided fine-needle aspiration in the suspicion of pancreatic metastases. *BMC Gastroenterol.* **2013**, *13*, 63. [CrossRef]
21. Porta, M.; Fabregat, X.; Malats, N.; Guarner, L.; Carrato, A.; de Miguel, A.; Ruiz, L.; Jariod, M.; Costafreda, S.; Coll, S.; et al. Exocrine pancreatic cancer: Symptoms at presentation and their relation to tumour site and stage. *Clin. Transl. Oncol.* **2005**, *7*, 189–197. [CrossRef] [PubMed]
22. Palazzo, L.; Borotto, E.; Cellier, C.; Roseau, G.; Chaussade, S.; Couturier, D.; Paolaggi, J.A. Endosonographic features of pancreatic metastases. *Gastrointest. Endosc.* **1996**, *44*, 433–436. [CrossRef] [PubMed]
23. Bechade, D.; Palazzo, L.; Fabre, M.; Algayres, J.P. EUS-guided FNA of pancreatic metastasis from renal cell carcinoma. *Gastrointest. Endosc.* **2003**, *58*, 784–788. [CrossRef] [PubMed]
24. Xu, M.M.; Sethi, A. Imaging of the Pancreas. *Gastroenterol. Clin. N. Am.* **2016**, *45*, 101–116. [CrossRef] [PubMed]
25. Shi, H.Y.; Zhao, X.S.; Miao, F. Metastases to the Pancreas: Computed Tomography Imaging Spectrum and Clinical Features: A Retrospective Study of 18 Patients With 36 Metastases. *Medicine* **2015**, *94*, e913. [CrossRef] [PubMed]
26. Vincenzi, M.; Pasquotti, G.; Polverosi, R.; Pasquali, C.; Pomerri, F. Imaging of pancreatic metastases from renal cell carcinoma. *Cancer Imaging* **2014**, *14*, 5. [CrossRef]
27. Boudghene, F.P.; Deslandes, P.M.; LeBlanche, A.F.; Bigot, J.M. US and CT imaging features of intrapancreatic metastases. *J. Comput. Assist. Tomogr.* **1994**, *18*, 905–910. [CrossRef]
28. Atiq, M.; Bhutani, M.S.; Ross, W.A.; Raju, G.S.; Gong, Y.; Tamm, E.P.; Javle, M.; Wang, X.; Lee, J.H. Role of endoscopic ultrasonography in evaluation of metastatic lesions to the pancreas: A tertiary cancer center experience. *Pancreas* **2013**, *42*, 516–523. [CrossRef]
29. Storm, A.C.; Lee, L.S. Endoscopic ultrasound-guided techniques for diagnosing pancreatic mass lesions: Can we do better? *World J. Gastroenterol.* **2016**, *22*, 8658–8669. [CrossRef]

Disclaimer/Publisher's Note: The statements, opinions and data contained in all publications are solely those of the individual author(s) and contributor(s) and not of MDPI and/or the editor(s). MDPI and/or the editor(s) disclaim responsibility for any injury to people or property resulting from any ideas, methods, instructions or products referred to in the content.

MDPI
St. Alban-Anlage 66
4052 Basel
Switzerland
www.mdpi.com

Journal of Clinical Medicine Editorial Office
E-mail: jcm@mdpi.com
www.mdpi.com/journal/jcm

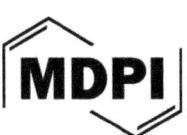

Disclaimer/Publisher's Note: The statements, opinions and data contained in all publications are solely those of the individual author(s) and contributor(s) and not of MDPI and/or the editor(s). MDPI and/or the editor(s) disclaim responsibility for any injury to people or property resulting from any ideas, methods, instructions or products referred to in the content.

www.ingramcontent.com/pod-product-compliance
Lightning Source LLC
LaVergne TN
LVHW070626100526
838202LV00012B/733